PROSTATE UNLOCKED

THE UROLOGIST'S GUIDE TO PSA, SCREENING, PROSTATE CANCER RISK, AND SEXUAL FUNCTION

THE UROLOGIST GUIDE

DAVID SHUSTERMAN

UroLongevity Press

ISBN (Paperback): 979-8-90649-005-6

ISBN (Hardcover): 979-8-90649-006-3

ISBN (E-Book): 979-8-90649-004-9

Published by UroLongevity Press New York, NY

A note on the author's interests. The author is a practicing urologist who performs many of the procedures discussed in this book, and his practice derives income from them — prostatic artery embolization in particular, where he diagnoses the patient, selects the case and manages the aftercare while an interventional radiology colleague performs the embolization itself. The same is true of Rezūm, of prostate biopsy, and of the office testing described throughout. So where he states a preference for one approach over another, that preference reflects his clinical judgement and his professional stake at the same time, and the reader is entitled to know both. Throughout the book the reasoning behind each recommendation is set out so it can be evaluated on its merits, along with the alternatives and the trade-offs. Readers should discuss any treatment decision with their own physician, who has no stake in this book — including a physician who disagrees.

Patient stories in this book are drawn from years of clinical practice. Identifying details have been changed, and in many instances several similar cases have been combined into one, so that no individual patient can be identified. Any resemblance to a specific person is unintended. Where a case is described, it is included because it illustrates a clinical pattern — not because it predicts what will happen to any particular reader.

Medicine changes. The guidance in this book reflects the evidence, guidelines, and clinical practice current as of its publication date, shown on the copyright page. Recommendations — particularly regarding medications, dosing, antibiotic selection, and screening intervals — are revised over time, and some of what follows will eventually be superseded. Readers should confirm current recommendations with their own physician rather than relying on any book, including this one, as the final word.

Formatted with Vellum

MEDICAL DISCLAIMER

CHAPTER 1

WHAT IS THE PROSTATE?

MOST MEN DO NOT THINK about the prostate until the prostate forces them to think about it. A man can go through childhood, adolescence, early adulthood, marriage, fatherhood, work, travel, sex, exercise, and life without once asking where his prostate is or what it does. Then one day something changes. He starts waking up at night to urinate. The stream is weaker. It takes longer to start. He feels like he is not emptying completely. His primary doctor tells him his PSA is elevated. A friend gets diagnosed with prostate cancer. Another friend has a catheter placed in the emergency room because he suddenly cannot urinate. Only then does the prostate become real.

That is one of the strange things about men's health. The prostate is a small gland, buried deep in the pelvis, but it can eventually affect urination, sleep, sex, fertility, cancer risk, bladder health, and quality of life. It is not an organ most men understand, yet it becomes one of the most important organs in male aging.

The prostate is not the penis. It is not the testicle. It is not the bladder. It is a gland that sits directly underneath the bladder, in front of the rectum, and around the urine channel that carries urine from the bladder out through the penis. That location explains almost everything.

When the prostate is small and quiet, urine flows normally. When the prostate enlarges, swells, becomes inflamed, or develops cancer, it can affect the urine channel, the bladder, PSA testing, ejaculation, and a man's sense of control over his own body. The prostate is small, but it sits in a powerful position.

THE PROSTATE'S ORIGINAL JOB

The prostate is part of the male reproductive system. Its main job is to produce fluid that becomes part of semen.

Sperm are made in the testicles. Much of the fluid in semen comes from the seminal vesicles, which sit behind the bladder. The prostate adds its own fluid and proteins to that mixture. During ejaculation, these fluids pass through the prostate area and out through the urine channel.

One of the most important proteins made by the prostate is PSA, which stands for prostate-specific antigen. Most men hear about PSA only as a blood test. They think of it as a cancer test, because PSA is commonly used to help evaluate prostate cancer risk. But PSA did not originally exist so doctors could order a blood test. PSA has a biological job.

PSA helps semen liquefy after ejaculation. Immediately after ejaculation, semen can become thicker or more gel-like. Over a short period of time, PSA helps break down proteins in that semen clot so the semen becomes more liquid and sperm can move more freely. In other words, PSA is part of the reproductive function of the prostate before it ever becomes a cancer-risk marker in a blood test.

That is an important distinction. The prostate is not a useless gland. It has a role in reproduction. It produces fluid. It contributes to semen. It produces PSA. It helps the semen behave properly after ejaculation.

But the prostate is not essential for survival. A man can live without a prostate. Men who have their prostate removed for prostate cancer can continue to live, work, exercise, and function, although removal can affect urinary control, erections, ejaculation, and quality of life.

That is what makes the prostate unusual. It has a meaningful reproductive function earlier in life, but later in life it can become one of the most troublesome organs in the male body.

It is useful when a man is young. It becomes clinically important when a man gets older.

WHY THE LOCATION MATTERS

The prostate would be far less important if it were sitting somewhere else. The problem is where it sits.

The bladder stores urine. The urine channel, called the urethra, carries urine out of the body. The prostate wraps around that channel just below the bladder. I often explain it to patients like this: imagine the bladder as a storage tank and the urethra as the drainpipe. The prostate sits around the drainpipe near the outlet.

When the prostate is small, the drainpipe stays open. Urine leaves the bladder freely. The stream starts easily, flows strongly, and ends cleanly.

When the prostate enlarges, the drainpipe can become compressed, stretched, narrowed, or distorted. The bladder then has to push harder to empty. At first, the man may barely notice. Maybe the stream is a little weaker. Maybe it takes a few seconds longer to start. Maybe he wakes up once at night. He tells himself it is normal aging.

Over time, the changes may become more obvious. He may stop and start. He may strain. He may feel like urine is left behind. He may urinate more often. He may wake up two or three times per night. He may begin planning his day around bathrooms.

That is why the prostate's location is so important. It sits at the exit of the bladder. When it grows, it does not grow in an empty space. It grows around the tube a man needs to urinate. A prostate problem becomes a urinary problem because anatomy makes it one.

THE PROSTATE AND THE BLADDER ARE A SYSTEM

FIGURE 1.1

The Prostate-Bladder Unit

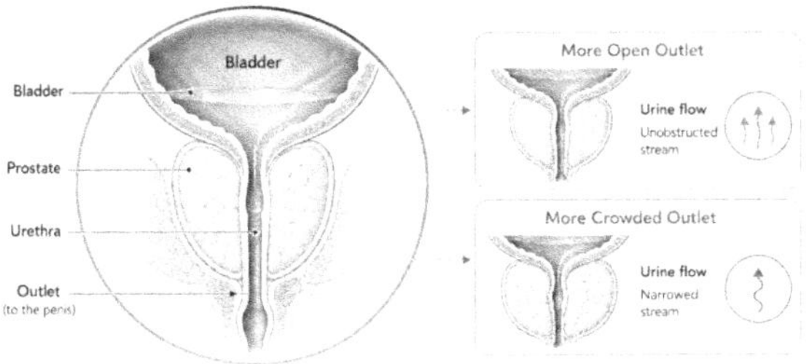

The prostate and bladder function as one urinary system: the prostate may narrow the outlet, but the bladder carries the workload.

Figure 1.1 - The Prostate-Bladder Unit. The prostate and bladder function as one urinary system.

One of the most important ideas in this book is that the prostate and bladder should not be thought of as completely separate organs. The prostate may create the blockage, but the bladder has to fight against it.

That is the prostate-bladder connection. When the prostate narrows the outlet, the bladder must generate more pressure to push urine through. At first, the bladder may compensate. It may work harder and still empty reasonably well. Later, it may become irritated. That irritation can create urgency, frequency, and waking up at night. Eventually, in some men, the bladder may weaken and stop emptying normally.

This is why prostate care is not just about making the stream a little better. It is about protecting the bladder.

A man can feel somewhat improved on medication and still have urine left behind after he finishes. He can be told he is "stable" while the bladder is slowly adapting to obstruction. He can be reassured for years and then suddenly end up in retention, unable to urinate, with a catheter in place.

The prostate may be the culprit, but the bladder is the organ we are trying to protect. That idea will appear throughout this book because it changes how men should think about urinary symptoms. A weak stream is not just a weak stream. Waking up at night is not just an annoyance. Taking medication is not automatically proof that the problem is controlled. The real question is whether the bladder is emptying safely and whether the prostate is creating resistance that should be treated earlier.

WHY MEN USUALLY NOTICE THE PROSTATE LATER IN LIFE

For many men, the prostate stays quiet for decades. Younger men can certainly have prostate-related problems. They can develop prostatitis, pelvic pain, urinary symptoms, sexually related discomfort, or, rarely, prostate cancer. But the classic age-related prostate problem — benign prostate enlargement — usually becomes much more common after age fifty.

Benign prostate enlargement is often called BPH, short for benign prostatic hyperplasia. The phrase sounds complicated, but the concept is simple. The prostate grows in a non-cancerous way. Because the prostate surrounds the urine channel, that growth can interfere with urination.

BPH is not cancer. That is important. But benign does not mean harmless. A benign prostate can still obstruct urine flow, damage sleep, cause bladder symptoms, lead to retention, and affect quality of life.

The reason this becomes more common with age is biological. The prostate is influenced by hormones, aging, inflammation, genetics, and local growth signals inside the gland. It is not simply a matter of "too much testosterone." That is an oversimplification. The prostate changes over time in a more complex way.

Modern longevity has also made prostate health more important. In earlier eras, many men did not live long enough to experience the full burden of prostate enlargement, long-term urinary obstruction, PSA screening, and prostate cancer detection. Today, men routinely live into their seventies, eighties, and nineties. That is a success of modern medicine and public health, but it also means the prostate has more time to become a clinical problem.

A man who lives long enough is likely to deal with his prostate in some way. The goal is not to fear that. The goal is to understand it early enough to make good decisions.

THE PROSTATE CAN AFFECT MORE THAN URINATION

Many men think prostate problems are only about the bathroom. That is not true.

Urination is often the first thing men notice, but the prostate sits at the center of several major male health issues. It can affect fertility and ejaculation because it contributes fluid to semen. It can affect PSA testing because prostate cells produce PSA. It can affect cancer risk because prostate cancer is one of the most common cancers in men. It can affect sleep because urinary symptoms may wake a man repeatedly at night. It can affect sexual confidence because urinary symptoms, prostate medications, prostate inflammation, and prostate cancer treatments can all intersect with erections, ejaculation, and performance.

The prostate does not create erections by itself. Erections are mainly about blood flow, nerves, hormones, and the brain. But prostate disease and prostate treatment can still affect a man's sexual life. A man who wakes up four times a night, worries about leakage, takes medications that change ejaculation, or faces prostate cancer treatment is not dealing with a purely urinary issue. He is dealing with a male function issue.

This is why I do not view the prostate as an isolated gland. It is part of a larger male health system that includes the bladder, hormones, sexual function, sleep, metabolism, vascular health, cancer risk, and aging. That is also why the old model of prostate care is not enough.

The old model was too narrow. It often reduced the prostate to a finger exam, a PSA number, and a medication refill. Modern prostate care has to be broader than that. It has to ask what is happening to the prostate, what is happening to the bladder, what is happening to the man's sleep, what is happening to his sexual function, and what risk signals are being missed.

WHY MEN IGNORE PROSTATE SYMPTOMS

Men ignore prostate symptoms for predictable reasons. They assume a weaker stream is just age. They assume waking up at night is normal. They assume urgency is not serious. They assume medication is enough because someone gave them a prescription. They assume a prostate evaluation means embarrassment. They assume that if they can still urinate, nothing dangerous is happening.

Those assumptions are common, but they are often wrong. The prostate usually gives warnings before it creates a crisis. The problem is that men normalize the warnings. A man may spend years waking up two or three times per night. He may avoid long car rides. He may choose restaurants based on bathroom access. He may stand at the toilet waiting for the stream to start. He may quietly accept that sex, sleep, and confidence are not what they used to be. Then one day he cannot urinate.

To him, it feels sudden. From a medical standpoint, it may have been building for years.

That is why measurement matters. A man should know how large his prostate is. He should know whether part of the prostate is growing up into the bladder and blocking the outlet like a ball valve. He should know how much urine is left behind after he finishes. He should know how fast the urine comes out. He should know whether his bladder is safe.

He does not need to memorize every medical abbreviation. He needs to understand the meaning.

Modern prostate care should not make the patient feel stupid. It should make the problem understandable.

THE FINGER EXAM AND THE MODERN UPGRADE

For generations, men associated prostate care with the digital rectal exam. That association has kept many men away from urologists.

The finger exam came first because doctors had limited tools. Before modern imaging, office ultrasound, MRI, PSA testing, bladder scans, flow testing, and cystoscopy, the finger exam was one of the few ways to estimate the prostate. It had a historical role.

But the fact that something came first does not mean it should remain central forever. If the question is how large the prostate is, ultrasound gives better information. If the question is whether prostate tissue is growing into the bladder, ultrasound gives better information. If the question is how much urine remains in the bladder after urination, a bladder scan or ultrasound gives better information. If the question is how fast the urine comes out, a urine flow test gives better information. If the question is whether the bladder is emptying safely, objective testing gives better information.

A finger exam may still have selected uses in medicine. But for modern evaluation of prostate enlargement and urinary obstruction, it should not be the centerpiece. A finger exam alone cannot build a modern prostate plan.

A man should not avoid care because he thinks prostate evaluation means only embarrassment. A modern evaluation should be about measurement, anatomy, bladder safety, and risk — not just tradition. If ultrasound had existed first, no one would have designed modern prostate care around a finger exam.

THE HISTORICAL LESSON

Severe urinary obstruction is not a new problem. Historical accounts suggest that Peter the Great, the Russian czar, suffered serious urinary tract and bladder problems near the end of his life. Some medical historians have suggested that urinary obstruction and kidney complications may have contributed to his decline. We cannot diagnose him with certainty centuries later, and it would be irresponsible to pretend otherwise. But the story is useful because it reminds us of a basic truth: when urine cannot leave the body properly, the consequences can become serious.

Today, men should not have to wait for urinary obstruction to become a catastrophe. We have tools that earlier generations did not have. We can measure the prostate. We can measure urine left behind. We can measure the speed of the stream. We can look inside the urinary channel with a small camera when needed. We can use MRI for cancer risk. We can use less invasive procedures for selected men. We can treat earlier and more intelligently.

The tragedy is not that prostate problems exist. The tragedy is when men ignore them, or when they are reassured without real measurement until the bladder has already been damaged.

THE MODERN WAY TO THINK ABOUT THE PROSTATE

The old way of thinking was reactive. Wait until symptoms are bad. Try medication. Keep refilling medication. Delay procedures as long as possible. Act when the man can barely urinate or goes into retention. The modern way is different.

The modern approach asks what the prostate is doing, what the bladder is doing, and what risk signals are present. It asks whether the prostate is enlarged, whether it is growing into the bladder, whether urine is being left behind, whether the stream is slow, whether the bladder is still strong, and whether PSA is appropriate for the man's age and risk. That is the difference between guessing and knowing.

This book is built around that difference. It is not enough to say, "Your prostate is enlarged." It is not enough to say, "Your PSA is high." It is not enough to say, "You are fine," when the patient is taking pills and still cannot urinate well.

A man deserves to understand what is happening. The prostate is not one disease. It can enlarge, inflame, obstruct, produce PSA, develop cancer, affect ejaculation, interact with the bladder, and become part of the larger aging male health picture. Treating it properly requires more than a label.

It requires measurement. It requires mechanism. It requires a plan.

DR. SHUSTERMAN'S MODERN PROSTATE TAKEAWAY

The prostate is a small reproductive gland with an enormous clinical impact because of where it sits. It lives directly under the bladder and surrounds the urine channel. Its original biological job is reproductive: it contributes fluid to semen and produces PSA, which helps semen liquefy after ejaculation. But as men age, the prostate can enlarge, obstruct urination, elevate PSA, become inflamed, develop cancer, and damage bladder function.

The most important point is simple: prostate care is not just about the prostate. It is about the prostate-bladder system and the man attached to it.

A modern man should not be afraid of his prostate. He should understand it before it controls his life.

CHAPTER 2

WHY THE PROSTATE BECOMES A PROBLEM WITH AGE

A MAN DOES NOT USUALLY THINK about his prostate when he is twenty-five. He urinates without planning around bathrooms. He sleeps through the night. His stream is strong. Sex is usually not something he has to analyze medically. PSA is not on his radar. The bladder empties, the body works, and the prostate is invisible.

That is exactly how the prostate is supposed to be. The prostate is one of those organs that does its job quietly for decades. It contributes to semen. It sits below the bladder. It surrounds the urinary channel. It participates in reproduction. For a younger man, the prostate usually creates no daily awareness at all. Then age changes the equation.

The prostate does not suddenly become evil. It does not wake up one morning and decide to ruin a man's life. What happens is slower, more mechanical, and more biological. The prostate continues to respond to hormones, inflammation, growth signals, genetics, and time. The bladder continues to push urine through the channel that passes through the prostate. The urinary system keeps adapting until it cannot adapt as well anymore. That is when a man begins to notice.

The stream is not quite as strong. The bathroom trip takes longer.

He wakes once at night, then twice, then three times. He stands at the toilet waiting for urine to start. He feels like he is done, zips up, and then dribbles. He starts choosing aisle seats, avoiding long drives, and checking where the bathroom is before a meeting or dinner.

At first, he may call it normal aging. That is partly true. But it is not the whole truth.

Aging is real. Neglect is optional.

THE PROSTATE IS BUILT IN A BAD LOCATION

The main reason the prostate becomes a problem with age is simple anatomy. The prostate sits directly below the bladder and surrounds the urinary channel. That means urine has to pass through the prostate area before leaving the body. If the prostate enlarges, stiffens, changes shape, or grows inward toward the urinary channel, the bladder has to work harder to empty.

This is not a small detail. It is the central design flaw.

If the prostate grew on the outside of the arm, most men would not care. If it enlarged slightly, it might be visible or annoying, but it would not affect urination. If it grew in the abdomen without touching the bladder or urinary channel, it might matter only if it became very large.

But the prostate grows around a tube. That tube carries urine.

This is why benign prostate enlargement can create such disruptive symptoms. The condition is not dangerous because the word "benign" is wrong. It is benign because it is not cancer. But it can still matter because it sits in the wrong place. A benign traffic jam is still a traffic jam.

THE PROSTATE DOES NOT HAVE TO BE HUGE TO CAUSE TROUBLE

FIGURE 2.1

Why Size Alone Is Not Enough

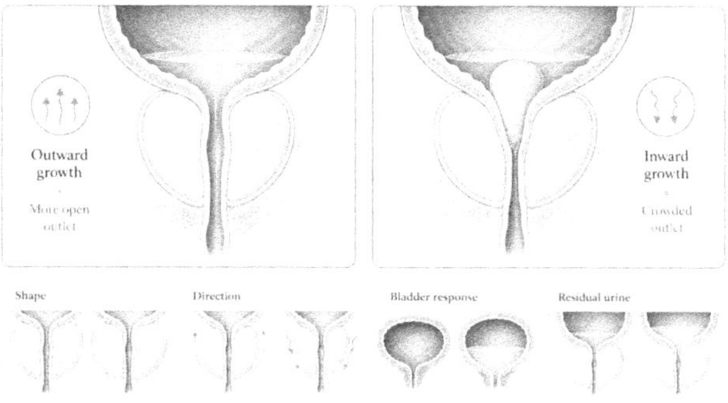

Prostate size matters, but shape, direction of growth, bladder response, and leftover urine often matter just as much.

Figure 2.1 - Why Size Alone Is Not Enough. Size, shape, direction of growth, and bladder response all matter.

Many men assume prostate problems are only about size. That is not true.

Size matters, but shape matters too. Direction of growth matters. The relationship between the prostate and the bladder opening matters. A prostate that grows outward may become quite large before it causes major obstruction. A smaller prostate that grows inward toward the urinary channel or upward into the bladder opening can create significant symptoms earlier.

This is one of the most important concepts in modern prostate care. A man can have a moderately enlarged prostate and still be very obstructed. Another man can have a larger prostate and surprisingly mild symptoms. The difference often comes down to anatomy, bladder response, and how the tissue affects the urinary channel.

That is why "your prostate is enlarged" is not enough information. The better questions are: How large is it?

Where is it growing? Is it narrowing the urinary channel? Is it growing into the bladder opening?

Is the bladder emptying safely? How fast does the urine come out? How much urine is left behind? Without those answers, treatment becomes guesswork.

HORMONES KEEP TALKING TO THE PROSTATE

The prostate is hormone-sensitive. Throughout adult life, prostate tissue responds to androgen signaling. Testosterone and its more potent derivative, DHT, influence prostate biology. This does not mean testosterone is bad, and it does not mean every man with testosterone has prostate trouble. Men need testosterone for muscle, mood, libido, sexual function, energy, bone health, and overall vitality. But the prostate lives in a hormonal environment.

As men age, the relationship between hormones, tissue growth, inflammation, and prostate remodeling becomes more complicated. The prostate may gradually enlarge. The internal architecture may change. The tissue around the urinary channel may become more obstructive. Some men are genetically more prone to this than others.

This is why prostate growth is not simply a lifestyle failure. A thin man can develop BPH. A healthy man can develop BPH. A man who eats well and exercises can still develop a prostate that blocks urine. Lifestyle matters, but it does not cancel anatomy, genetics, hormones, or aging.

This is important because men should not blame themselves for every prostate issue. But they also should not use aging as an excuse to ignore it.

The right response is not guilt. The right response is measurement.

THE BLADDER COMPENSATES BEFORE IT COMPLAINS

One reason prostate problems are often missed is that the bladder is strong. At least at first.

When the prostate begins to create resistance, the bladder does not immediately fail. It adapts. It squeezes harder. It develops more force. It pushes against the resistance and still manages to empty reasonably well.

During this early period, a man may have very few symptoms. He may think everything is fine. Even if he notices changes, they may seem minor. But the bladder is not a machine with unlimited reserve.

Over time, if it keeps pushing against resistance, the bladder muscle can become thicker, more irritable, and less efficient. Some men develop urgency and frequency because the bladder becomes sensitive. Others begin leaving urine behind because the bladder cannot fully overcome the blockage. Some develop both problems at the same time. This is why symptoms can be misleading.

A man may not feel severely obstructed until the bladder has already been struggling for years. Another man may have urgency and nighttime urination that everyone labels "overactive bladder," when the real trigger is a prostate blockage forcing the bladder to work too hard.

The prostate may start the problem, but the bladder often pays the price. That is why the question is not only, "How do I improve the stream?" The better question is, "Is my bladder safe?"

THE SLOW CREEP OF URINARY CHANGE

Prostate symptoms often appear gradually. That makes them easy to normalize.

A man does not usually go from perfect urination to severe urinary dysfunction overnight. He adapts without realizing it. He spends a little longer at the toilet. He wakes once at night. He starts urinating before leaving the house even when he does not feel an urgent need. He chooses the bathroom before the car ride. He stops drinking water before events. He avoids sitting in the middle of a theater row.

At first, these adjustments seem minor. Then they become lifestyle.

This is one of the most damaging parts of prostate enlargement. It trains men to shrink their lives around the bathroom.

They do not always call it suffering. They call it being careful. They call it being practical. They call it getting older. But when a man plans travel, sleep, exercise, sex, meetings, and social events around urination, the prostate has already become a quality-of-life issue.

A man should compare his urination not only to other men his age, but to himself at twenty-five. That comparison is often more honest.

NIGHTTIME URINATION IS NOT A SMALL PROBLEM

Many men tolerate nighttime urination for years. They should not be so casual about it.

Waking up once may not be a major issue. Waking up three or four times a night is different. That is not just a urinary symptom. It is sleep fragmentation. It affects recovery, mood, concentration, testosterone, metabolism, cardiovascular health, and daily performance.

A man who wakes up repeatedly to urinate may not realize how much of his fatigue is coming from broken sleep. He may blame aging. He may blame stress. He may blame low testosterone. He may blame poor motivation. He may ask for sleeping pills. He may ask for hormone therapy. But if the bladder is waking him all night, the prostate-bladder system needs to be evaluated.

Nighttime urination can come from several causes. It may be

prostate obstruction. It may be overactive bladder. It may be sleep apnea. It may be diabetes, evening fluids, alcohol, leg swelling, medications, or kidney-related urine production. Sometimes more than one factor is involved.

That is exactly why it should be evaluated rather than dismissed. A man cannot optimize longevity while waking up all night to urinate. Sleep is not optional.

THE PROSTATE AGES DIFFERENTLY IN DIFFERENT MEN

Not every man ages the same way. Some men develop major prostate enlargement in their fifties. Others reach their seventies with mild symptoms. Some men have small prostates but severe urinary complaints. Others have large prostates and function surprisingly well. Some men develop cancer risk without urinary symptoms at all.

There is no single prostate-aging pattern. Genetics matter. Family history matters. Hormones matter. Metabolic health matters. Inflammation matters. Anatomy matters. Bladder strength matters. Prior infections, procedures, medications, and neurologic health can all matter. This is why prostate care must be individualized.

A guideline can describe populations. It cannot understand one man's bladder. It cannot know whether his prostate is growing into the bladder opening. It cannot know whether he is leaving urine behind. It cannot know how much sleep he is losing. It cannot know whether his sexual function is important to him. It cannot know whether he is a healthy seventy-eight-year-old with a decade of meaningful life ahead or a frail man whose care goals are different.

Modern prostate care cannot be based only on age. It must be based on the man.

PSA BECOMES PART OF THE AGING CONVERSATION

As men age, PSA also enters the conversation. PSA is not a diagnosis. It is not a verdict. It is not automatically cancer. It is a signal from the prostate that must be interpreted in context.

The prostate can produce more PSA for several reasons. Benign enlargement can raise PSA. Inflammation can raise PSA. Infection can raise PSA. Urinary retention can raise PSA. Procedures and manipulation can affect PSA. Prostate cancer can raise PSA.

The problem is not PSA itself. The problem is poor interpretation.

Some men are terrified of PSA because they think one elevated number means cancer and immediate treatment. Other men ignore PSA because they have heard screening is controversial. Both reactions are too simplistic.

Checking PSA does not mean automatic biopsy. Biopsy does not mean automatic treatment. Finding low-risk prostate cancer does not mean a man automatically needs surgery or radiation.

Modern urology has MRI, biomarkers, targeted biopsy, active surveillance, genomic testing, better staging, and more nuanced treatment decisions. The older problem was not information. The older problem was overreaction to information.

The answer is not ignorance. The answer is smarter interpretation.

CANCER AND URINATION ARE NOT THE SAME CONVERSATION

A major source of confusion is the belief that urinary symptoms and prostate cancer move together. Most of the time, they do not.

A man can have terrible urinary symptoms from benign enlargement and no prostate cancer. Another man can urinate perfectly and still have clinically significant prostate cancer. This is because most prostate cancers begin in areas of the prostate that do not immediately block the urinary channel.

This is why a strong stream does not prove the prostate is cancer-free. It is also why urinary symptoms do not automatically mean cancer.

The prostate can create two separate aging problems: benign enlargement affecting urination, and cancer risk affecting long-term survival. They can overlap, but they are not the same disease. A modern evaluation should keep both questions in view.

Is the prostate affecting urination and bladder safety? Is there a prostate cancer-risk signal that needs evaluation?

Those are different questions. Both matter.

LIFESTYLE MATTERS, BUT IT DOES NOT REPLACE ANATOMY

Lifestyle affects prostate and urinary health, but it is not a cure-all. Weight, insulin resistance, diabetes, alcohol, sleep quality, physical activity, constipation, hydration patterns, caffeine, medications, and cardiovascular health can all influence urinary symptoms and sexual function.

A man who drinks several glasses of wine at night may worsen nighttime urination. A man with untreated sleep apnea may wake repeatedly and urinate more. A man with constipation may worsen pelvic pressure and urinary symptoms. A man with diabetes may urinate frequently because of blood sugar. A man with poor vascular health may develop ED before he develops obvious heart symptoms. These factors matter.

But lifestyle should not be used to dismiss structural obstruction. A man with a large prostate blocking the bladder opening cannot kale-smoothie his way out of a mechanical problem. Weight loss may improve inflammation, sleep, testosterone, and metabolic health. Better hydration habits may help. Reducing alcohol may reduce nighttime urination. Treating constipation may improve pelvic symptoms. But if the prostate is physically blocking the urinary channel, anatomy still has to be addressed.

Lifestyle is part of the plan. It is not a substitute for diagnosis.

THE PROBLEM WITH "YOU'RE GETTING OLDER"

Few phrases are more dangerous in men's health than "you're just getting older." It may be true, but it is incomplete. Aging explains why prostate problems become more common. It does not prove that symptoms should be ignored. It does not prove that the bladder is safe. It does not prove that PSA is irrelevant. It does not prove that ED is harmless. It does not prove that fatigue is normal. It does not prove that waking four times a night is acceptable.

Aging should prompt better evaluation, not lower standards. A man who is fifty-five and waking three times a night should not be dismissed. A man who is sixty-five and leaving urine behind should not be told to just refill medication forever. A man who is seventy-two and healthy should not have his PSA ignored because he crossed an age line. A man who is eighty-one and active should be treated differently from a frail eighty-eight-year-old with limited life expectancy.

Aging changes the conversation. It should not end the conversation.

EARLY EVALUATION CREATES MORE OPTIONS

One of the biggest advantages of earlier prostate evaluation is choice. When a man comes in early, before retention, before bladder damage, before repeated infections, before stones, before severe sleep disruption, there are usually more options. Medication may be reasonable. Observation may be reasonable. Lifestyle adjustment may be enough for a while. Minimally invasive treatment may fit. PAE or Rezūm may be considered before the bladder is in crisis.

When a man waits too long, the choices narrow. A bladder that has been pushing against resistance for years may not recover fully. A man in retention may need urgent catheterization. Recurrent infections may complicate care. Bladder stones may require treatment. Severe obstruction may require more aggressive intervention. The patient who wanted to avoid procedures may end up needing a bigger one because the problem was ignored too long.

This is the irony. Men often delay evaluation because they fear treatment. But delay can lead to more treatment, not less.

The goal is not to rush every man into a procedure. The goal is to identify who is safe, who can be watched, who can use medication, who needs a modern procedure, and who is at risk if nothing changes.

THE MODERN PROSTATE MINDSET

The old mindset was passive. Wait until symptoms are severe. Try pills indefinitely. Use a finger exam and vague reassurance. Treat PSA like a panic button or ignore it completely. Offer whatever procedure the doctor happens to do most often. The modern mindset is different.

Measure the prostate. Measure bladder emptying. Measure urine flow.

Interpret PSA intelligently. Use MRI before biopsy when appropriate. Protect sexual function.

Think about sleep. Think about testosterone. Think about metabolic health.

Match treatment to anatomy. This is not overtesting. It is precision.

Men are used to tracking heart rate, sleep scores, steps, glucose, cholesterol, testosterone, and body composition. Yet many still do not know the size of the organ sitting around their urinary channel. That makes no sense. A modern man should know his prostate the way he knows the rest of his health.

DR. SHUSTERMAN'S TAKEAWAY

The prostate becomes a problem with age because biology and anatomy collide. The gland grows. Hormones keep signaling. Inflammation and tissue remodeling accumulate. The urinary channel runs through the prostate. The bladder compensates until it struggles. PSA becomes part of the cancer-risk conversation. Sexual function, sleep, metabolism, and urinary health begin to overlap.

None of this means a man should panic. It means he should pay attention.

Prostate aging is common, but common does not mean harmless. A weak stream, nighttime urination, incomplete emptying, urgency, rising PSA, and sexual changes are not just annoyances to be tolerated indefinitely. They are signals. They deserve interpretation. The goal is not to fear the prostate.

The goal is to understand it early enough to stay ahead of it. Aging is real. Neglect is optional.

CHAPTER 3

UNDERSTANDING BPH: THE MOST COMMON PROSTATE CONDITION

A MAN COMES in holding a piece of paper from another office. It says his prostate is enlarged.

He wants to know two things. Is it cancer, and is he going to need surgery. Nobody has told him either answer, so for three weeks he has assumed the worst on both counts.

The paper is not wrong. His prostate is enlarged. But by itself that sentence tells him almost nothing about what is happening to him, because an enlarged prostate is one of the most common findings in medicine and one of the least informative on its own. By eighty, most men have one. Many of them will never have a problem because of it.

What matters is not the size of the gland. What matters is what the gland is doing to the bladder sitting on top of it.

That is the distinction this chapter is built around, and it is the one most men are never given. A man can walk out of an office with a diagnosis, a prescription, and no idea whether his bladder is safe. Those are different questions, and only one of them determines what happens to him over the next twenty years.

If there is one prostate diagnosis that almost every man will hear about as he gets older, it is BPH. BPH stands for benign prostatic hyperplasia. The term may sound intimidating, but it simply refers to a noncancerous enlargement of the prostate gland. As men age, the prostate often continues to grow. For many men, this growth causes little trouble. For others, it gradually begins to interfere with the normal flow of urine and can significantly affect daily life.

One of the most important facts to understand is that BPH is not prostate cancer. It is not an infection, and it is not a condition that spreads throughout the body. Nevertheless, because of the way the prostate is positioned around the urinary channel, even a benign enlargement can create meaningful urinary problems.

Millions of men live with symptoms related to BPH. Some notice only minor changes, such as a slightly weaker stream or an occasional nighttime trip to the bathroom. Others find themselves constantly searching for restrooms, waking multiple times each night, or feeling frustrated by the sensation that their bladder never fully empties. The impact can range from a mild inconvenience to a major disruption of quality of life.

The condition becomes increasingly common with age. By middle age, many men already have microscopic evidence of prostate enlargement. As the decades pass, enlargement becomes more prevalent, and by the age of eighty, most men have some degree of BPH whether they have symptoms or not. The presence of enlargement alone is not necessarily the problem. What matters most is whether that enlargement is affecting urinary function.

WHAT ACTUALLY HAPPENS IN BPH

To understand BPH, it helps to understand the anatomy. The prostate sits just below the bladder and surrounds the urethra, the tube that carries urine out of the body. Because the urethra passes directly through the prostate, any increase in prostate tissue has the potential to narrow that channel.

A useful analogy is to imagine gently squeezing a garden hose.

Water can still pass through, but the flow becomes slower and requires greater pressure. In a similar way, an enlarging prostate can create resistance to urine flow. The bladder must work harder to push urine through the narrowed passage.

Initially, the bladder is remarkably capable of adapting. The bladder muscle contracts more forcefully and often compensates for the increased resistance. During this stage, symptoms may be minimal or absent. Over time, however, the bladder may become irritated, overworked, or less efficient. When that happens, urinary symptoms become more noticeable and often more bothersome.

WHAT "ENLARGED" ACTUALLY MEANS

Enlarged is a word, not a measurement. It is worth knowing what the numbers behind it are.

A young adult prostate is often described as roughly walnut-sized and commonly measures around twenty to twenty-five grams. Prostate volume tends to increase with age, but the range is wide and a single size does not determine whether a man has obstruction or needs treatment. Glands of eighty or one hundred grams, and occasionally larger, are seen in clinical practice.

But here is what the number does not tell you. Prostate volume correlates only loosely with symptoms, and hardly at all with whether a man is in danger. I have seen men with hundred-gram prostates urinating well and sleeping through the night, and men with thirty-gram prostates in retention.

The reason is direction. A prostate that grows outward, away from the channel, can become very large and cause little obstruction. A prostate that grows inward, or that pushes a lobe up into the bladder opening like a ball sitting on a drain, can be modest in size and block almost completely.

So when a man is told his prostate is enlarged, the useful follow-up questions are not about the number. They are: which direction is it growing, is it narrowing the channel, is a lobe intruding into the bladder, and is the bladder still emptying?

Those questions can be answered. Size alone cannot answer them.

COMMON SYMPTOMS OF BPH

Many men associate BPH with only one symptom: a weak urinary stream. While a weak stream is certainly common, prostate enlargement can produce a much broader range of urinary complaints.

A man with BPH may notice that it takes longer to begin urinating after reaching the bathroom. He may find that the stream stops and starts during urination or that he needs to strain to empty his bladder. Some men feel as though urine remains behind even after they have finished. Others experience frequent urination throughout the day, sudden urgency that is difficult to postpone, or repeated awakenings at night to urinate. Dribbling after urination is also common.

Not every man experiences symptoms in the same way. Some men have substantial enlargement with surprisingly few complaints, while others develop significant symptoms despite only modest enlargement. This variation is one reason why symptoms alone do not always provide a complete picture of what is happening inside the urinary tract.

WHY SYMPTOMS AND SIZE DO NOT ALWAYS MATCH

One of the most common misconceptions about BPH is the belief that larger prostates automatically cause worse symptoms. In reality, the relationship between prostate size and symptom severity is often more complicated.

The location and pattern of growth frequently matter as much as the overall volume of the gland. A prostate that expands outward may become quite large without significantly affecting urine flow. In contrast, a smaller prostate that grows inward toward the urethra or protrudes into the bladder can create substantial obstruction.

As a result, two men with similar prostate measurements may have dramatically different experiences. One may have minimal symptoms and little disruption to daily life, while the other struggles with urinary difficulties every day. This is why objective evaluation is so important. Imaging studies, flow measurements, and other diagnostic tools often provide information that symptoms alone cannot.

THE BLADDER'S RESPONSE TO OBSTRUCTION

The bladder is designed to store urine and then empty efficiently when appropriate. When the prostate creates resistance to urine flow, the bladder initially responds by working harder. Stronger contractions help overcome the obstruction and maintain adequate emptying.

For a period of time, this compensation can be effective. A man may notice only subtle changes or may not recognize any symptoms at all. Eventually, however, the increased workload begins to affect the bladder itself.

The bladder muscle may become thicker and more irritable. As this occurs, urgency and frequency often develop. Men may find themselves rushing to the bathroom more often during the day and waking repeatedly at night. If obstruction persists for many years, the bladder can eventually lose some of its strength and efficiency.

When the bladder no longer empties completely, urine remains behind after urination. Physicians refer to this as post-void residual urine. Increasing residual urine can contribute to infections, bladder dysfunction, and other complications. For this reason, evaluating bladder function is an important part of assessing men with BPH.

WHAT THE BLADDER CAN AND CANNOT TAKE

The bladder is a muscle, and like any muscle it can be trained by resistance and it can be ruined by it. A healthy bladder holds around five hundred millilitres comfortably. Somewhere between four hundred and six hundred is the normal working range. When a man is habitually holding more than six hundred — because he cannot empty, or because he has learned to ignore the signal for hours at a stretch — the bladder is being stretched beyond what it was built for, and that stretch is where the damage begins.

Early on, obstruction makes the bladder stronger. The muscle thickens and contracts harder to force urine past the narrowing, and it succeeds. This is why a man can have significant obstruction for years and describe his stream as fine. His bladder is compensating, and compensation is invisible.

Then the wall becomes thick and irritable rather than strong. This is the stage where urgency and frequency appear, and it is the stage where most men finally mention it to someone. Somewhat counterintuitively, the symptoms that bring a man in — the rushing to the bathroom, the waking at night — are not signs of a weak bladder. They are signs of a bladder still fighting.

The dangerous stage is quieter. After long enough, an over-stretched bladder stops fighting. The urgency settles. The man may say he is better. What has actually happened is that the muscle has lost the ability to generate a useful contraction, and urine now simply accumulates. That is the stage worth understanding, because it is the one that does not reverse.

POTENTIAL COMPLICATIONS OF UNTREATED BPH

Many men view urinary symptoms as little more than an annoyance. In some cases, that may be true. However, significant obstruction can sometimes lead to more serious consequences if left unaddressed.

One of the most dramatic complications is urinary retention, a condition in which a man suddenly becomes unable to urinate despite having a full bladder. The discomfort can be severe, and emergency catheter placement is often necessary to relieve the pressure. For many patients, urinary retention becomes the event that finally prompts them to seek medical attention.

Other complications may include recurrent urinary tract infections, bladder stones, blood in the urine, progressive bladder dysfunction, and, in severe situations, damage to kidney function. Although these outcomes are not inevitable, they illustrate why persistent urinary symptoms should not simply be ignored. The goal of modern prostate care is to identify problems early, understand their cause, and intervene before complications develop.

HOW BPH IS DIAGNOSED

Diagnosing BPH involves much more than asking a patient whether he urinates frequently. A thorough evaluation seeks to determine not only whether the prostate is enlarged but also whether that enlargement is affecting bladder function and urinary health.

The process typically begins with a detailed medical history and discussion of symptoms. Physicians often use standardized questionnaires to better understand how urinary issues are affecting daily life. A physical examination may provide additional clues, while laboratory testing such as urinalysis and, when appropriate, PSA testing can help evaluate other potential concerns.

Imaging studies and specialized testing frequently play an important role. Ultrasound can provide information about prostate size and bladder emptying. Measurements of post-void residual urine help determine whether urine remains in the bladder after urination. Flow-rate testing can assess how effectively urine passes through the urinary tract. In selected situations, cystoscopy allows direct visualization of the urethra, prostate, and bladder.

Each piece of information contributes to a more complete understanding of the situation. The objective is to answer several critical questions. How large is the prostate? Is it causing obstruction? Is the bladder functioning properly? Could another condition be contributing to the symptoms? Without these answers, treatment decisions become far less precise.

NOT EVERY URINARY PROBLEM IS BPH

Although BPH is extremely common, it is not the only cause of urinary symptoms in men. Assuming that every urinary complaint is caused by prostate enlargement can lead to missed diagnoses and ineffective treatment.

A variety of conditions can mimic or coexist with BPH. Overactive bladder may cause urgency and frequency even when the prostate is not significantly obstructing urine flow. Urinary tract infections can produce burning, urgency, and frequent urination. Bladder stones, neurologic disorders, diabetes, sleep apnea, pelvic floor dysfunction, and certain medications can all contribute to urinary symptoms.

In many cases, more than one factor is involved. A man may have both BPH and an overactive bladder. Another may have mild prostate enlargement but severe sleep apnea that contributes to nighttime urination. Understanding the true source of symptoms is essential because successful treatment depends on an accurate diagnosis.

HOW MUCH A MAN DRINKS IS PART OF THE DIAGNOSIS

Before any extensive bladder workup, I ask a question that sounds too simple to matter. How much do you drink in a day?

The answers are often remarkable. Men arrive convinced they have a prostate problem while drinking four, five, six litres a day — a large water bottle refilled all afternoon, coffee through the morning, a habit picked up from a trainer or a podcast telling them hydration is health. They are urinating frequently because they are producing an extraordinary volume of urine. The prostate is a bystander.

For most men, around two litres a day is sufficient. A little more with heat, sweating, or hard exercise. Drinking substantially beyond that is not a health strategy, and in a man with any degree of outlet obstruction it turns a manageable situation into a miserable one.

Timing matters as much as volume. A man who takes in most of his fluid after six in the evening will be up three times a night regardless of the state of his prostate.

None of this means the symptoms are imaginary or that the prostate is innocent. It means that some of what gets labelled a prostate problem is a drinking pattern, and that is worth knowing before anyone measures anything or writes a prescription. It is the cheapest test in urology, and it is skipped constantly.

TREATMENT IS NOT ONE-SIZE-FITS-ALL

One of the most encouraging developments in modern urology is the wide range of treatment options available for BPH. Not every enlarged prostate requires intervention, and not every patient benefits from the same approach.

For men with minimal symptoms and no evidence of complications, careful observation may be entirely appropriate. Monitoring allows physicians to track changes over time while avoiding unnecessary treatment.

Lifestyle modifications can also be helpful. Reducing fluid intake before bedtime, limiting alcohol consumption, managing constipation, improving sleep quality, and addressing metabolic health may lessen symptoms for some individuals.

Medications remain an important option for many patients. Alpha blockers help relax the muscles around the prostate and bladder neck, improving urine flow. Other medications can gradually reduce prostate size in selected men. Additional therapies may target bladder-related symptoms when they are present.

When symptoms become more significant or when complications arise, procedural treatment may offer the best solution. Advances in technology have expanded the number of minimally invasive therapies available, while surgical approaches continue to provide excellent results for appropriately selected patients. The ideal treatment depends on prostate anatomy, symptom severity, bladder function, overall health, and personal preferences.

WHY MEN DELAY EVALUATION

Despite the prevalence of BPH, many men postpone seeking medical attention for years. Some feel embarrassed discussing urinary symptoms. Others assume that frequent urination and nighttime awakenings are simply unavoidable parts of aging.

Fear also plays a role. Some men worry that evaluation will inevitably lead to surgery, while others believe that nothing can be done to improve their symptoms. These assumptions often prevent men from learning about the many effective treatment options now available.

Unfortunately, delaying evaluation can allow manageable problems to progress. Earlier assessment often provides more choices and greater flexibility in treatment planning. Understanding what is happening empowers patients to make informed decisions rather than reacting only when symptoms become severe.

BPH AND QUALITY OF LIFE

The effects of BPH extend far beyond the bathroom. Repeated nighttime awakenings can disrupt sleep and contribute to fatigue, reduced concentration, and diminished productivity. Constant urgency may interfere with travel, social activities, and professional responsibilities.

Many men gradually adapt to these limitations without realizing how much their daily lives have changed. They plan outings around restroom availability, avoid long drives, or accept poor sleep as normal. Over time, these adjustments can affect mood, relationships, and overall well-being.

Improving urinary function often produces benefits that reach well beyond the urinary tract. Better sleep, increased energy, greater confidence, and improved quality of life are frequently among the most meaningful outcomes of successful treatment.

THE ONE COMPLICATION THAT CANNOT BE UNDONE

Most of what goes wrong with a prostate can be fixed. Retention can be relieved. Infections can be treated. Stones can be removed. Obstruction can be opened by any number of routes. There is one exception, and in my experience it is the hardest situation in this entire field.

Long-standing obstruction can weaken the bladder muscle, reduce its ability to contract, and in some men lead to persistent incomplete emptying even after the outlet is opened. Treating the obstruction may still improve flow and emptying, especially when pressure-flow testing confirms obstruction, but recovery is variable and some men continue to need catheterization or other bladder-directed management. At that point the clinical problem is no longer explained by the prostate alone; bladder contractility and outlet resistance both matter.

These men live with a catheter. Either a tube through the urethra or one through the lower abdomen, changed on a schedule, indefinitely. Not because they had bad surgery or bad luck, but because they were told for a decade that their symptoms were a normal part of getting older, and they believed it.

This is the reason I am insistent about measuring bladder emptying rather than asking a man how he feels he is doing. Feeling fine is not evidence that the bladder is safe. It is often the last thing a man reports before it isn't.

Severe loss of bladder contractility is one of the most consequential problems that can accompany prolonged outlet obstruction, but it is not uniformly permanent and it is not the only potentially lasting harm in prostate care. The practical lesson is to measure residual urine and determine why emptying is poor before years of dysfunction narrow the available options. Looking early does not commit a man to treatment; it protects the chance to act while bladder function may still be better preserved.

DR. SHUSTERMAN'S MODERN BPH TAKEAWAY

BPH is the most common prostate condition men encounter as they age. Although it is a benign condition, it should not be dismissed because it is not cancer.

The central issue is not whether the prostate has become larger. The real question is whether that enlargement is affecting bladder function, urinary health, sleep quality, or overall quality of life. Symptoms provide important clues, but objective measurements and a thorough evaluation are equally important.

Modern prostate care focuses on understanding the individual patient rather than treating every enlarged prostate the same way. By identifying problems early, measuring them accurately, and selecting the most appropriate strategy, men can often avoid unnecessary suffering and reduce the risk of future complications.

Knowledge leads to better decisions. When men understand what BPH is, how it affects the urinary system, and what treatment options are available, they are better equipped to protect both their urinary health and their quality of life for years to come.

CHAPTER 4

THE PROSTATE-BLADDER CONNECTION

A MAN WALKS into the office after a frightening weekend. He had been urinating poorly for years, but he had adapted to it. His stream was slower than it used to be. He woke up several times a night. He stood at the toilet longer. Sometimes he had to wait before the urine started. Sometimes he felt like he was finished, then had to go again a few minutes later.

He had seen doctors. He had been told his prostate was enlarged. He had been placed on medication. The medication helped a little. At follow-up visits, he was told things were stable. Then, one night, he could not urinate at all.

Not a weak stream. Not difficulty starting. Not waking up more often. He simply could not get urine out. His bladder filled. The pressure became unbearable. He went to the emergency room, where a catheter was placed to drain the bladder. Now he is sitting in my office with a reasonable question.

"How did this happen if I was being followed?" That question is at the center of modern prostate care. Many men are not ignored. They are seen. They are prescribed medication. They return for follow-up. They are reassured. But the wrong thing is often being followed. The conversation focuses on the prostate, the pill, or the symptom score, while the bladder is quietly doing the hard work in the background.

The prostate may be the part causing the blockage, but the bladder is the organ that has to fight through it. That is the prostate-bladder connection.

If you understand that connection, you will understand why BPH should not be treated casually. You will understand why "better" is not always enough. You will understand why a man can take medication and still be at risk. You will understand why the most important question is not only, "How large is my prostate?" but also, "Is my bladder safe?"

THE PROSTATE DOES NOT ACT ALONE

The prostate sits directly below the bladder and surrounds the urine channel. That anatomy creates a simple mechanical relationship. If the prostate enlarges or changes shape in a way that narrows the outlet, the bladder has to push harder to empty.

At first, the bladder can often compensate. The bladder is a muscle, and like other muscles, it can work harder for a period of time. A man may notice that urination is slower, but he still gets the urine out. He may wake up at night, but he gets used to it. He may stand longer at the toilet, but he does not think of it as dangerous.

This stage can last a long time. That is one reason prostate obstruction can be deceptive. The man is not suddenly sick. He is slowly adapting. The bladder is adapting too.

When the bladder pushes against resistance for months or years, it may become thicker, more irritable, and less efficient. At first, the symptoms may be urgency and frequency. The man feels like he has to go all the time. He wakes up at night. He may be told he has an overactive bladder.

Sometimes that is true. But sometimes the bladder is overactive because it is fighting a blocked outlet.

That distinction matters. If the bladder is reacting to a prostate blockage, calming the bladder without addressing the blockage is not a full solution. It may quiet the alarm while the fire continues.

WHEN THE BLADDER STARTS LOSING THE FIGHT

The bladder's job is not only to store urine. It must also empty effectively. A healthy bladder fills at low pressure, holds urine comfortably, and then contracts strongly enough to empty when the time is right.

When the prostate creates resistance, the bladder has to generate more pressure to push urine through the narrowed channel. In the beginning, it may succeed. Later, it may struggle. Eventually, in some men, it starts leaving urine behind.

This leftover urine after urination is one of the most important measurements in prostate care. Doctors call it the post-void residual, but the plain-English meaning is more important than the term: after the man urinates, how much urine is still sitting in the bladder?

A man may feel empty and still not be empty. That is a key point. Sensation is not always reliable. The bladder can stretch over time. The patient can adapt. A man may finish urinating, zip up, and believe the bladder is empty, while a significant amount of urine remains behind.

That leftover urine matters. It can worsen urgency. It can increase the risk of infection. It can contribute to bladder stones. It can indicate that the bladder is working too hard or no longer working well enough. If it continues to rise, it may become a warning sign that the patient is moving toward retention.

This is why modern prostate care cannot rely only on symptoms. The patient tells us what he feels. Measurement tells us what the bladder is doing.

BETTER IS NOT FIXED

FIGURE 4.1

Medication Improvement vs Bladder Safety

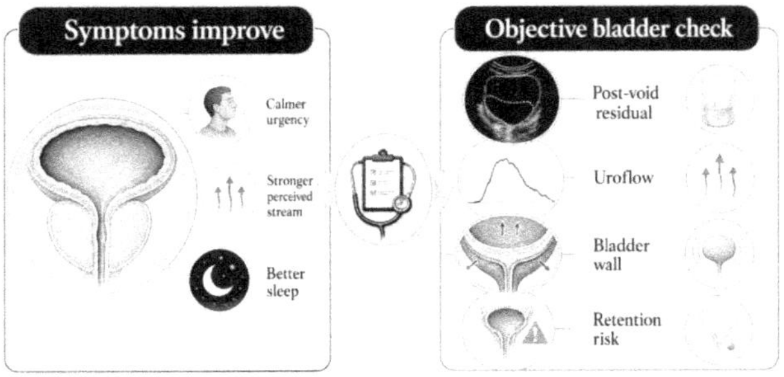

Feeling better on medication does not always prove the bladder is emptying safely.

Figure 4.1 - Medication Improvement vs Bladder Safety. Feeling better does not always prove the bladder is emptying safely.

One of the most dangerous moments in BPH care is when medication helps a little. That may sound strange. Improvement should be good, and often it is. Medication can be useful in properly selected men. If a man has early symptoms, a reasonably small prostate, no major blockage, a bladder that empties well, and a good response to medication, that may be an appropriate plan.

The problem is partial improvement being mistaken for control. A man starts medication. His stream is slightly better. He wakes up two times instead of three. He is less bothered. Everyone feels encouraged. The medication is refilled.

But nobody checks how much urine is left in the bladder. Nobody measures how fast the urine comes out. Nobody measures the prostate. Nobody looks to see whether part of the prostate is growing up into the bladder and blocking the outlet like a ball valve.

The man is better, but he may not be fixed. That phrase matters. Better is not fixed.

If the bladder is still leaving urine behind, the medication has not solved the whole problem. If the stream remains very slow, the medication has not solved the whole problem. If the prostate is physically blocking the bladder opening, relaxing the prostate muscle may not be enough. If the man still structures his life around bathrooms, he should not be told everything is fine because the prescription was renewed.

The question is not whether the medication did something. The question is whether it did enough.

THE MEDICATION ILLUSION

Many prostate medications work by relaxing muscle around the prostate and bladder opening. That can make urination easier. For the right patient, this can be helpful. But relaxing is not the same as removing an obstruction.

If the prostate is acting like a tight collar around the urine channel, relaxing that collar may improve flow. If the prostate is large, protruding, or physically blocking the outlet, medication may give only partial relief. It can reduce some resistance but leave the main anatomical problem in place.

Patients need to understand this distinction because medication can create the illusion that the problem is being fully treated. A man may say, "I'm on something for my prostate."

That does not tell me whether his bladder is safe. It does not tell me whether he is emptying. It does not tell me whether his stream is strong enough. It does not tell me whether the prostate is growing into the bladder. It does not tell me whether he is moving closer to retention.

A prescription is not a measurement. A refill is not a plan.

Medication should be judged by what it accomplishes. Does the man sleep better? Does he urinate more freely? Does the bladder empty? Is there less urine left behind? Is the top speed of urination improved? Is the patient's life actually better? Is the bladder protected? If those questions are not being answered, the treatment plan is incomplete.

THE BALL-VALVE PROSTATE

FIGURE 4.2

Ball-Valve Prostate

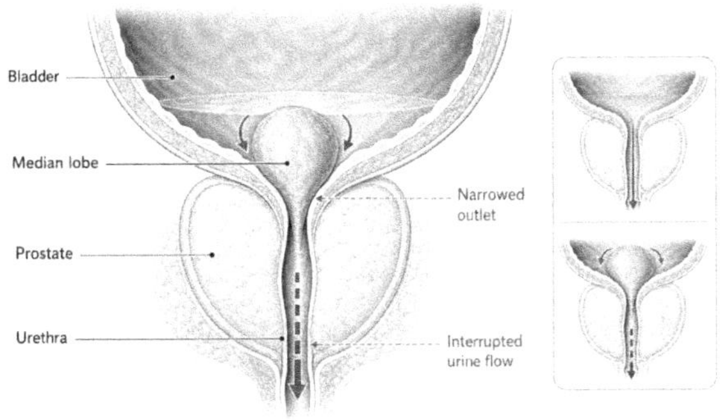

Intravesical prostate growth can act like a ball valve at the bladder outlet, blocking urine flow disproportionately to overall prostate size.

Figure 4.2 - Ball-Valve Prostate. Intravesical growth can block the outlet out of proportion to size.

Some men have a prostate that does not simply squeeze the urine channel from the sides. Instead, part of the prostate grows upward into the bladder opening. Doctors call this intravesical prostatic protrusion, but most patients do not need that phrase. They need the concept.

Think of it as prostate tissue bulging into the bladder outlet. When the bladder tries to empty, that tissue can act like a ball valve. Urine is trying to leave, but the prostate tissue sits at the exit and interferes with flow. This can happen even when the total prostate size is not enormous.

This is why prostate size alone can be misleading. A moderately enlarged prostate growing in the wrong direction can cause more trouble than a larger prostate growing outward. The shape and position of the tissue matter.

This also helps explain why medication sometimes disappoints. A pill can relax muscle, but it cannot make a ball-valve blockage disappear. It cannot make prostate tissue stop protruding into the bladder. It cannot guarantee the bladder is emptying.

When a man is told his prostate is enlarged, he should ask a more specific question: is any part of the prostate growing into the bladder opening? That answer can change the entire treatment conversation.

THE STREAM TELLS A STORY, BUT IT SHOULD BE MEASURED

Patients describe their urinary stream in everyday language. They say it is weak, slow, hesitant, or not what it used to be. That information is useful, but it is subjective. Some men understate their symptoms. Others have adapted so much that they no longer realize how abnormal the stream has become. That is why measuring the urine stream matters.

A urine flow test measures how fast the urine comes out. The medical term for the maximum speed of urination is Qmax, but in a patient book, the meaning is what matters. We want to know whether the urine comes out with good force or whether it trickles through a narrowed outlet.

A slow stream can mean several things. It can mean the prostate is blocking the outlet. It can mean the bladder muscle is weak. It can mean both.

That is why the urine flow test has to be interpreted with the rest of the evaluation. If the stream is slow and a lot of urine is left behind, the bladder is not emptying well. If the prostate is enlarged and bulging into the bladder opening, obstruction becomes more likely. If the prostate is not very enlarged but the stream is slow and the bladder is weak, the problem may be more about bladder function.

The number matters because it moves the conversation away from guessing. A man should not spend years saying, "My stream is not great," while nobody ever measures how slow it really is.

THE BLADDER CAN BECOME THE DISEASE

The tragedy in BPH is not simply that the prostate becomes enlarged. The tragedy is when the bladder is damaged by years of pushing against obstruction.

There is a point where the prostate is still the original problem, but the bladder has become the bigger problem. The bladder may be stretched. It may not contract well. It may leave urine behind. It may become irritable and overactive. It may fail voiding trials after a catheter is removed. Some men end up needing a catheter for longer than expected. Some may need to catheterize themselves to empty. This is the stage we want to avoid.

When men hear the word "procedure," many assume the doctor is being aggressive. But sometimes the more aggressive decision is doing nothing while the bladder continues to struggle. Sometimes the conservative decision is to protect the bladder before it fails. That is a different way of thinking about BPH.

The old model was to delay procedures as long as possible. Keep the man on medication. Wait until symptoms are severe. Wait until retention. Wait until the bladder proves it is in trouble. The modern model is to ask earlier whether the bladder is safe.

That does not mean every man needs a procedure. It means every man deserves to know where he stands.

URGENCY MAY BE A BLADDER CRY FOR HELP

Many men with prostate obstruction develop urgency and frequency. They feel like they need to urinate often. They may rush to the bathroom. They may wake up repeatedly at night.

Because these symptoms feel like bladder symptoms, the diagnosis may be called overactive bladder. Sometimes that is correct. But sometimes the bladder is overactive because it is reacting to obstruction.

This distinction is clinically important. If the bladder is overactive because the prostate is blocking the outlet, the root problem is not simply a bladder that needs to be calmed. The bladder is responding to pressure, resistance, incomplete emptying, or chronic irritation.

Treating urgency without checking the outlet is like turning off a smoke alarm without checking for smoke. Before a man is placed on bladder-calming medication, the doctor should know whether he is emptying. If a large amount of urine is already being left behind, some bladder medications can make emptying worse. They may reduce urgency but increase retention risk in the wrong patient.

Again, the issue is not that bladder medications are bad. They can be useful. The issue is using them without understanding why the bladder is irritated in the first place.

SLEEP IS PART OF THE BLADDER STORY

One of the most common ways the prostate-bladder connection shows up is nighttime urination. A man wakes up once, then twice, then three or four times per night. He may call it annoying, but the true cost is bigger than inconvenience. He is losing sleep. Chronic sleep disruption affects energy, mood, weight, metabolism, testosterone, heart health, focus, and sexual function.

If a bladder problem is destroying sleep, it is no longer just a bladder problem. It is a whole-body problem.

This is especially important in a modern men's health and longevity framework. Men want to live longer, but they also want to function longer. They want energy, strength, sexual performance, mental clarity, and independence. A man who is up all night urinating is not recovering. He is not optimizing health. He is being controlled by his bladder. That bladder may be reacting to the prostate.

This is why urinary symptoms should not be dismissed as minor because they are common. Common does not mean harmless.

"STABLE" COMPARED TO WHAT?

Patients are often told they are stable. That word can be reassuring, but it can also be vague.

Stable symptoms? Stable prostate size? Stable PSA? Stable left-over urine in the bladder? Stable urine flow? Stable bladder function? If none of those things were measured, "stable" may only mean the conversation sounded the same as last time.

A man can be stable at a poor level of function. He can be stable waking up three times a night. He can be stable with a weak stream. He can be stable leaving too much urine behind. He can be stable on a medication that is only partly working.

Stable is not the same as safe. That distinction is important. Modern prostate care should not be satisfied with vague stability. It should ask whether the man is improving, whether the bladder is protected, and whether the current treatment is achieving its goal. A man who is still struggling should not be told he is fine just because his symptoms are familiar.

WHAT A MODERN EVALUATION SHOULD TELL YOU

A modern evaluation of prostate-related urinary symptoms should answer practical questions in language the patient understands. How large is the prostate? Is part of it growing into the bladder opening? How much urine is left behind after urination? How fast does the urine come out? Does the bladder appear to be working too hard or weakening? Is the patient's nighttime urination damaging sleep? Is medication truly working, or is it only partially masking the problem?

These questions are not academic. They guide treatment.

If the prostate is only mildly enlarged, the bladder empties well, and the stream is reasonable, medication or monitoring may be appropriate. If the prostate is growing into the bladder, the stream is slow, and urine is left behind, the conversation should become more serious. If the bladder appears weak or the patient has already gone into retention, additional testing may be needed to understand whether the bladder can still recover.

This is not about ordering every test on every patient. It is about asking the right question before choosing the treatment.

THE PATIENT'S MOST IMPORTANT QUESTION

If a man remembers only one question from this chapter, it should be this: Is my bladder safe? That question cuts through vague reassurance. It forces the conversation to move beyond "your prostate is enlarged" and "keep taking the medication." It asks whether the urinary system is functioning.

A man should not need to know every technical term to advocate for himself. He does not need to walk into the office speaking like a urologist. He should be able to ask in plain English: "Am I emptying my bladder? Is urine being left behind? Is my stream dangerously slow? Is the prostate blocking the bladder opening? Are we protecting the bladder, or just treating symptoms?" Those are fair questions. A modern urologist should be able to answer them.

DR. SHUSTERMAN'S MODERN PROSTATE TAKEAWAY

The prostate and bladder are connected. The prostate may create resistance, but the bladder has to fight against it. Over time, that fight can lead to urgency, frequency, nighttime urination, leftover urine in the bladder, infections, stones, retention, and eventually bladder weakness.

Medication can be helpful, especially early. But partial improvement does not always mean the bladder is safe. A man can feel better and still be obstructed. He can take medication and still leave urine behind. He can be told he is stable while the bladder is slowly losing ground.

Better is not fixed. Modern prostate care is not just about the size of the prostate. It is about what the prostate is doing to the bladder. The question every man should ask is simple: is my bladder safe?

CHAPTER 5

THE PROSTATE IS NOT ONE DISEASE

ONE OF THE biggest mistakes men make is using the word "prostate" as if it means one thing. A man comes into the office and says, "Doctor, I have a prostate problem."

That sounds specific, but medically it is not specific at all. A "prostate problem" could mean many different things. It could mean benign enlargement. It could mean inflammation. It could mean a urinary blockage. It could mean a rising PSA. It could mean prostate cancer. It could mean pelvic pain. It could mean the bladder is not emptying. It could mean the bladder is overactive. It could mean constipation is making urinary symptoms worse. It could even mean the prostate is being blamed for something that is not primarily a prostate problem. That distinction matters.

The prostate is an organ. It is not a diagnosis. When a man says his prostate is the problem, the next question should always be: what kind of prostate problem are we talking about?

This is where many men get confused. They hear the word prostate and immediately think of cancer. Or they hear the word enlarged and assume it is harmless. Or they have urinary symptoms and assume every symptom must be coming from the prostate. Or their PSA rises and they assume that means cancer.

All of those assumptions can be wrong. Modern prostate care begins by separating the possibilities. A man may have benign enlargement. He may have inflammation. He may have prostate cancer risk. He may have bladder dysfunction. He may have more than one problem at the same time. The treatment depends on knowing which problem is present.

A vague diagnosis leads to vague treatment. A precise diagnosis leads to a plan.

THE FEAR AROUND THE WORD "PROSTATE"

For many men, the word prostate creates anxiety before the doctor even explains what is happening. That fear usually comes from cancer. Almost every man knows someone who had prostate cancer, had a biopsy, had radiation, had surgery, or struggled with sexual or urinary side effects after treatment. Prostate cancer is common, and the fear around it is real. But most prostate complaints are not prostate cancer.

A man with a weak stream usually does not have urinary symptoms because of cancer. A man waking up at night to urinate is usually not waking up because of cancer. A man who feels urgency or incomplete emptying is often dealing with benign enlargement, bladder irritation, obstruction, inflammation, or a combination of issues.

At the same time, early prostate cancer often causes no urinary symptoms at all. That is the part men often miss.

A man can urinate normally and still have prostate cancer. Another man can have terrible urinary symptoms and have no cancer. Urinary symptoms and cancer risk overlap in the same organ, but they are not the same thing.

This is why the prostate must be approached with calm precision. Fear is not a strategy. Reassurance without testing is not a strategy either. The goal is to understand which problem is present.

BENIGN ENLARGEMENT IS NOT CANCER

The most common prostate condition men hear about with age is benign prostate enlargement, often called BPH. The medical name is benign prostatic hyperplasia, but patients do not need to get lost in the phrase. The simple meaning is that the prostate has enlarged in a noncancerous way.

That distinction is important. BPH is not prostate cancer. It does not spread through the body. It does not mean a man has cancer. It does not automatically turn into cancer. But benign does not mean meaningless.

Because the prostate surrounds the urine channel, even noncancerous growth can create a real urinary problem. The prostate can narrow the channel, distort the outlet of the bladder, and force the bladder to work harder to empty. That can cause weak stream, urgency, frequency, nighttime urination, incomplete emptying, infections, bladder stones, and urinary retention.

This is one of the central misunderstandings in men's health. Men hear "not cancer" and think the problem does not matter. But a benign prostate can still damage quality of life and bladder function. Cancer is not the only prostate problem worth taking seriously.

CANCER AND ENLARGEMENT OFTEN BEGIN IN DIFFERENT AREAS

Part of the confusion comes from the fact that both BPH and prostate cancer involve the same organ. But they often begin in different areas of that organ.

Benign enlargement usually develops closer to the urine channel, in the part of the prostate that surrounds the passage where urine exits the bladder. That is why BPH causes urinary symptoms. It grows near the plumbing.

Prostate cancer often begins more toward the outer portion of the prostate. That is one reason early prostate cancer can be silent. It may not press on the urine channel at all. The man may feel perfectly fine while a cancer-risk signal appears only on a PSA blood test, MRI, or biopsy.

This does not mean the separation is absolute. Cancer can appear in different zones, and a man can have both benign enlargement and cancer. In fact, older men commonly have some degree of enlargement while also needing cancer-risk evaluation.

But the concept is useful. Urinary symptoms usually tell us about the prostate-bladder system. PSA tells us about cancer risk. They are related, but they are not the same. A man should not assume he has cancer because he urinates poorly. He also should not assume he is cancer-free because he urinates well.

PSA IS A SIGNAL, NOT A DIAGNOSIS

PSA is one of the most misunderstood blood tests in medicine. PSA stands for prostate-specific antigen. It is a protein made by prostate cells. Doctors use it as a tool to help assess prostate cancer risk, but PSA itself is not cancer.

A man can have an elevated PSA for several reasons. A larger benign prostate can produce more PSA because there is more prostate tissue. Inflammation can raise PSA. Infection can raise PSA. Urinary retention can raise PSA. Recent procedures or irritation of the prostate can raise PSA. Cancer can raise PSA as well.

This is why PSA should not be treated like a panic button. It should also not be ignored.

The correct approach is thoughtful risk assessment. How old is the man? What was the PSA last year? Is the number rising quickly? How large is the prostate? Has there been infection, inflammation, or retention? Is there a family history of prostate cancer? Is the man at higher risk? Would a more advanced blood test help clarify risk? Is an MRI appropriate? Does he need a biopsy?

A single number rarely tells the story. PSA starts a conversation. It does not finish it.

The mistake is reacting blindly. Some men panic and rush into procedures they may not need. Other men dismiss a rising PSA because they feel fine. Both responses can be dangerous.

Modern prostate care lives between fear and denial. It interprets the signal.

PROSTATE CANCER IS NOT ONE DISEASE EITHER

Even prostate cancer is not one disease in the way men often imagine. The word cancer creates immediate fear, but prostate cancer exists on a spectrum. Some prostate cancers are very low risk and may never threaten the man's life. Others are aggressive and need timely treatment. The name alone does not tell the story.

This is why pathology matters. The biopsy result, Grade Group, Gleason pattern, number of positive cores, PSA level, MRI findings, genomic testing, and imaging all help define risk. A tiny low-grade cancer found in an older man is not the same as a high-grade cancer in a younger man with many positive biopsy cores and concerning imaging.

The treatment should match the risk. Some men are best managed with active surveillance, meaning careful monitoring rather than immediate treatment. Other men need radiation, focal therapy, hormone therapy, surgery, or combinations of treatment depending on the situation. The word cancer is emotionally powerful, but the risk category is what guides the plan.

A man should never be treated only for the word. He should be treated for the biology of the disease.

PROSTATITIS: THE CONFUSING DIAGNOSIS

Prostatitis means inflammation of the prostate. That sounds straightforward, but in real practice it can be one of the most confusing diagnoses in urology.

Sometimes prostatitis is bacterial. The patient may have burning, urinary symptoms, fever, pelvic discomfort, a positive urine culture, or recurrent infections. When bacterial prostatitis is suspected, antibiotics can be appropriate and important. But not every prostatitis-like symptom is a bacterial infection.

Some men have pelvic pain, discomfort with ejaculation, urinary frequency, or pressure without clear evidence of bacteria. In those patients, the problem may involve inflammation, pelvic floor muscle tension, bladder sensitivity, constipation, nerve irritation, stress physiology, or a combination of factors.

This is where men often get stuck. One doctor gives antibiotics. The patient feels a little better, then symptoms return. Another round is given. Then another. Eventually the patient has taken multiple antibiotics but still does not understand what is wrong.

The problem is not that antibiotics are always wrong. Bacterial prostatitis is real. The problem is repeating a treatment without reassessing the diagnosis.

If the clinical picture suggests infection, treat it. If the patient improves clearly, that is useful information. But if symptoms persist or recur, the doctor must step back and ask whether something else is being missed.

Is there a stone? Is the bladder not emptying? Is there a prostate blockage? Is constipation worsening pelvic pressure? Is the pelvic floor involved? Is the PSA elevated because of inflammation, or is cancer risk still present?

Prostatitis is not a trash-can diagnosis. It should be explained, evaluated, and followed.

THE BLADDER CAN IMITATE THE PROSTATE

Not every urinary symptom in a man is caused by the prostate. This is obvious when you think about women. Women do not have prostates, yet they can have urgency, frequency, nighttime urination, bladder pain, infections, leakage, pelvic floor dysfunction, and incomplete emptying.

Men can have those issues too. The prostate is common, but it is not always guilty.

A man with urgency and frequency may have an overactive bladder. Or he may have a bladder that is overactive because the prostate is blocking the outlet. A man with slow urination may have prostate obstruction. Or he may have a weak bladder muscle that cannot push strongly. A man waking up at night may have prostate enlargement. Or he may have sleep apnea, diabetes, excess nighttime urine production, evening alcohol intake, heart disease, kidney issues, or medication effects. This is why diagnosis matters.

If a bladder problem is mislabeled as prostate enlargement, treatment may fail. If prostate obstruction is mislabeled as overactive bladder, the blockage may continue while the bladder is simply medicated into silence. If sleep apnea is causing nighttime urination, a prostate pill will not fix the real problem.

Symptoms are the entry point. They are not the diagnosis.

CONSTIPATION AND THE CROWDED MALE PELVIS

The pelvis is a crowded space. The bladder, prostate, rectum, pelvic floor muscles, nerves, and urine channel all sit close together. When one part of that system is irritated, the others may feel it. Constipation is a good example.

Men often do not connect bowel habits with urinary symptoms, but they should. A full rectum sits directly behind the prostate and bladder area. Chronic straining can tighten the pelvic floor. Constipation can increase pelvic pressure, worsen urgency, aggravate prostatitis-like discomfort, and make a man feel that he is not emptying normally.

Constipation may not be the entire diagnosis, but it can be an amplifier. If a man has urinary symptoms, pelvic discomfort, pressure, or recurrent irritation, bowel habits should be part of the conversation. How often does he move his bowels? Does he strain? Does he feel incomplete evacuation? Do urinary symptoms worsen when he is constipated?

A prostate evaluation that ignores the bowel can miss an important contributor. Modern urology should not treat the pelvis as separate rooms with locked doors. The organs interact.

PELVIC FLOOR DYSFUNCTION

The pelvic floor is a group of muscles that helps coordinate urination, bowel function, sexual function, and pelvic support. When these muscles are too tight, irritated, or poorly coordinated, they can create symptoms that feel like prostate disease. Men may have pelvic pain, testicular discomfort, urinary frequency, urgency, hesitancy, pain after ejaculation, rectal pressure, or a sensation of incomplete emptying.

Pelvic floor dysfunction is real, but it should be used carefully as a diagnosis. It should not become an excuse to ignore obvious obstruction. A man with a prostate bulging into the bladder, a very slow urine stream, and a large amount of urine left behind should not be told everything is pelvic floor tension. At the same time, a man with normal emptying, no major prostate obstruction, pelvic pain, constipation, and muscle tension may absolutely have a pelvic floor component.

The modern approach is balanced. Do not blame every symptom on the prostate. Do not blame every symptom on the pelvic floor. Measure the system, then decide.

BLADDER STONES AND RECURRENT INFECTIONS

Sometimes the problem is hidden until someone looks inside. A man may have recurrent urinary infections and receive antibiotic after antibiotic. Each course may help temporarily. Then the infection returns. The assumption is that he simply keeps getting infections. But why?

If the bladder does not empty well, urine sits behind. That left-over urine can increase infection risk. Over time, bladder stones may form. A bladder stone can act like a hiding place for bacteria. Antibiotics may reduce the infection temporarily, but if the stone remains, the bacteria can return.

In that situation, the diagnosis is not just "urinary infection." The real problem may be prostate blockage, incomplete bladder emptying, a bladder stone, and recurrent infection all connected. A camera test of the bladder can answer questions antibiotics cannot.

This is why repeated infections in a man deserve evaluation. The goal is not only to treat the bacteria. The goal is to find out why the infections are happening.

SEXUAL SYMPTOMS AND THE PROSTATE

The prostate also gets blamed for sexual problems, sometimes correctly and sometimes not. The prostate does not create erections by itself. Erections are mainly about blood flow, nerves, hormones, and the brain. But the prostate can still be connected to sexual function in several ways.

Prostate medications can affect ejaculation. Some men notice reduced semen volume or retrograde ejaculation, where semen goes backward into the bladder instead of out through the penis. Prostate inflammation can cause pain with ejaculation. Prostate cancer treatments can affect erections, ejaculation, orgasm, and urinary control. Urinary symptoms themselves can reduce confidence and sexual comfort. A man who is exhausted from waking up all night to urinate may not feel sexually well.

At the same time, erectile dysfunction can be a sign of vascular or metabolic disease, not simply a prostate issue. A man with ED may need blood pressure evaluation, diabetes screening, cholesterol management, testosterone assessment, cardiovascular risk review, and lifestyle intervention.

The prostate may be part of the sexual health story. It is not always the story. That is another reason vague labels fail.

MIXED PROBLEMS ARE COMMON

Many men do not have one clean diagnosis. A man can have benign prostate enlargement and an overactive bladder. He can have prostate enlargement and prostatitis. He can have a rising PSA and a large benign prostate. He can have urinary obstruction and constipation. He can have erectile dysfunction, low testosterone, poor sleep, and nighttime urination at the same time.

Medicine is often mixed. That is why one-size-fits-all care fails. A man with mild enlargement and bladder overactivity should not be treated the same way as a man with a ball-valve prostate blockage and urine left behind. A man with a rising PSA should not be reassured only because his urinary stream is good. A man with pelvic pain should not receive endless antibiotics if repeated testing does not support infection.

The diagnosis must be specific enough to guide treatment. A good prostate evaluation should identify the main driver of symptoms and also recognize secondary contributors.

THE DANGER OF TREATING THE WRONG PROBLEM

Wrong diagnosis leads to wrong treatment. If prostate obstruction is mistaken for overactive bladder, the man may receive bladder medication while the outlet remains blocked. If pelvic floor dysfunction is mistaken for infection, he may receive repeated antibiotics without lasting improvement. If constipation is ignored, urinary symptoms may persist despite prostate treatment. If prostate cancer risk is dismissed because the man urinates normally, a silent cancer may be missed. If elevated PSA is assumed to be cancer without context, the patient may undergo unnecessary anxiety and procedures.

The point is not that every patient needs every test. The point is that the treatment should match the mechanism.

What problem are we treating?Why is it happening?What measurement supports the diagnosis?What endpoint tells us the treatment worked? Those questions apply to everything in this book.

WHAT A MAN SHOULD ASK

A man does not need to speak like a urologist to advocate for himself. If he is told he has a prostate problem, he should ask what kind of problem it is. Is the prostate enlarged? Is it blocking urine? Is urine being left behind after he finishes? Is the bladder overactive, or is it reacting to a blockage? Is there inflammation or infection? Is the PSA appropriate for his age and risk? Is cancer being evaluated properly? Could constipation, sleep apnea, medication, diabetes, or pelvic floor issues be contributing?

The language can be simple. The thinking should be precise. The question is not, "Do I have a prostate problem?" The better question is, "Which prostate problem are we actually treating?" That question protects the patient from vague medicine.

DR. SHUSTERMAN'S MODERN PROSTATE TAKEAWAY

The prostate is not one disease. It is an organ that can enlarge, obstruct, inflame, produce PSA, develop cancer, affect ejaculation, interact with the bladder, and confuse the entire pelvic system.

BPH is not cancer, but it can still damage urinary function. Prostate cancer is often silent early. PSA is a risk signal, not a diagnosis. Prostatitis means inflammation, but not always infection. The bladder can create symptoms that look like prostate symptoms. Constipation and pelvic floor dysfunction can amplify urinary complaints. Sexual dysfunction may overlap with prostate disease but is not always caused by the prostate.

The goal is not to label everything as "prostate." The goal is to identify the real mechanism. A man should not leave the office with a vague phrase. He should leave with an explanation, a measurement, and a plan.

The prostate is not one disease. And if the diagnosis is not specific, the treatment will not be either.

CHAPTER 6

WHY MEN START PEEING DIFFERENTLY

MOST MEN KNOW when their urination has changed, even if they do not know what to call it. They may not walk into the office using medical language. They usually do not say, "Doctor, I have lower urinary tract symptoms." They say it the way real men say it.

"My stream is not what it used to be." "I have to wait before it starts." "I wake up too much at night." "I feel like I just went, and then I have to go again." "I always need to know where the bathroom is." "I thought this was just part of getting older." That last sentence is the one that concerns me. A change in urination may be common with age, but common does not always mean normal. It may be the first sign that the prostate-bladder system is changing. Sometimes the prostate is the main issue. Sometimes the bladder is the main issue. Sometimes the problem is sleep, diabetes, constipation, inflammation, medication, alcohol, caffeine, or a combination of factors. But when urination changes, the answer should not be casual dismissal.

The way a man urinates is one of the simplest windows into his aging male health. A man does not need to panic because his stream is slower than it used to be. But he should not ignore it either. A weak stream, nighttime urination, urgency, and incomplete emptying are not just annoyances. They are signals. The job of modern urology is to understand what those signals mean.

THE SLOW CHANGE MEN NORMALIZE

Most prostate-related urinary changes do not happen overnight. A man usually does not go from urinating perfectly to being in trouble in one day. The change is often gradual. At first, he may notice that the stream takes a little longer to start. Then the stream becomes weaker. Then he wakes once at night. Then once becomes twice. He starts standing closer to the bathroom at events. He chooses the aisle seat. He avoids long car rides without planning stops. He tells himself he is just getting older. That slow adaptation is part of the danger.

If a man had the urinary function of a seventy-year-old suddenly at age twenty-five, he would think something was wrong immediately. But when the change happens over years, he adjusts. He lowers his expectations. He begins to compare himself not to his younger normal, but to other men his age who are also struggling. That is the wrong comparison.

A man should ask himself how his urination compares to when he was twenty or twenty-five. Not because every older man must urinate like a college athlete, but because the comparison reveals the direction of change. Did the stream lose force? Does it take longer to start? Does he wake up when he never used to? Does he need to return to the bathroom soon after finishing? That simple self-check often tells us there is a real change worth evaluating.

THE STREAM TELLS A STORY

FIGURE 6.1

The Stream Tells a Story

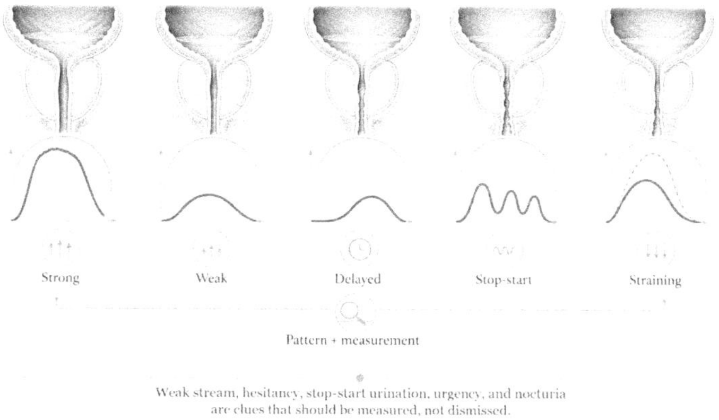

Figure 6.1 - The Stream Tells a Story. Urinary patterns should be measured, not dismissed.

The urinary stream is one of the first things men notice. A healthy stream usually starts easily, flows with force, and ends cleanly. When the stream becomes weak, slow, hesitant, or interrupted, it suggests that something in the system is no longer working freely.

For many men, the prostate is the reason. The prostate sits around the urine channel. As it enlarges, it can narrow or distort that channel. If part of the prostate grows upward into the bladder opening, it may block the exit like a ball valve. The bladder then has to push through resistance.

But a weak stream does not always mean the prostate is the only problem. A man can also have a weak bladder muscle. He can have a narrowing in the urine channel. He can have a tight bladder neck. He can have a neurologic problem. He can have more than one issue at the same time.

That is why the stream should not only be described. It should be measured.

A urine flow test can measure the maximum speed of urination. Doctors may call this number Qmax, but patients do not need to obsess over the abbreviation. The plain-English question is: how fast does the urine come out?

That number matters. A man may say his stream is "not terrible," but the test may show that urine is coming out very slowly. Another man may feel his stream is weak, but testing may show reasonable flow and point us toward a different cause of symptoms. Without measurement, everyone is guessing.

WAITING TO START

Many men notice that urination does not begin immediately. They stand at the toilet and wait. Sometimes they need to relax. Sometimes they shift position. Sometimes they push with their abdomen. Eventually the stream starts, but it no longer feels automatic.

This delay is called hesitancy, but the name is less important than the experience. Urination has become a negotiation.

In a healthy system, the bladder contracts and the outlet opens. The process should be relatively smooth. When a man has to wait, the body may be telling us there is resistance at the outlet, poor coordination, or a bladder that is struggling to generate enough force.

Prostate enlargement is a common reason. A tight bladder neck, a narrowed urine channel, or a weak bladder can also contribute. The symptom points us toward the problem, but it does not prove the cause.

That is why a man with hesitancy should not simply be handed medication and forgotten. He should know whether the bladder is emptying, whether urine is being left behind, whether the stream is dangerously slow, and whether the prostate is physically blocking the bladder opening. A symptom is the beginning of the conversation, not the end of it.

THE STOP-AND-START STREAM

Another common complaint is the stream that starts and stops. A man begins to urinate, then the flow weakens or cuts off. He waits. It starts again. He may need to push. He may think he is finished, then more urine comes out. The process feels inefficient and frustrating.

This stop-and-start pattern can happen when the outlet is obstructed. It can also happen when the bladder muscle does not contract smoothly or strongly enough. Sometimes the prostate creates resistance and the bladder is still strong. Sometimes the bladder is weak. Sometimes years of resistance have created a mixed picture.

This distinction matters because treatment depends on the mechanism. If the prostate is blocking and the bladder is strong, opening the outlet may help significantly. If the bladder is already weak, treating the prostate may still be necessary, but expectations must be different. If both problems are present, the plan has to account for both.

The patient experiences one symptom: a stream that stops and starts. The doctor must figure out why.

STRAINING IS NOT NORMAL URINATION

Some men push to urinate. They tighten the abdomen. They bear down. They use pressure from the belly to help the bladder empty. That should not be normal.

The bladder is designed to empty by contracting. A man should not have to use his abdominal muscles like he is forcing out a bowel movement just to urinate. When he strains, it usually means the system is not emptying freely.

Straining can mean the prostate is blocking the outlet. It can mean the bladder is weak and the man is trying to compensate. It can mean both.

It can also be dangerous because straining may give the man a false sense that he is managing. He gets urine out, but only by forcing the system. He may not realize that urine is still being left behind. He may not realize the bladder is under stress.

A man who has to push to urinate deserves an objective evaluation. How much urine remains after he finishes? How fast does the urine come out? Is the prostate enlarged? Is prostate tissue growing into the bladder opening? Does the bladder still appear strong? Those questions matter more than simply asking whether the patient can still get urine out.

FEELING EMPTY DOES NOT MEAN BEING EMPTY

One of the most important lessons in prostate care is that feeling empty is not the same as being empty. A man can finish urinating and feel done. He may not feel pressure. He may not feel discomfort. He may believe the bladder is empty.

Then we check with ultrasound or a bladder scan and find a significant amount of urine still sitting there. Doctors call this post-void residual urine. I prefer to explain it in plain language: it is the urine left behind after you pee.

That leftover urine is a critical measurement. It tells us whether the bladder is emptying. If the amount is low, that is reassuring. If the amount is rising or high, the conversation changes.

Leftover urine can increase the risk of infection. It can contribute to bladder stones. It can worsen frequency because the bladder never truly starts from empty. It can be a sign of blockage, bladder weakness, or both. If it becomes severe, the patient may be approaching retention.

This is why a man should not be reassured only because he says he feels empty. The bladder should be measured.

URGENCY: THE BLADDER'S ALARM

Urgency is the sudden strong need to urinate. For many men, urgency is more disruptive than a weak stream. A weak stream is annoying, but urgency controls behavior. Men with urgency scan every room for a bathroom. They avoid long meetings. They worry on the highway. They plan their day around access to a restroom. Some men begin to withdraw from activities because the bladder feels unpredictable.

Urgency feels like a bladder problem, and sometimes it is. The bladder may be overactive on its own. But urgency can also be the bladder's response to obstruction.

A bladder pushing against a blocked outlet can become irritated. Over time, it may begin sending signals too early and too often. The man feels urgency, but the root problem may still be the prostate.

This is why treating urgency without checking emptying can be a mistake. If the bladder is already leaving urine behind, some bladder-calming medications may worsen emptying in the wrong patient. They may reduce the alarm while the underlying obstruction remains. Before calming the bladder, make sure the bladder is not reacting to a blocked exit.

FREQUENCY: GOING OFTEN DOES NOT ALWAYS MEAN MAKING TOO MUCH URINE

Frequency means urinating often during the day. Some men truly make too much urine because of fluid intake, diabetes, medications, caffeine, alcohol, or other medical issues. But many men urinate frequently because the bladder is not emptying well or because it has become irritated.

If the bladder never fully empties, it may fill again quickly. The man may feel like he just went, then needs to go again soon after. The problem is not that the bladder is producing urine too quickly. The problem is that the bladder never truly reset to empty. This is another reason leftover urine matters.

A man may think he has a small bladder. He may think he drinks too much water. He may think he has anxiety. Those things may contribute, but if he is leaving urine behind after each trip to the bathroom, the explanation is different.

Frequency should not be treated blindly. It should be understood.

NIGHTTIME URINATION IS A SLEEP PROBLEM

Nighttime urination is one of the most common complaints in aging men. Doctors call it nocturia, but the simple meaning is waking up at night to urinate.

Many men minimize it. They say they get up "only" two or three times. They say they are used to it. They say it is part of aging.

But waking up several times every night is not a small issue. It fragments sleep. Poor sleep affects energy, mood, weight, metabolism, testosterone, cardiovascular health, mental focus, and sexual performance. In a modern healthspan model, sleep is not optional. It is one of the pillars of function.

Nighttime urination can come from the prostate, but not always. A man may wake because the prostate is blocking emptying. He may wake because the bladder is irritated. He may produce too much urine at night because of sleep apnea, leg swelling, heart or kidney issues, diabetes, evening alcohol, excess fluids, or certain medications.

This is why nighttime urination deserves evaluation rather than assumption. If a man wakes once occasionally, that may not be a major concern. But new, worsening, persistent, or never-evaluated nighttime urination should not be dismissed. A man waking three or four times per night is not simply "getting older." His sleep is being injured, and the cause should be understood.

MODERATE SYMPTOMS CAN STILL BE A MAJOR PROBLEM

Medicine often uses symptom scores to classify urinary symptoms as mild, moderate, or severe. These tools can be useful. They help track progress and give structure to the discussion. But patients should be careful with the word "moderate."

Moderate does not mean acceptable. A man with moderate urinary symptoms may wake up every night, rush to the bathroom, strain to urinate, stop and start, and feel that his bladder is never fully empty. On paper, he may be called moderate. In real life, he may be miserable.

This becomes especially important when medication improves symptoms only slightly. A man may start with severe symptoms and improve into the moderate range. That is progress, but it may not be success. If he is still bothered, still sleeping poorly, still leaving urine behind, or still urinating slowly, the treatment may not be enough.

Better is not fixed. A symptom score is useful, but it should not replace common sense. The real question is whether the man is functioning well and whether the bladder is safe.

WHEN SYMPTOMS ARE NOT FROM THE PROSTATE

Because prostate enlargement is so common, men and doctors sometimes blame the prostate too quickly. Not every urinary symptom in a man is caused by the prostate.

Diabetes can increase urination. Sleep apnea can cause nighttime urination. Diuretics can make a man urinate more often. Alcohol and caffeine can irritate the bladder. Urinary tract infections can cause urgency, frequency, and burning. Bladder stones can cause irritation and blood in the urine. Constipation can worsen urgency, frequency, and pelvic pressure. Pelvic floor muscle problems can mimic prostate symptoms. Neurologic conditions can affect bladder function.

The prostate is a common suspect, but it is not the only suspect. This is one reason modern evaluation matters. If a man has a weak stream, prostate obstruction must be considered. If he has urgency and frequency, the bladder must be considered. If he wakes all night, sleep and medical causes must be considered. If he has burning, infection and inflammation must be considered. The right diagnosis prevents the wrong treatment.

THE BATHROOM STARTS CONTROLLING LIFE

Many men do not realize how much they have adapted until symptoms improve. They had stopped going to movies unless they had an aisle seat. They avoided long car rides. They checked where the bathroom was in every restaurant. They woke up tired every morning. They avoided drinking water before meetings. They carried anxiety around travel. They accepted slow urination as normal.

Then, after proper treatment, they sleep better, travel more comfortably, and feel less controlled. That is when they realize how much the prostate-bladder problem had taken from them.

Urinary symptoms are not just plumbing. They affect confidence, sleep, relationships, work, travel, exercise, and independence. A man may not be dying from BPH, but he may be living a smaller life because of it.

That matters. Quality of life is not a minor endpoint.

WHAT A MODERN EVALUATION SHOULD CLARIFY

When a man starts peeing differently, the goal is to answer a few practical questions. Is the prostate enlarged? Is it blocking the urine channel? Is part of it growing into the bladder opening? How much urine is left behind after urination? How fast does the urine come out? Is the bladder overactive because it is irritated, or because it is fighting obstruction? Is nighttime urination coming from the prostate, the bladder, sleep apnea, metabolic issues, or another cause? Is the bladder safe?

A man should not leave the office with only the phrase "your prostate is enlarged." That does not tell him enough. He should understand what is happening in ordinary language.

If the doctor uses technical terms, the doctor should translate them. The patient does not need to memorize abbreviations. He needs to understand whether the system is working.

THE QUESTION MEN SHOULD ASK EARLIER

Most men wait too long. They wait until the stream is terrible. They wait until they are waking up all night. They wait until medication fails. They wait until they cannot travel comfortably. Some wait until they cannot urinate at all. The better approach is to ask earlier: why am I peeing differently?

That question is not dramatic. It is not fearful. It is responsible.

A man does not need to demand treatment for every mild symptom. But he should understand what is changing. If everything is safe, he can monitor. If the prostate is starting to obstruct, he can plan. If the bladder is leaving urine behind, he can act before retention. If the issue is sleep apnea or diabetes, he can address the real cause.

Early evaluation does not force aggressive treatment. It creates options.

DR. SHUSTERMAN'S MODERN PROSTATE TAKEAWAY

Men start peeing differently for many reasons. The prostate is common, but it is not the only cause. A weak stream may suggest blockage. Urgency may be the bladder's alarm. Frequency may reflect incomplete emptying or bladder irritation. Nighttime urination may be a prostate issue, a bladder issue, a sleep issue, or a metabolic issue.

The mistake is not noticing symptoms. The mistake is normalizing them without understanding them. A man should know whether his prostate is enlarged, whether it is blocking the bladder opening, how much urine is left behind after he urinates, how fast the urine comes out, and whether the bladder is safe.

The way a man urinates is one of the earliest signals that the prostate-bladder system may be changing. Do not wait until weak stream becomes retention. Do not wait until poor sleep becomes normal. Common aging is not the same as healthy function.

CHAPTER 7

THE PROSTATE SIZE GAUGE

ONE OF THE least helpful things a man can be told in a urology office is, "Your prostate is enlarged." That may sound like information, but by itself it does not tell the patient enough. Enlarged compared to what? Slightly enlarged? Moderately enlarged? Very large? Is the prostate growing outward, where it may not cause much blockage, or is it growing upward into the bladder opening, where it can act like a ball valve? Is urine being left behind after the man finishes urinating? Is the stream slow? Is the bladder still emptying safely?

The word enlarged is too vague. Patients deserve numbers. They deserve explanations. They deserve to understand what those numbers mean in real life.

This is why I like the idea of a prostate size gauge. Men understand gauges. They understand a speedometer. They understand blood pressure numbers. They understand when a tire is low, when a tank is empty, or when a warning light comes on. The prostate should not be discussed in language so vague that the patient leaves with no idea where he stands.

A man should know whether his prostate is normal-sized, mildly enlarged, moderately enlarged, severely enlarged, or very large. He should also understand that size is only the beginning. The shape of the prostate, the direction of growth, the speed of the urine stream, and the amount of urine left behind after urination may matter just as much as the size itself.

The prostate size gauge is not meant to scare men. It is meant to replace vague reassurance with useful understanding.

WHY "ENLARGED" IS NOT ENOUGH

Imagine a patient being told his blood pressure is "a little high," but nobody gives him the number. He would not know whether the pressure is mildly elevated or dangerously high. He would not know whether he needs lifestyle changes, medication, urgent treatment, or simple monitoring.

The same problem happens with the prostate. A man hears, "Your prostate is enlarged," but he is not told whether it is thirty grams, sixty grams, ninety grams, or one hundred and fifty grams. He is not told whether the prostate is growing into the bladder. He is not told whether the bladder is emptying. He is not told whether the urine stream is acceptable or dangerously slow.

Then he is given a pill. That is not modern prostate care.

A patient should not need to become a urologist, but he should know the basic facts about his own anatomy. If a man is going to make decisions about medication, procedures, cancer testing, sleep disruption, and bladder protection, he needs more than the word enlarged. He needs a map.

WHAT PROSTATE SIZE ACTUALLY MEANS

FIGURE 7.1

The Prostate Size Gauge

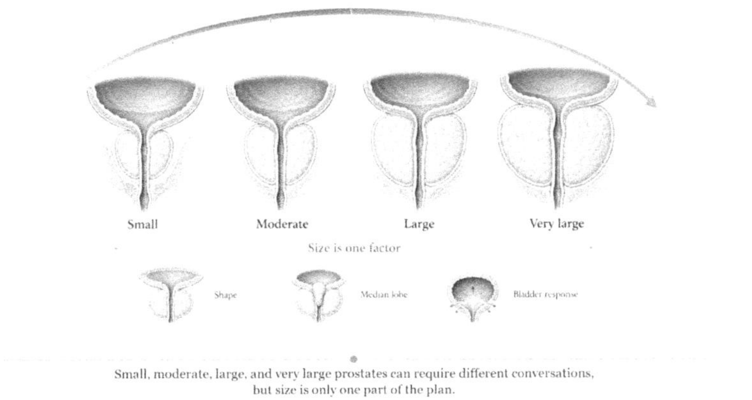

Figure 7.1 - The Prostate Size Gauge. Prostate volume is useful, but never the whole story.

Prostate size is usually measured in grams or cubic centimeters. For patient understanding, those numbers are close enough that men can think of them in a similar way. A prostate measured at forty cubic centimeters is often discussed as roughly forty grams. The exact technical conversion is less important than the general category.

A normal or small prostate is usually around twenty grams or less. Once the prostate grows above that, we begin to describe degrees of enlargement. A prostate in the twenty-to-forty-gram range is mildly enlarged. A prostate in the forty-to-sixty-gram range is moderately enlarged. A prostate between sixty and one hundred grams is severely enlarged. A prostate over one hundred grams is very large.

Those categories are not absolute laws. They are a practical framework.

A thirty-five-gram prostate can cause serious symptoms if it grows in the wrong direction. A seventy-gram prostate may cause fewer symptoms if it grows outward and the bladder empties well. A one-hundred-gram prostate may be surprisingly tolerated for a while, but it still deserves a serious discussion because the bladder may be compensating under strain.

Size matters, but size is not the entire diagnosis. It is the beginning of the conversation.

A NORMAL-SIZED PROSTATE

A young healthy prostate is often around twenty grams or less. In that range, the prostate is usually small enough that it should not be assumed to be the main cause of severe urinary obstruction.

If a man has major urinary symptoms with a small prostate, the doctor should think carefully. The problem may be a tight bladder neck, a narrowing in the urine channel, a weak bladder muscle, overactive bladder, pelvic floor dysfunction, inflammation, infection, constipation, diabetes, sleep apnea, medication effects, or another condition.

That is why knowing prostate size matters. It prevents lazy diagnosis. If the prostate is small and the patient is miserable, the answer should not automatically be, "It is just your prostate." The doctor should ask what else may be happening.

This is one of the major benefits of measuring the prostate. It tells us when the gland is large enough to explain symptoms, and it also tells us when we need to look elsewhere.

MILD ENLARGEMENT

A prostate between twenty and forty grams is mildly enlarged. Many men in this range can be managed with observation, lifestyle changes, or medication if symptoms are mild and the bladder is emptying well. But the word mild should not make everyone relax automatically. A mildly enlarged prostate can still cause trouble if it grows in a strategically bad direction.

The most important example is prostate tissue growing upward into the bladder opening. Doctors may call this intravesical prostatic protrusion, but the patient-friendly explanation is simpler: part of the prostate is bulging into the bladder outlet and may block the exit like a ball valve.

That can happen even when the overall prostate size is not enormous. This is why a man with a thirty-five-gram prostate may still have significant symptoms, a slow stream, or urine left behind after urination. The prostate may not be huge, but it may be growing in the wrong place. The question is not only, "How big is it?" The question is, "What is it doing?"

MODERATE ENLARGEMENT

The forty-to-sixty-gram range is where the conversation often becomes more serious. This is not a tiny prostate anymore. It may not be massive, but it is large enough to cause meaningful blockage, especially if the prostate is growing around the urine channel or upward into the bladder opening. At this size, medication may help some men, but it should not be used blindly without knowing how the bladder is doing.

A man in this range should understand whether urine is being left behind after he finishes. He should know how fast the urine comes out. He should know whether the prostate is simply enlarged or whether it is bulging into the bladder outlet. He should know whether medication is truly helping or only partially masking the problem.

This is also the range where patients are often undertreated. The prostate may be described as "not that big," but the symptoms can be substantial. The patient may wake up repeatedly at night, have urgency, and struggle with a slow stream. He may be on medication and still not feel right.

When the size is moderate and the symptoms are persistent, the doctor should not dismiss the patient. The anatomy and bladder function should be measured. A moderate prostate can still create a major quality-of-life problem.

SEVERE ENLARGEMENT

A prostate between sixty and one hundred grams is severely enlarged. At this point, the gland is large enough that the patient deserves a more strategic discussion. Some men may still do reasonably well on medication if the bladder empties, the stream is acceptable, and symptoms are controlled. But medication becomes less convincing when the stream is slow, urine is left behind, the prostate is growing into the bladder, or the patient remains significantly bothered.

The danger is that a man with severe enlargement may adapt for years. He may say he is "okay" because he has learned to live with poor urination. He wakes up at night. He avoids certain activities. He stands longer at the toilet. He takes medication. He tells himself this is aging.

Meanwhile, the bladder may be doing extra work every day. Severe enlargement should not automatically mean a procedure, but it should mean careful evaluation. The patient should understand whether the prostate is simply large or whether it is actively threatening bladder function. There is a difference between a large prostate that is being watched safely and a large prostate that is being ignored.

VERY LARGE PROSTATES

A prostate over one hundred grams is very large. These glands require a serious conversation. They are not rare in a urology practice, but many patients are shocked when they hear the number. A man may have been told for years that his prostate was enlarged, but nobody explained that it had become three, four, or five times the size of a young normal prostate.

A very large prostate does not always mean immediate danger, but it changes the strategy. Medication may provide some symptom relief, but it is often not enough if the patient has poor flow, urine left behind, repeated nighttime urination, bladder stones, infections, or retention.

Historically, very large prostates were often treated with more invasive surgical procedures. Those procedures still have a role in selected patients. But modern urology has expanded the discussion. Prostate artery embolization, for example, can be an important option for larger glands because it treats the prostate through its blood supply rather than cutting through the urine channel.

The point is not that every large prostate should be treated the same way. The point is that very large prostates deserve modern planning, not casual reassurance.

SIZE IS ONLY PART OF THE STORY

The prostate size gauge is useful, but it has to be interpreted correctly. The size of the prostate is like the size of a house. It tells you something, but it does not tell you the entire layout. Two houses can have the same square footage and different floor plans. One may feel open and functional. Another may feel cramped because of the way the walls are arranged.

The prostate is similar. Two men can have the same prostate size and different urinary function. One prostate may grow outward and create little blockage. Another may grow inward around the urine channel. Another may push upward into the bladder opening. The total size may be similar, but the effect on urination can be different. That is why the direction of growth matters.

The most important question is often whether the prostate is bulging into the bladder opening. If it is, the prostate may create a ball-valve type blockage. The bladder tries to empty, but the tissue sits at the exit and interferes with the flow.

A pill can relax muscle. It cannot make a ball-valve blockage disappear.

This is why patients need more than size. They need shape, position, bladder emptying, and flow.

WHY THE BLADDER MUST BE PART OF THE GAUGE

A prostate size number without bladder information is incomplete. A man may have a large prostate but still empty well. Another man may have a moderately enlarged prostate and leave a significant amount of urine behind after every trip to the bathroom. Those two men should not be treated the same way.

The bladder tells us whether the prostate is causing functional damage. One of the most important measurements is how much urine remains after urination. This is the urine left behind after a man thinks he is finished. If very little remains, that is reassuring. If a large amount remains, the bladder is not emptying normally.

The speed of the urine stream also matters. A man may describe his stream as "not great," but the flow test may show that urine is coming out very slowly. That slow flow may mean the prostate is blocking the outlet, the bladder is weak, or both.

The prostate size gauge should therefore be paired with two bladder questions: is the bladder emptying, and is the stream strong enough? Without those answers, the size number can be misleading.

THE FINGER EXAM CANNOT GIVE THE WHOLE ANSWER

For generations, men associated prostate evaluation with a finger exam. That exam may give a rough impression of the prostate in selected situations, but it cannot provide the information needed for a modern prostate size gauge.

A finger exam cannot accurately measure prostate volume. It

cannot show whether the prostate is growing into the bladder. It cannot measure urine left behind after urination. It cannot measure the speed of the urine stream. It cannot show whether the bladder is under strain.

That does not mean the exam has no role in medicine. It means it should not be the centerpiece of modern evaluation for urinary obstruction when better tools are available.

If the question is prostate size and shape, ultrasound is far more useful. If the question is bladder emptying, a bladder scan or ultrasound is needed. If the question is flow, the stream should be measured. If the question is internal anatomy, a small camera test may be appropriate.

A man with urinary symptoms deserves objective information. A finger and a guess are not enough.

WHY ULTRASOUND MATTERS

Prostate ultrasound is one of the most useful tools in modern BPH evaluation. It can measure prostate size. It can help show the shape of the gland. It can identify when the prostate is bulging into the bladder opening. It can help determine how much urine is left behind after the patient urinates. It gives the doctor and patient a better understanding of the anatomy.

This is not exotic testing. In a modern office, ultrasound should be practical, fast, and extremely informative. A man who has urinary symptoms, rising PSA, poor flow, nighttime urination, or concern about prostate enlargement should not be managed for years without someone measuring the gland.

The difference between "your prostate is enlarged" and "your prostate is about eighty grams and part of it is pushing into the bladder opening" is enormous. The first statement is vague. The second statement helps guide treatment.

PROSTATE SIZE AND PSA

Prostate size also helps interpret PSA. PSA is made by prostate cells. If a man has more prostate tissue, he may produce more PSA even without cancer. That does not mean a high PSA in a large prostate is automatically harmless. It means size gives context.

A PSA of four in a very large prostate may mean something different than a PSA of four in a very small prostate. The doctor still has to look at age, PSA trend, family history, inflammation, infection, retention, MRI findings, and other risk factors. But without knowing prostate size, the PSA story is incomplete.

This is another reason vague prostate care fails. A man may be told his PSA is elevated, but no one measures the prostate. Or he may be told his prostate is enlarged, but no one explains how that affects PSA interpretation. Modern care connects the dots. The prostate size, PSA trend, urinary symptoms, bladder emptying, and cancer-risk evaluation should all be part of one conversation.

SIZE AND MEDICATION

The prostate size gauge also helps explain why medication works better for some men than others. A pill that relaxes the prostate opening may help when the main problem is muscle tightness and mild obstruction. It may help a man with early symptoms, a smaller prostate, and a bladder that empties well. But medication has limits.

If the gland is very large, medication may not be enough. If prostate tissue is bulging into the bladder outlet, medication may not be enough. If urine is being left behind, medication may not be enough. If the stream is very slow, medication may not be enough.

This does not mean medication is bad. It means medication must be judged honestly.

The question is not whether the pill did something. The question is whether it solved enough of the problem to protect the bladder and improve the man's life. If the prostate is large and the bladder is struggling, endless refills are not a modern plan.

SIZE AND PROCEDURE CHOICE

Knowing prostate size also helps match a man to the right procedure. Different treatments work in different ways. Some relax tissue. Some heat tissue. Some remove tissue. Some pull tissue aside. Some treat the blood supply to the prostate. Some are better suited for smaller glands. Some are better suited for larger glands. Some are more appropriate when the prostate is bulging into the bladder. Some preserve ejaculation better than others. Some are more likely to cause irritation during recovery.

A man should not ask only, "What is the best procedure?" The better question is, "What is the best procedure for my prostate size, prostate shape, bladder function, and goals?" That is the modern way to think. A smaller or moderately enlarged prostate may be suited to one set of options. A very large prostate may require a different conversation. A prostate that grows into the bladder opening may need a strategy that addresses that specific anatomy. A bladder that is weak or leaving a lot of urine behind may require additional testing before choosing a procedure. Treatment should follow anatomy.

WHAT A PATIENT SHOULD KNOW

A man does not need to memorize every medical detail, but he should understand the basics of his own prostate. He should know whether the prostate is small, mildly enlarged, moderately enlarged, severely enlarged, or very large. He should know whether the prostate is growing into the bladder opening. He should know whether his bladder empties after he urinates. He should know whether the urine comes out with reasonable speed. He should know whether his PSA makes sense for his age, prostate size, and risk.

These are not advanced questions. They are basic ownership of one's health.

A man who knows his numbers is harder to dismiss. He is also better able to make decisions. He can understand why medication may be reasonable, why a procedure may be appropriate, or why observation may be safe.

The goal is not to create anxiety. The goal is to create clarity.

THE DANGER OF NOT KNOWING

The danger of not knowing prostate size is that treatment becomes generic. A man gets the same pill as every other man. He gets the same reassurance. He gets the same follow-up interval. He is told he is stable, but nobody has measured what matters.

Stable compared to what? Stable symptoms? Stable prostate size? Stable urine left behind? Stable stream speed? Stable bladder function? Stable PSA? If nobody measures those things, "stable" may not mean much.

This is how men drift into trouble. The prostate grows slowly. The bladder adapts slowly. The stream weakens slowly. Urine left behind increases slowly. The patient adjusts slowly. Then, one day, he cannot urinate.

He thinks it happened suddenly, but often the warning signs were there for years. They were just not measured.

DR. SHUSTERMAN'S MODERN PROSTATE TAKEAWAY

The phrase "enlarged prostate" is not enough. A man should know the size of his prostate, whether it is growing into the bladder opening, how much urine is left behind after urination, how fast the urine comes out, and whether the bladder is safe.

The prostate size gauge gives men a practical way to understand where they stand. A prostate around twenty grams or less is usually small or normal. Twenty to forty grams is mildly enlarged. Forty to sixty grams is moderately enlarged. Sixty to one hundred grams is severely enlarged. Over one hundred grams is very large. But size is only part of the story.

Shape matters. Direction of growth matters. Bladder emptying matters. Urine flow matters. Symptoms matter. PSA context matters. A prostate growing into the bladder can behave more dangerously than its size suggests.

Modern prostate care should not be vague. Once the prostate is measured, the conversation changes from guessing to planning.

CHAPTER 8

TESTING BEFORE TREATMENT

FIGURE 8.1

Testing Before Treatment

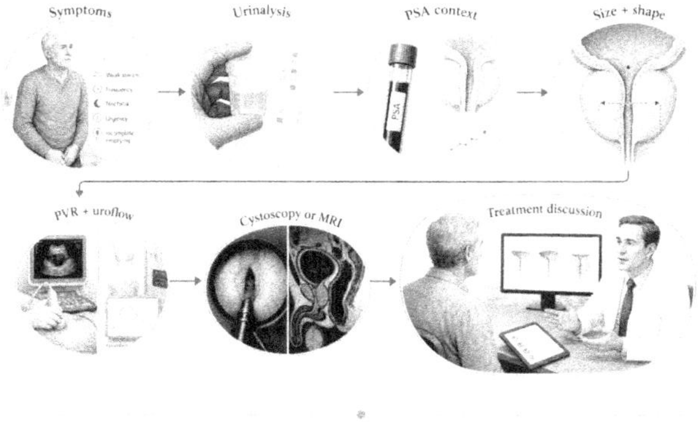

Modern prostate care asks what the prostate and bladder are doing and what risk signals are present before treatment is chosen.

FIGURE 8.1 - TESTING BEFORE TREATMENT. *Modern prostate care starts with measurement before treatment choice.*

One of the most common mistakes in prostate care is starting treatment before understanding the problem. A man walks into a urology office because he is urinating differently. He is waking up at night. His stream is weaker. He feels like he does not empty completely. Maybe he has urgency. Maybe he has to stand at the toilet and wait. Maybe he is embarrassed and only admits half of what is happening.

Too often, the visit ends with a prescription. The medication may help. It may not. But the deeper problem is that no one has clearly answered the most important questions. How large is the prostate? Is it actually blocking the bladder opening? Is urine being left behind after the man finishes? How fast does the urine come out? Is the bladder still working well? Is the PSA appropriate for the patient's age and risk? Is this truly a prostate problem, or is the bladder, sleep, diabetes, infection, constipation, or another issue contributing?

Without those answers, treatment becomes guesswork. A prescription is not a diagnosis. A refill is not a plan. A procedure should not be chosen before the anatomy is understood. A bladder medication should not be given before knowing whether the bladder is already struggling to empty.

The principle is simple: Treating without measuring is guessing. And when the bladder is at risk, guessing is not good enough.

SYMPTOMS ARE IMPORTANT, BUT THEY ARE NOT ENOUGH

A patient's story matters. I want to know when symptoms started, how quickly they changed, and how much they affect the man's life. Does he wake up once at night or four times? Does the stream start immediately or does he have to wait? Does he push to urinate? Does he stop and start? Does he feel empty? Does he return to the bathroom ten minutes later? Has he ever been unable to urinate? Has he seen blood? Has he had infections? Is he taking prostate medication already? Does he have diabetes, sleep apnea, constipation, neurologic disease, or take medications that affect urination?

Those questions are essential. They tell me what the patient experiences. But symptoms do not always tell me why they are happening.

A man with urgency may have an overactive bladder. Or he may have a bladder that is irritated because the prostate is blocking the outlet. A man with a weak stream may have prostate enlargement. Or he may have a weak bladder muscle. A man waking up all night may have prostate obstruction. Or he may have sleep apnea, excess night-time urine production, diabetes, alcohol-related bladder irritation, or a combination of causes.

The same symptom can come from different mechanisms. That is why symptoms should guide testing, not replace testing.

THE DANGER OF SYMPTOM-ONLY TREATMENT

Symptom-only treatment often sounds reasonable in the beginning. A man says he urinates frequently, so he is treated for overactive bladder. A man says his stream is weak, so he is given a prostate pill. A man says he wakes up at night, so the problem is assumed to be BPH. A man has an elevated PSA, so anxiety rises and biopsy is discussed immediately.

Sometimes the first assumption is correct. Often it is incomplete.

If a man has urgency because the bladder is reacting to a blocked prostate, calming the bladder without addressing the blockage may miss the root cause. If a man has a weak stream because the bladder muscle has become weak, simply relaxing the prostate may not solve the problem. If a man wakes at night because of sleep apnea, a prostate pill may do very little. If a man's PSA is elevated because of infection or retention, the next step may not be immediate panic.

Symptoms open the door. They do not finish the evaluation.

Modern prostate care should not be built on assumptions that sound plausible. It should be built on measurements that show what is happening.

THE FIRST MEASUREMENT IS THE STORY

Before any machine, scan, or test, the first diagnostic tool is still the conversation. A good history can separate different problems. A man who has had slowly worsening urinary symptoms for ten years is different from a man who developed burning and frequency over three days. A man who wakes up at night but urinates normally during the day may have a different problem from a man who has a weak stream, incomplete emptying, and daytime frequency. A man with diabetes, sleep apnea, and leg swelling may have nighttime urination for reasons that are not purely prostate-related.

The story also reveals how much the symptoms are affecting life. Some men minimize. They say they are "fine," but then admit they wake up every two hours, avoid long drives, and know every bathroom in every restaurant they visit. Other men are more bothered by mild symptoms because those symptoms interfere with their work, sleep, travel, or sexual confidence.

A good urologist listens carefully. But listening should lead to the right measurements.

THE SYMPTOM SCORE

One useful tool is a urinary symptom questionnaire. The best-known version is often called the International Prostate Symptom Score. Patients do not need to remember that name. What matters is that the questionnaire asks about the problems men commonly experience: incomplete emptying, frequent urination, stopping and starting, urgency, weak stream, straining, and waking up at night.

A symptom score helps because it puts numbers on the patient's experience. It makes follow-up more meaningful. If a man starts treatment, we can compare how he felt before and after. Did nighttime urination improve? Did urgency improve? Did the stream improve? Is quality of life better? But the symptom score has limits.

It does not measure prostate size. It does not show whether the prostate is growing into the bladder opening. It does not tell us how much urine remains after urination. It does not measure the maximum speed of the urine stream. It does not show whether the bladder is strong or weak. It does not rule out cancer.

A symptom score is the patient's report. It is not the whole diagnosis.

URINE TESTING: THE BASIC STEP THAT MATTERS

A simple urine test can reveal important information. If a man has blood in the urine, that may require further evaluation. If there are signs of infection, the treatment changes. If glucose is spilling into the urine, diabetes may be part of the urinary frequency. If there is protein or other abnormality, the kidneys or broader medical issues may need attention.

This is why a urinalysis should not be skipped casually. Not every urinary symptom is BPH. Infection, stones, blood, diabetes, and kidney-related issues can all appear through urine testing. A man with urgency and frequency may not need only a prostate medication. He may need evaluation for infection, blood, bladder irritation, or metabolic disease. The urine test is not glamorous, but it is one of the basic ways we avoid missing something obvious.

PSA: A RISK SIGNAL, NOT A VERDICT

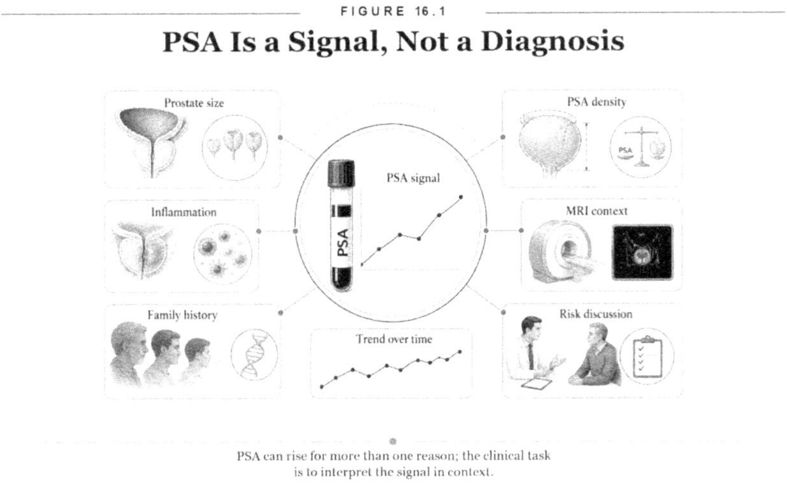

Figure 8.2 - PSA Is a Signal, Not a Diagnosis. PSA should be interpreted in context, not treated as a verdict.

PSA testing is often part of prostate evaluation, but it must be interpreted correctly. PSA is a protein made by prostate cells. Doctors use it to help assess prostate cancer risk, but PSA is not cancer. A larger benign prostate can produce more PSA. Inflammation can raise PSA. Infection can raise PSA. Urinary retention can raise PSA. Recent procedures or irritation can raise PSA. Cancer can raise PSA as well.

This is why a PSA number should never be interpreted in isolation. The real question is context. How old is the patient? What was the PSA last year? Is it rising slowly or quickly? How large is the prostate? Has there been infection, inflammation, or recent retention? Is there family history? Is the patient in a higher-risk group? Should a more advanced blood test or MRI be used before deciding on biopsy?

PSA should not create automatic panic, but it should not be

ignored. It is a signal. Modern medicine's job is to interpret the signal intelligently.

MEASURING THE PROSTATE

If a man has urinary symptoms, the prostate should not remain a mystery. A modern evaluation should measure the prostate. Ultrasound is one of the most practical tools for this. It can help determine how large the gland is and whether the size is mild, moderate, severe, or very large. It can also help show whether prostate tissue is growing upward into the bladder opening. That last point is critical.

A man may be told his prostate is "not that big," but if part of the gland is bulging into the bladder outlet, it can still create a major blockage. This ball-valve type growth may explain why medication does not work well enough. A pill may relax muscle, but it cannot remove tissue sitting in the wrong place.

This is why the prostate measurement should not be reduced to one number. Size matters, but shape and direction of growth also matter. A forty-five-gram prostate growing into the bladder may cause more trouble than a larger prostate growing outward.

The patient-friendly question is simple: is the prostate just enlarged, or is it blocking the bladder opening? That answer can change the plan.

MEASURING WHAT IS LEFT BEHIND

One of the most important tests in urinary evaluation is measuring how much urine remains in the bladder after the man urinates. Doctors call this the post-void residual. Patients can think of it simply as the urine left behind after peeing. This number matters because a man can feel empty and still not be empty.

When urine is left behind, it may mean the prostate is blocking the outlet. It may mean the bladder muscle is weak. It may mean both. It may increase the risk of infection, bladder stones, worsening frequency, and eventually retention.

A small amount of leftover urine may be acceptable, depending on the situation. A rising amount is concerning. A large amount changes the conversation completely.

This is one of the measurements that separates vague prostate care from modern prostate care. Without it, a doctor may reassure a patient who is retaining urine. With it, the patient can understand whether the bladder is emptying safely. If a man is being treated for prostate symptoms and no one has checked how much urine is left behind, the evaluation is incomplete.

MEASURING THE SPEED OF URINATION

FIGURE 8.2

Uroflow + PVR

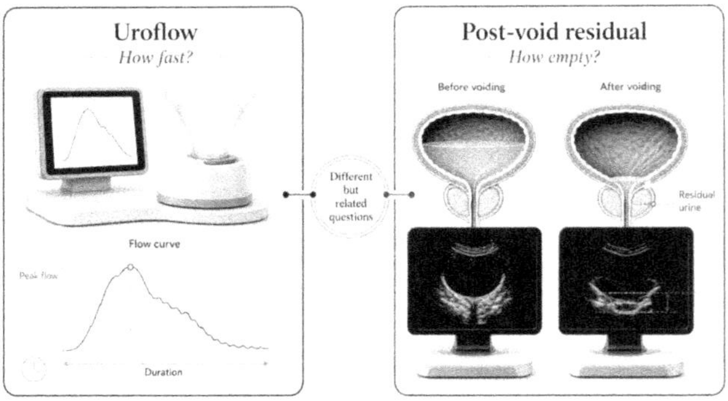

Uroflow shows how the stream behaves; post-void residual shows whether the bladder actually emptied.

Figure 8.3 - Uroflow + PVR. Flow and residual urine answer different but related questions.

The urinary stream should also be measured when symptoms suggest obstruction or poor emptying. A urine flow test is simple. The patient urinates into a special device that measures how fast the urine comes out. The medical term for the top speed is Qmax, but the patient does not need to focus on the abbreviation. The plain-English concept is maximum speed of urination.

This number gives useful information. A very slow stream may suggest a blockage, a weak bladder, or both. A reasonable stream may point the evaluation in another direction. The result is especially useful when interpreted together with prostate size, urine left behind, symptoms, and bladder function.

The flow test also gives patients a reality check. Men often adapt to poor urination. They may say, "It is not that bad," because the decline happened slowly. But a measured flow can show that the stream is much slower than it should be.

Again, the point is not to bury patients in numbers. The point is to replace impressions with evidence. A man should know whether his urine comes out with reasonable force.

WHEN PRESSURE MATTERS

Sometimes flow alone does not tell the full story. A slow stream can happen because the prostate is blocking the outlet, but it can also happen because the bladder is too weak to push well. Those are different problems. A man with a strong bladder pushing against blockage may benefit from opening the outlet. A man with a weak bladder may still need treatment, but the expectations and planning are different. This is where pressure-based testing can help.

Some offices use noninvasive pressure-flow testing, which estimates how hard the bladder is pushing during urination. I often explain it to patients as something like a blood-pressure test for urination. More formal bladder pressure testing, called urodynamics, may be needed in selected cases, especially when the patient has very high leftover urine, retention, failed voiding trials, neurologic disease, or symptoms that do not match the basic findings.

Patients do not need every advanced test automatically. But when the central question is whether the bladder is strong enough, pressure testing can be extremely valuable.

The wrong procedure in a man with a weak bladder can lead to disappointment. Testing helps prevent false promises.

CYSTOSCOPY: LOOKING INSIDE

Cystoscopy is a small camera test that allows the doctor to look inside the urine channel, the prostate channel, the bladder opening, and the bladder itself. Many patients fear cystoscopy before they have it. They imagine something much worse than the actual procedure. In a modern office, it is usually brief and well tolerated. Numbing jelly is used. The scope is small. The purpose is to see the anatomy directly.

Cystoscopy can answer questions that other tests cannot. It can show whether there is a narrowing in the urine channel. It can show how the prostate is blocking from the inside. It can show whether the bladder neck is tight. It can show stones, tumors, inflammation, or signs that the bladder has been working against obstruction for a long time.

Not every man needs cystoscopy at the first visit. But when the question is internal anatomy, when a procedure is being considered, when symptoms are severe, when there is blood in the urine, recurrent infection, bladder stones, retention, or failed treatment, cystoscopy can be one of the most useful tests in urology.

A procedure should not be chosen blindly. The doctor should understand the channel before changing it.

MRI AND CANCER-RISK EVALUATION

MRI has transformed prostate cancer evaluation. It is not the first test for every man with simple urinary symptoms. If the main question is urinary obstruction, ultrasound, urine flow testing, leftover urine measurement, and cystoscopy may be more directly useful. But when the question is prostate cancer risk, MRI becomes important.

If PSA is elevated or rising, if prior biopsy was negative but suspicion remains, or if the risk picture does not make sense, MRI can help identify suspicious areas in the prostate. It can help decide whether biopsy is needed and where tissue should be sampled.

MRI does not replace biopsy when biopsy is necessary. It does, however, make the biopsy decision smarter. The old model was too crude: PSA goes up, patient panics, biopsy happens.

The modern model is more thoughtful. PSA rises, the risk is interpreted, prostate size and clinical context are considered, advanced blood tests may be used when appropriate, MRI is obtained when indicated, and biopsy is performed when the risk justifies it.

The goal is not to avoid biopsy at all costs. The goal is to avoid unnecessary biopsy while still detecting meaningful cancer.

ADVANCED BLOOD TESTS

In some patients, advanced blood tests can help refine prostate cancer risk. One example is IsoPSA, which looks at structural information related to PSA rather than only measuring the amount of PSA in the blood. The details matter less to most patients than the purpose: it can help clarify risk when the decision about biopsy is uncertain.

This fits the larger theme of the book. Modern prostate care should not rely on one number or one tradition. It should use better tools to make better decisions. If the PSA is concerning, the question is not automatically, "How fast can we biopsy?" The question is, "What is this man's actual risk, and what is the smartest next step?"

Sometimes that step is repeat testing. Sometimes it is advanced blood testing. Sometimes it is MRI. Sometimes it is biopsy. The plan should match the risk.

TESTING BEFORE MEDICATION

Medication can be useful in BPH, but it should not be used blindly. Before a man is placed on long-term medication, he should understand the target. Is the medication supposed to relax the prostate opening? Is it supposed to slowly shrink the prostate? Is it mainly helping urinary symptoms and erections? How quickly should it work? What side effects matter? How will success be measured?

If the goal is symptom improvement, the symptom score should improve. If the goal is better emptying, less urine should be left behind. If the goal is better stream, the flow should improve. If the man is still waking up all night, still straining, still leaving urine behind, or still living around bathrooms, the medication may not be enough.

A medication trial is reasonable when it has a plan. It becomes weak medicine when it turns into indefinite refills without measurement.

TESTING BEFORE BLADDER MEDICATION

This point is important enough to repeat. A man with urgency and frequency may be treated as if the bladder is the main problem. Sometimes that is correct. But before calming the bladder, the doctor should know whether the bladder is irritated because the prostate is blocking the exit.

If a man already leaves too much urine behind, some bladder-calming medications can make emptying worse. That does not mean these medications are bad. They can be helpful in properly selected patients. But selection matters. Before quieting the bladder, make sure the bladder is not reacting to obstruction. That is the kind of thinking that prevents complications.

TESTING BEFORE PROCEDURES

Procedures should be matched to anatomy. This should be obvious, but it is often not how patients experience the medical system. A procedure may be recommended because a doctor likes it, because a facility owns the equipment, because it is marketed heavily, or because it is the procedure most familiar to that practice. That is not the right way to choose.

The right procedure depends on prostate size, whether prostate tissue is growing into the bladder opening, how much urine is left behind, how fast the urine comes out, whether the bladder is strong, whether the patient wants to preserve ejaculation, how severe the symptoms are, how much recovery he can tolerate, and what future options should remain open. A man should not ask only, "What is the newest procedure?" He should ask, "What procedure fits my anatomy?" That is the modern question.

TESTING BEFORE BIOPSY

Biopsy is how prostate cancer is diagnosed, but biopsy should answer a real risk question. A man should not be biopsied because everyone became nervous. He also should not avoid biopsy when the risk is significant.

The decision should consider age, PSA level, PSA trend, prostate size, family history, MRI findings, advanced blood tests, prior biopsy history, overall health, and life expectancy. If MRI shows a clearly suspicious lesion in a man who is healthy enough to benefit from diagnosis and treatment, biopsy may be appropriate. If the findings are borderline, the decision may require more discussion. This is another example of testing before treatment.

The biopsy is not the first thought. Risk assessment is the first thought.

THE FINGER EXAM IS NOT ENOUGH

For generations, men associated prostate evaluation with the finger exam. That exam has a history, and it may still have selected uses. But for modern evaluation of urinary symptoms, it is not enough.

A finger exam cannot accurately measure prostate size. It cannot show whether the prostate is bulging into the bladder opening. It cannot tell how much urine is left behind. It cannot measure how fast the urine comes out. It cannot determine whether the bladder is weak. It cannot replace ultrasound, flow testing, bladder scanning, cystoscopy, MRI, or appropriate cancer-risk evaluation.

If a man has urinary symptoms and the entire evaluation is a finger exam and a prescription, that is not modern care. That is flying blind.

A man should not avoid urology because he fears the exam. Modern prostate care is about measurement, imaging, function, and risk assessment. The old symbolic prostate exam should not define the entire field.

WHAT THE PATIENT SHOULD LEAVE KNOWING

A man should not leave the urologist's office with only vague language. He should understand what is known and what still needs to be clarified. He should know whether the prostate is enlarged and whether that enlargement appears to be blocking the bladder opening. He should know whether the bladder empties after urination. He should know whether the urine stream is slow. He should know whether PSA is appropriate for his age and risk. He should know whether medication is likely to be enough. He should know what the next step is if symptoms persist.

The patient does not need to memorize every abbreviation. He does not need to speak like a urologist. But he should understand his own situation in ordinary language. That is what good prostate care should provide.

DR. SHUSTERMAN'S MODERN PROSTATE TAKEAWAY

Testing before treatment is not overcomplication. It is responsible medicine.

Symptoms tell us what the patient feels. Testing tells us what the prostate, bladder, urine stream, and cancer-risk signals are doing.

A man with urinary symptoms should not be treated blindly. The prostate should be measured. The bladder should be checked. The urine stream should be evaluated. PSA should be interpreted in context. A bladder medication should not be used to ignore obstruction. A procedure should match anatomy. A biopsy should answer a risk question.

The future of prostate care is not more guessing. It is measurement, mechanism, and treatment that makes sense. Treating without measuring is guessing. And guessing is not good enough when the bladder is at risk.

CHAPTER 9

BPH MEDICATIONS: USEFUL EARLY, LIMITED BY ANATOMY

MEDICATION HAS an important place in prostate care. That needs to be said clearly because patients sometimes hear a discussion about modern procedures and assume medication is being dismissed. It should not be. Many men benefit from prostate medication. For the right patient, at the right stage, with the right anatomy, medication can improve urinary symptoms and delay or avoid procedures.

The problem is not that prostate medication exists. The problem is when medication becomes the entire plan.

A man starts a pill because his stream is weak or he wakes up at night. At first, he feels a little better. The prescription is refilled. Then it is refilled again. Years pass. He is still waking up. The stream is still not normal. He still has urgency. He still plans around bathrooms. No one has measured how much urine is left behind after he finishes. No one has checked how fast the urine comes out. No one has shown him whether the prostate is growing into the bladder opening. No one has answered the real question: is the bladder safe? That is where medication can become misleading.

A pill can improve symptoms without fixing the underlying

anatomy. A man can feel somewhat better while still being obstructed. He can be on medication and still leave urine behind. He can be "treated" on paper while the bladder continues to work against resistance every day. Medication should be used as a tool, not as a substitute for diagnosis.

WHAT MEDICATION CAN AND CANNOT DO

FIGURE 9.1

BPH Medication Jobs

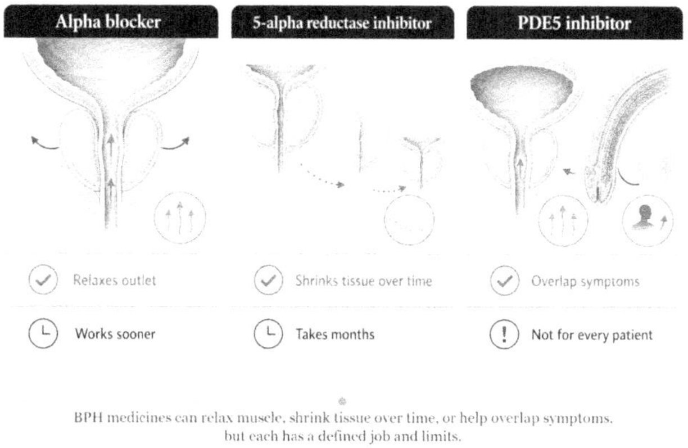

Figure 9.1 - BPH Medication Jobs. Each medication has a job, a timeline, and limits.

The first thing a man needs to understand is that prostate medications do different things. Some medications relax the prostate opening and bladder neck so urine can pass more easily. Some medications can slowly shrink selected enlarged prostates over time. Some medications, especially daily tadalafil, may help both erections and urinary symptoms in selected men.

Those mechanisms are real. But each mechanism has limits.

Relaxing the prostate opening is not the same as removing a blockage. Slowly shrinking a prostate is not the same as immediately relieving severe obstruction. Helping urinary symptoms and erections is not the same as fixing a large gland that is physically blocking the bladder exit.

This is where the conversation must become practical. The patient should not simply ask, "Am I on medication?" He should ask what the medication is supposed to accomplish.

Is it supposed to relax the outlet? Is it supposed to shrink the prostate? Is it supposed to improve the stream? Is it supposed to reduce nighttime urination? Is it supposed to help the bladder empty? How will we know if it worked?

A medication without a clear target becomes a ritual. A medication with a target becomes a treatment plan.

THE MEDICATION TRIAL

A medication trial can be useful. If a man starts a prostate-relaxing medication and his stream improves quickly, that tells us something. It suggests that part of the problem may be related to muscle tone at the prostate opening or bladder neck. If his symptoms improve, his sleep improves, and the bladder empties well, medication may be a reasonable approach. But the trial should be judged honestly.

Some men improve a little and are then left on medication indefinitely. That is not enough. The question is not whether the medication did something. The question is whether it did enough.

If the man wakes up three times per night instead of four, that may be improvement, but it may not be success. If his stream is slightly better but still slow, that may be improvement, but it may not be success. If he feels less urgency but still leaves a large amount of urine behind, that is not bladder protection.

Better is not fixed. That line is important because it prevents false reassurance. Partial improvement should lead to reassessment, not automatic celebration. The man should be asked how his life has changed. The doctor should check whether the bladder is emptying. The urine stream should be measured when appropriate. The prostate anatomy should be understood.

If the medication works well and the bladder is safe, that is a good outcome. If the medication helps a little but the system remains unsafe, the plan needs to change.

THE MOST COMMON PROSTATE-RELAXING PILLS

The most common prostate medications are often called alpha blockers. Patients do not need to remember the drug class name as much as they need to understand what the pills do.

These medications relax smooth muscle around the prostate and bladder opening. When that area relaxes, urine may pass more easily. Common examples include tamsulosin, alfuzosin, silodosin, doxazosin, and terazosin. Many men know tamsulosin by the brand name Flomax.

These medications can work relatively quickly. Some men feel improvement within days. Others need a few weeks. They may notice that it is easier to start urinating, that the stream is stronger, or that they strain less. For the right patient, this can be helpful.

But these medications do not shrink the prostate. They do not remove prostate tissue. They do not make a large gland small. They do not erase a middle portion of the prostate that is pushing into the bladder. They do not prove the bladder is emptying safely.

They relax. That is their job.

A man should understand that difference. If the main problem is a tight, muscular outlet, relaxation may help. If the main problem is a large piece of tissue physically blocking the bladder opening like a ball valve, relaxation may only help partially.

That does not make the medication useless. It means the medication has a limit.

THE DOORWAY ANALOGY

I often explain it this way. Imagine a doorway that is hard to open because the hinges are stiff. If you oil the hinges, the door opens better. That is a good use of a relaxing medication.

Now imagine the doorway is blocked by a couch. You can oil the hinges all day, but the couch is still in the way.

Some prostate problems are more like stiff hinges. Some are more like furniture blocking the doorway. Many are a combination of both. A relaxing pill may help the hinge part of the problem, but it will not move the couch.

This is why anatomy matters. A man with early symptoms, mild enlargement, and good bladder emptying may do well with medication. A man with a larger prostate, a very slow stream, significant urine left behind, and prostate tissue growing into the bladder opening may not.

The pill is not wrong. It may simply be insufficient.

SIDE EFFECTS MATTER

Prostate-relaxing medications are generally well known and commonly prescribed, but they are still medications. They can cause side effects.

Some men feel lightheaded or dizzy, especially when standing up. This matters more in older patients, men on blood pressure medication, or men at risk of falls. Some medications in this group can affect blood pressure more than others.

Ejaculation changes are also common with certain prostate-relaxing pills. Some men notice less semen coming out during orgasm. Others may experience semen going backward into the bladder instead of out through the penis, a condition called retrograde ejaculation. This is usually not dangerous, but it can be bothersome and can matter for fertility or sexual satisfaction.

These side effects should be discussed before the patient is surprised by them. A man should not be told only, "Take this pill." He should understand why he is taking it, what benefit to expect, what side effects may occur, and how long the trial should last before reassessment. If a man accepts side effects but still does not urinate well, that is a poor trade.

THE REFILL VISIT SHOULD BE A CHECKPOINT

The six-month refill visit is one of the most important missed opportunities in prostate care. A patient comes back and says the medication is helping "a little." The prescription is renewed. Another six months pass. The same thing happens again. Nobody measures the urine left behind. Nobody measures the stream. Nobody revisits the anatomy. Nobody asks whether the patient is truly satisfied or simply used to living poorly. That is not how medication should be managed.

A refill visit should be a checkpoint. The doctor should ask whether the man is sleeping better, whether the stream is meaningfully stronger, whether urgency is controlled, whether sexual side effects matter, and whether the bladder is emptying safely. If the symptoms persist, the plan should not be "just keep taking it" forever.

"Just keep taking it" may be reasonable when the patient is doing well. It is not reasonable when he is still struggling. A prescription refill should not replace clinical thinking.

PILLS THAT CAN SLOWLY SHRINK THE PROSTATE

Another group of medications can slowly shrink selected enlarged prostates. These medications include finasteride and dutasteride. They work by affecting the hormone pathway that converts testosterone into a stronger hormone called DHT, which plays an important role in prostate growth. These medications are different from prostate-relaxing pills.

A relaxing pill may work quickly. A shrinking pill works slowly.

It may take months before the patient notices benefit. It is usually most useful in men with larger prostates, where reducing gland size can make a meaningful difference.

For selected patients, this can be a reasonable treatment. These medications can reduce prostate volume over time and may lower the risk of retention or future surgery in appropriately selected men. But they are not for everyone.

If a man is already severely bothered, has a very slow stream, leaves a lot of urine behind, or is close to retention, waiting months for partial shrinkage may not be enough. If the prostate is not very large, the benefit may be limited. If the main issue is prostate tissue growing into the bladder opening like a ball valve, slow shrinkage may not solve the mechanical problem adequately. Again, the medication must match the mechanism.

PSA AND SHRINKING PILLS

Finasteride and dutasteride can lower PSA. That is important because PSA is used to help assess prostate cancer risk. If a medication changes the PSA number, the doctor must interpret the PSA differently.

A patient taking one of these medications should always make sure any doctor reviewing his PSA knows he is taking it. The absolute PSA number may be lower, but that does not mean cancer risk disappears. In fact, a rising PSA while on one of these medications can be especially important.

This is one reason these medications should not be prescribed casually. They affect urinary symptoms, prostate size, sexual function in some men, and PSA interpretation.

That does not mean they are bad medications. It means they require monitoring. A prostate medication that affects a cancer-risk marker deserves respect.

SEXUAL SIDE EFFECTS AND PATIENT PRIORITIES

Some men tolerate finasteride and dutasteride well. Others do not.

Potential side effects may include decreased libido, erectile difficulties, ejaculation changes, breast tenderness, mood changes, and concerns about persistent sexual side effects in a subset of patients. Not every man experiences these problems, but they should be discussed.

This conversation is especially important because men often care deeply about sexual function, but may not bring it up unless the doctor does. A man may accept mild dizziness more easily than loss of libido. Another man may care more about avoiding urinary retention than about ejaculation changes. A third man may be highly sexually active and unwilling to accept certain risks unless the expected benefit is significant.

There is no one answer for every man. That is why the treatment discussion must include priorities. What matters most to the patient? Better sleep? Stronger stream? Preserving ejaculation? Avoiding procedures? Avoiding sexual side effects? Protecting the bladder? Minimizing medication?

The best treatment is not only the one that works biologically. It is the one that fits the man's anatomy and his life.

DAILY TADALAFIL: WHEN ED AND URINARY SYMPTOMS OVERLAP

Daily tadalafil, commonly known by the brand name Cialis, can help some men with urinary symptoms. It is better known as an erectile dysfunction medication, but at a low daily dose it may also improve urinary complaints in selected patients.

This makes sense because erectile function and urinary function share some biological pathways involving blood flow, smooth muscle, nitric oxide signaling, vascular health, and overall male aging. Many men with prostate symptoms also have erectile dysfunction. In the right patient, daily tadalafil can address both issues.

This can be a good option when the man has mild to moderate urinary symptoms and erectile dysfunction. But tadalafil is not an anatomy fix.

It does not remove tissue. It does not shrink a large prostate in a meaningful way. It does not eliminate a ball-valve blockage at the bladder opening. It does not prove the bladder is emptying.

For a man with erectile dysfunction and mild urinary symptoms, tadalafil may be reasonable. For a man with a large obstructing prostate, a very slow stream, and significant urine left behind, tadalafil should not be used as a way to avoid proper evaluation. It may help, but it may not be enough.

TADALAFIL SAFETY

Tadalafil is generally well tolerated, but it has important safety considerations. The most important is that it should not be used with nitrates, because that combination can cause a dangerous drop in blood pressure. Men with significant heart disease, unstable symptoms, recent major cardiac events, or complex medication regimens need appropriate medical review before using it.

Common side effects can include headache, flushing, nasal congestion, heartburn, back discomfort, or muscle aches. Many men tolerate the medication well, but the discussion should still be individualized. This is another example of a broader rule. Even helpful medications should be prescribed with a reason.

COMBINATION THERAPY

Some men take more than one prostate medication. A common combination is a prostate-relaxing pill plus a prostate-shrinking pill.

The logic is understandable. One medication may help sooner by relaxing the outlet, while the other may slowly reduce prostate size over time. For selected men with larger glands and bothersome symptoms, this can be appropriate. But combination therapy should not become a way to delay necessary treatment when the bladder is at risk.

If a man is taking two medications and still waking up all night, still urinating slowly, still leaving urine behind, and still has prostate tissue blocking the bladder opening, the answer is not automatically another refill. The answer may be that medication has reached its limit.

A man on multiple pills who still cannot urinate well is not fine. He is undertreated.

MEDICATION FAILURE DOES NOT MEAN ZERO BENEFIT

Medication failure does not always mean the medication did nothing. It may mean the medication did not do enough.

This distinction matters because doctors and patients sometimes disagree about whether a drug "worked." The patient may say, "It helped a little." The doctor may hear that as success. But if the patient is still living around bathrooms, still sleeping poorly, still straining, or still retaining urine, then partial benefit is not the same as adequate treatment.

A medication has failed when symptoms remain unacceptable. It has failed when side effects are worse than the benefit. It has failed when the bladder still does not empty. It has failed when the stream remains severely slow. It has failed when the prostate anatomy is too obstructive for the medication to overcome. The endpoint is not "some improvement." The endpoint is meaningful improvement and bladder protection.

THE BIGGEST MISTAKE WITH PROSTATE MEDICATION

The biggest mistake is not starting medication. The biggest mistake is staying on medication too long when it is clearly not enough.

This happens because the old model of prostate care trained everyone to delay procedures as long as possible. That made more sense when the main procedures were more invasive and more difficult to recover from. But modern prostate care has changed. We have better testing, better imaging, better minimally invasive options, and better ways to match treatment to anatomy.

A properly selected procedure is not a failure. Sometimes the failure is waiting too long.

If the bladder is leaving urine behind, if the stream is very slow, if the prostate is growing into the bladder opening, if the patient has recurrent infections or stones, if sleep is destroyed, or if retention is approaching, staying on medication indefinitely may not be conservative. It may be risky. True conservative care protects the patient before damage occurs.

MEDICATION AND THE BLADDER

The bladder is the judge. A man may feel better. The symptom score may improve. The medication may be easy to take. But if the bladder is still not emptying, the treatment is incomplete. That is why medication follow-up should not rely only on the question, "How are you doing?" The patient's answer matters, but it should be paired with measurement when there is concern.

How much urine remains after urination? Is the stream stronger? Is the bladder emptying safely? Are nighttime symptoms improving? Is the prostate anatomy stable or worsening? If the bladder is safe and the patient feels well, medication may be a good plan. If the bladder is not safe, medication alone is not enough.

WHEN MEDICATION MAKES SENSE

Medication makes sense when the problem fits the medication. A man with mild or moderate symptoms, reasonable urine flow, little urine left behind, no major prostate tissue growing into the bladder opening, and a preference to avoid procedures may be an excellent medication candidate. A man whose main problem is both erectile dysfunction and mild urinary symptoms may do well with daily tadalafil. A man with a larger prostate and low-risk symptoms may be considered for a shrinking medication if he understands the time course and side effects.

Medication also makes sense when the patient is monitored properly. The plan should define success. If the drug works, continue it. If it does not, reassess.

This is not anti-medication. This is intelligent medication use.

WHEN MEDICATION IS NOT ENOUGH

Medication may not be enough when the patient remains significantly bothered, when sleep remains disrupted, when the stream remains very slow, when a large amount of urine is left behind, when the prostate is physically blocking the bladder opening, when infections or bladder stones develop, when retention occurs, or when side effects are unacceptable. At that point, the conversation should move beyond pills.

That does not mean the patient automatically needs the most aggressive surgery. It means the doctor and patient should revisit the anatomy, the bladder, the treatment goals, and the available options.

Modern prostate care is not one-size-fits-all. Some men may be candidates for minimally invasive treatments. Some may benefit from prostate artery embolization. Some may need a tissue-removing procedure. Some may need bladder testing first. Some may need a different diagnosis entirely. But the key point is that the decision should be active.

Not passive. A man should not drift for years on medication while the bladder pays the price.

WHAT A MAN SHOULD ASK ABOUT HIS MEDICATION

A man does not need to memorize drug classes, but he should understand his own treatment. He should be able to ask: what is this medication supposed to do? Does it relax the prostate opening, shrink the prostate, or help erections and urinary symptoms together? How soon should I notice improvement? What side effects should I watch for? How will we know if it worked? Are we checking whether urine is still being left behind? Are we measuring the speed of urination? Do we know whether the prostate is growing into the bladder opening? What happens if the medication only helps a little?

These are not difficult questions. They are responsible questions.

A patient who asks them is not being difficult. He is participating in his care.

DR. SHUSTERMAN'S MODERN PROSTATE TAKEAWAY

BPH medications can be useful, especially early and in properly selected men. Prostate-relaxing pills can improve flow by relaxing muscle around the prostate and bladder opening. Prostate-shrinking pills can reduce selected larger prostates over time. Daily tadalafil can help men who have both erectile dysfunction and urinary symptoms. But medication has limits.

A pill cannot remove a ball-valve blockage at the bladder opening. A pill cannot always protect a bladder that is leaving urine behind. A pill cannot replace measuring the prostate, checking bladder emptying, or understanding why the stream is slow. Medication should have a mechanism, a goal, and a follow-up plan.

If the medication works and the bladder is safe, that is good medicine. If the man is better but not fixed, if he is still struggling, or if the bladder remains at risk, it is time to move beyond refills. The right question is not, “Is the patient taking medication?” The right question is, “Is the medication protecting the bladder and giving the man the life he wants?”

CHAPTER 10

SUPPLEMENTS AND "PROSTATE HEALTH" CLAIMS

THE PROSTATE SUPPLEMENT aisle is built on one very powerful emotion: hope. A man does not want to wake up all night to urinate. He does not want to talk about a weak stream. He does not want to think about retention, catheters, PSA, cancer, biopsies, or procedures. He does not want to be told that the prostate may be growing in a way that is starting to affect the bladder.

So when he sees a bottle that promises to "support prostate health," the message is attractive. It sounds simple. It sounds natural. It sounds private. It sounds like something he can do on his own without a doctor, without testing, and without confronting the real possibility that his urinary symptoms may need a more serious evaluation.

I understand why men are drawn to that. But understanding the appeal does not mean accepting the claim.

The prostate is not a vague wellness concept. It is a real gland in a real location, wrapped around the urine channel and sitting under the bladder. When the prostate enlarges, becomes inflamed, raises PSA, or blocks the bladder opening, the consequences are not theoretical. The stream slows. The bladder works harder. Urine may be left behind. Sleep may be damaged. Cancer risk may need evaluation.

A supplement label cannot tell the difference between mild urinary symptoms and dangerous bladder retention. It cannot tell whether the prostate is growing into the bladder opening. It cannot measure how much urine is left behind after urination. It cannot tell whether PSA is elevated because of benign enlargement, inflammation, retention, or cancer. That is the problem.

I am not against nutrition. I am not against healthy food. I am not against correcting deficiencies. I am not against intelligent supplementation when there is a real reason, a plausible mechanism, and a measurable goal. I am against vague marketing replacing diagnosis.

"PROSTATE HEALTH" IS NOT A DIAGNOSIS

The phrase "prostate health" sounds helpful, but it often means very little unless it is defined. Does the product improve the urinary stream? Does it reduce nighttime urination? Does it help the bladder empty? Does it reduce urine left behind after urination? Does it shrink the prostate? Does it reduce inflammation? Does it lower the risk of urinary retention? Does it lower prostate cancer risk? Does it improve PSA interpretation? Does it do anything measurable at all?

If those questions cannot be answered, "supports prostate health" is not a medical explanation. It is a marketing phrase.

That does not mean every product using that phrase is harmful. It means the phrase itself should not be accepted as evidence.

A man with urinary symptoms should not ask only whether something is "good for the prostate." He should ask what problem he is trying to solve. A weak stream is not the same as a rising PSA. Benign enlargement is not the same as prostatitis. Nighttime urination is not always a prostate problem. Prostate cancer risk is not treated with a bottle from a vitamin shelf. If the problem is not clearly defined, the treatment cannot be judged honestly.

A PROSTATE SUPPLEMENT DOES NOT HAVE GPS

FIGURE 10.1

The Supplement Evidence Filter

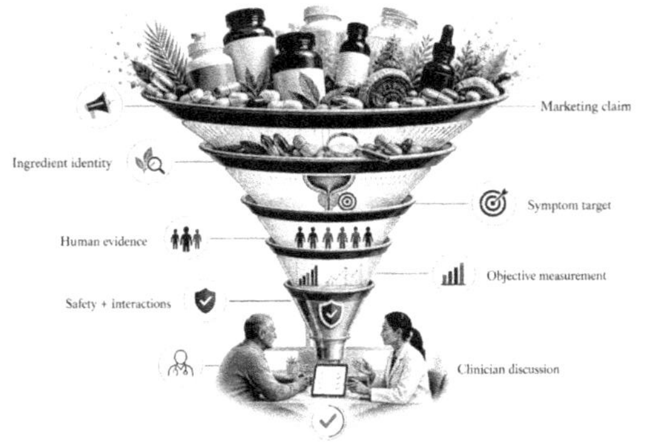

A supplement should not replace diagnosis, objective measurement, or cancer-risk evaluation.

Figure 10.1 - The Supplement Evidence Filter. Supplements should not replace diagnosis or objective measurement.

One of the simplest ways to understand the problem is this: a prostate supplement does not have GPS. When a man swallows a capsule, it goes through the digestive system. It is absorbed, metabolized, distributed through the bloodstream, processed by the liver and kidneys, and exposed to many tissues in the body. It does not travel directly to the prostate, identify the exact problem, and repair it.

If a supplement affects hormones, it may affect more than the prostate. If it affects inflammation, the question is which inflammatory pathway and whether that matters clinically. If it affects smooth muscle, it may not be prostate-specific. If it affects bleeding, that may matter before a procedure. If it affects metabolism, it may interact with medications.

The body is not fooled by the word "prostate" on the label. That is why mechanism matters. A real treatment should be able to explain how it works, where it works, and what it improves. If the claim is that a supplement helps urinary symptoms, then the stream should improve, nighttime urination should improve, or bladder emptying should improve. If the claim is cancer prevention, then meaningful cancer outcomes should support the claim. If the claim is inflammation reduction, then the patient should know what kind of inflammation and how improvement will be measured. Magic is not a mechanism of action.

THE DIFFERENCE BETWEEN FOOD AND SUPPLEMENTS

Patients often combine food, nutrition, vitamins, and supplements into one category. They are not the same.

A healthy diet is one of the foundations of men's health. A man who eats better, loses weight, improves insulin resistance, reduces alcohol, treats constipation, exercises, sleeps better, and improves cardiovascular health may improve many systems that overlap with urinary and sexual function. That is real.

But eating a healthier diet is not the same as taking a high-dose isolated extract sold as a prostate treatment. Food exists in a broader biological context. It contains fiber, micronutrients, structure, and a pattern of intake that affects metabolism over time. A capsule is a concentrated intervention, and concentrated interventions should be judged by evidence.

A tomato is food. A pill claiming to prevent prostate cancer is making a medical claim. Those should not be treated the same way.

This is why I encourage serious lifestyle improvement but remain skeptical of vague supplement promises. The first "natural" prostate strategy should not be a bottle. It should be the man's overall health: weight, sleep, alcohol, bowel habits, metabolic health, exercise, blood pressure, diabetes control, and hydration patterns.

None of that replaces medical evaluation when the prostate is obstructing the bladder. A healthy diet will not erase a large prostate bulging into the bladder opening. But improving the body's terrain matters.

Good nutrition supports the man. It does not replace measurement.

SAW PALMETTO: THE CLASSIC PROSTATE SUPPLEMENT

Saw palmetto is probably the most famous prostate supplement. Many men have tried it. Many have heard that it is natural, that it may help urinary symptoms, or that it may work like a mild version of prostate medication. It has been marketed for years to men with benign prostate enlargement.

The appeal is obvious. If a plant extract could meaningfully improve urinary symptoms without prescription medication or procedures, men would want that option.

The problem is that the evidence has not been strong enough to make saw palmetto a substitute for proper evaluation or established treatment. Some studies have suggested possible modest benefit, but higher-quality evidence has generally been disappointing. The National Center for Complementary and Integrative Health summarizes that a 2023 review of 27 studies found saw palmetto alone provides little or no benefit for symptoms of benign prostate enlargement. Other rigorous studies have also failed to show meaningful improvement compared with placebo.

That does not mean every man who takes saw palmetto is harmed. It means men should be realistic. If a man has mild symptoms, has been properly evaluated, empties his bladder well, has a reasonable stream, and wants to try it with full understanding that benefit is uncertain, that is one conversation.

If a man has severe symptoms, a slow stream, urine left behind, a prostate growing into the bladder opening, recurrent infections, bladder stones, or rising PSA, saw palmetto is not a plan. It should not delay diagnosis. It should not replace measurement.

THE PROBLEM WITH "NATURAL"

The word natural carries enormous power in health marketing. Many patients hear "natural" and immediately assume safer, gentler, and better. Sometimes natural approaches are helpful. Often a healthy lifestyle is exactly what a patient needs. But the word natural does not prove effectiveness or safety.

Tobacco is natural. Poisonous mushrooms are natural. Hemlock is natural. The body does not care whether something came from a plant if it does not solve the problem, if it interacts with medications, or if it delays proper treatment.

The better question is not whether a product is natural. The better question is whether it works for the specific problem, whether it is safe for the specific patient, whether the dose is reliable, and whether the claimed benefit can be measured.

A man with a slow stream needs to know why the stream is slow. A man waking up all night needs to know whether the prostate, bladder, sleep apnea, diabetes, alcohol, or another issue is involved. A man with rising PSA needs appropriate cancer-risk evaluation. The word natural does not answer any of those questions.

THE LONG INGREDIENT LIST

Many prostate supplements contain a long list of ingredients. The label may include saw palmetto, beta-sitosterol, pygeum, pumpkin seed oil, zinc, selenium, vitamin E, lycopene, nettle root, green tea extract, quercetin, or other compounds.

A long label can look scientific. It can also hide uncertainty.

When ten ingredients are combined in one product, the patient may have no idea which ingredient is supposed to do what. If symptoms improve, was it the product, a placebo effect, less evening fluid, less alcohol, natural fluctuation, or another change? If side effects occur, which ingredient caused them? If one ingredient has weak evidence and another has no evidence, what does the combination mean?

Combination products often create the appearance of sophistication without the clarity of a real treatment plan. A modern prostate plan should not be built on mystery mixtures.

This is especially important because supplement quality can vary. Products may differ by brand, extraction method, active ingredient concentration, purity, and manufacturing consistency. Two bottles with the same ingredient name may not be biologically equivalent.

Patients often assume the label equals the science. That is not always true.

THE PLACEBO EFFECT IS REAL, BUT THE BLADDER STILL MATTERS

Some men feel better when they take supplements. That should not be dismissed automatically. Symptoms are partly subjective, and the placebo effect is real. Expectation, attention, behavior change, and increased confidence can affect how a patient feels. A man who starts a supplement may also reduce evening fluids, drink less alcohol, think more about his health, or track symptoms more closely.

Feeling better matters. But feeling better is not the same as proving the bladder is safe.

This is the central danger. A man may feel slightly improved while still leaving too much urine behind after he finishes urinating. He may wake less often but still have a dangerously slow stream. He may believe he is treating his prostate while the obstruction continues.

The bladder does not care whether the improvement came from hope or chemistry. The bladder cares whether it can empty. If a supplement is being used, the patient should still know the basic measurements: prostate size, whether the prostate is growing into the bladder opening, how much urine is left behind, and how fast the urine comes out. Without those answers, reassurance is premature.

SUPPLEMENTS AND PSA ANXIETY

PSA anxiety drives many supplement purchases. A man gets a blood test. The PSA is higher than expected. He searches online. He finds products claiming to support prostate health or healthy PSA. He buys a bottle and hopes the problem will go away. That is not risk management.

PSA is a prostate-made protein used to help assess prostate cancer risk. It can rise for many reasons, including benign enlargement, inflammation, infection, urinary retention, recent procedures, and cancer. Because the causes vary, the response has to be thoughtful. A supplement does not explain the PSA.

It does not tell whether the prostate is large. It does not rule out cancer. It does not replace repeat testing, risk assessment, advanced blood tests, MRI, or biopsy when those are appropriate.

If a man wants to take a supplement while being properly evaluated, that is one thing. If he takes a supplement to avoid evaluation, that is dangerous. A rising PSA deserves interpretation, not wishful thinking.

ANTIOXIDANTS AND THE CANCER PREVENTION TRAP

The supplement industry has long promoted antioxidants as protective. The theory sounds simple. Oxidative stress can damage cells. Antioxidants reduce oxidative stress. Therefore antioxidants should reduce cancer. Human biology is not that simple.

Cancer does not develop from one pathway. It involves genetics, cell signaling, immune surveillance, tissue environment, inflammation, metabolism, hormones, and many other factors. A substance that sounds protective in theory may fail when tested in real people. Sometimes it may even create harm.

Selenium and vitamin E are cautionary examples. For years, they were promoted as possible prostate cancer prevention supplements. But large clinical trial evidence did not show prostate cancer prevention benefit, and vitamin E supplementation was associated with increased prostate cancer risk in later findings from the SELECT trial. That is the lesson.

A plausible theory is not enough. The endpoint matters.

If a supplement claims to prevent prostate cancer, the question is not whether the theory sounds good. The question is whether high-quality human outcomes show fewer meaningful cancers, less aggressive disease, or better survival without unacceptable risks.

Marketing loves theory. Medicine needs outcomes.

THE BIGGEST RISK MAY BE DELAY

For many prostate supplements, the biggest risk may not be direct toxicity. The biggest risk may be delay.

A man starts waking up at night. He buys a prostate supplement. The stream continues to weaken. He buys another bottle. He feels slightly better for a while, or he convinces himself he is being proactive. Months pass. Then years. No one measures his prostate. No one checks how much urine is left behind. No one measures the speed of urination. No one evaluates PSA properly.

Then he presents with retention, infection, bladder stones, or a much more advanced problem than he needed to have. That is the danger.

Supplements can create the illusion of action. The man feels he is doing something, but the disease process may not be understood. A bottle can make a patient feel proactive while the bladder quietly loses ground.

That is not prevention. That is delay disguised as wellness.

WHEN SUPPLEMENTS MAY BE REASONABLE

There are situations where supplements may be reasonable. If a man has been properly evaluated, has mild symptoms, empties his bladder well, has no concerning PSA pattern, and understands that the benefit is uncertain, he may decide to try a supplement as an adjunct. If he has a documented deficiency, correcting that deficiency may be appropriate. If a supplement is low risk, does not interact with medications, does not affect planned procedures, and does not delay real care, the discussion can be individualized.

The key phrase is as an adjunct. Not as a substitute.

A man with significant urinary obstruction should not use supplements instead of evaluation. A man with a rising PSA should not use supplements instead of cancer-risk assessment. A man with recurrent infections or bladder stones should not use supplements instead of finding out why urine is not emptying.

Supplements may have a place at the edge of care. They should not replace the center of care.

QUESTIONS TO ASK BEFORE TAKING A PROSTATE SUPPLEMENT

In the main chapters of this book, I try to avoid turning every section into a checklist. But this is one area where a man should develop a habit of questioning the claim.

Before taking a prostate supplement, he should ask himself what problem he is trying to treat. Is it a weak stream? Waking at night? PSA anxiety? Inflammation? Cancer prevention? Sexual function? General health? Those are not the same.

He should ask what the product is supposed to do and how he would know if it worked. Would his sleep improve? Would the stream improve? Would the bladder empty better? Would PSA risk become clearer? Would cancer risk actually decrease?

He should also ask whether he is using the supplement to avoid seeing a doctor. That last question is the most important. If the supplement delays diagnosis, it may be harmful even if the capsule itself is not.

THE DOCTOR SHOULD ASK TOO

Patients often do not mention supplements unless the doctor asks. They may not think of them as medications. They may assume they are harmless. They may forget. They may be embarrassed. Some may worry the doctor will dismiss them. A modern urologist should ask without judgment.

What are you taking? Why are you taking it? How long have you been taking it? What dose? Any side effects? Are you taking blood thinners? Are you planning a procedure? Are you using this instead of a medical evaluation? That conversation matters.

Supplements can interact with medications. Some may affect bleeding risk. Some may confuse the clinical picture. Some may simply waste money. But the doctor cannot advise the patient if the doctor does not know what the patient is taking. The goal is not to shame patients. The goal is to make the plan safer and smarter.

THE BETTER "NATURAL" STRATEGY

If a man wants to support prostate health naturally, the first step should not be the supplement aisle. It should be his overall health.

Weight matters. Exercise matters. Resistance training matters. Sleep matters. Alcohol matters. Constipation matters. Diabetes control matters. Blood pressure matters. Smoking matters. Hydration patterns matter. Metabolic health matters.

These factors do not replace prostate treatment when anatomy is obstructive, but they support the system around the prostate. They affect inflammation, vascular function, sexual function, hormone health, bladder behavior, sleep quality, and long-term resilience. A serious natural strategy looks less like a bottle and more like a program.

Improve the body. Measure the prostate. Protect the bladder. Evaluate PSA intelligently. Treat the actual problem. That is a modern approach.

DR. SHUSTERMAN'S MODERN PROSTATE TAKEAWAY

Supplements are not automatically bad, but prostate supplement marketing is often much stronger than the evidence behind it. "Supports prostate health" is not enough. A prostate supplement does not know whether a man has benign enlargement, inflammation, a bladder problem, a ball-valve blockage at the bladder opening, urine left behind after urination, a slow stream, or prostate cancer risk.

Natural does not mean effective. A plausible theory is not proof. A long ingredient list is not a treatment plan.

The biggest danger is often not the pill itself. The biggest danger is delay.

A man should not take capsules for years while his bladder quietly loses function or while PSA risk goes unevaluated. If a supplement is used, it should be used only after the real questions have been answered: what is the prostate doing, what is the bladder doing, and what outcome are we trying to improve?

Mechanism first. Endpoint second. Marketing last. Magic is not a mechanism of action.

CHAPTER 11

WHEN MEDICATION IS NOT ENOUGH

ONE OF THE most important moments in prostate care is knowing when to stop pretending that medication is enough. That does not mean medication is bad. It means medication has a job, and sometimes the job becomes too big for a pill.

A man may start medication for a weak stream, nighttime urination, urgency, or difficulty emptying. At first, he may feel better. Maybe the stream improves. Maybe he wakes up less often. Maybe he feels more comfortable leaving the house. That is a real benefit, and it should not be dismissed.

But years later, the situation may look different. The prostate may be larger. The bladder may be working harder. More urine may be left behind after urination. The stream may be slowing again. Nighttime urination may return. The patient may be taking one pill, then two, and still planning his life around the bathroom. This is where men get trapped.

They think that because they are on medication, they are being fully treated. They think that because the medication once helped, it must still be the right plan. They think that moving beyond medication means they have failed or that their doctor is jumping too quickly to something aggressive.

That is the wrong way to look at it. Medication is not a moral victory. A procedure is not a moral defeat. The only real question is whether the treatment is protecting the man's bladder, sleep, function, and quality of life. If the answer is no, medication is not enough.

THE OLD LAST-RESORT MENTALITY

For decades, men were trained to think of prostate procedures as a last resort. That attitude came from an older era. Historically, the main procedural options for prostate enlargement were more invasive. Many men were told to stay on medication as long as possible and only consider a procedure when they had severe symptoms, repeated retention, bladder stones, infections, or could no longer tolerate life as it was.

That thinking made some sense when the main options were more difficult to recover from. If the only meaningful choices were major surgery or living with symptoms, many men understandably chose to wait. But prostate care has changed.

We now have better ways to evaluate the prostate and bladder. We can measure the size of the prostate. We can see whether prostate tissue is growing into the bladder opening. We can measure how much urine is left behind after urination. We can measure the speed of the urine stream. We can look inside the urinary channel. We can evaluate whether the bladder is still strong.

We also have more treatment options than men had in the past. Some procedures are less invasive. Some preserve more anatomy. Some are better suited for certain prostate sizes or shapes. Some treat the prostate through the blood supply rather than cutting through the urine channel. Some can reduce obstruction while preserving future options.

Because the tools have changed, the timing conversation should change too. The question should not be, "How long can we delay doing anything?" The question should be, "At what point does waiting begin to put the bladder and the man's quality of life at risk?"

THE PROBLEM WITH WAITING TOO LONG

Waiting can feel safe. A man says, "I can live with it." He wakes up twice a night, then three times. He sits through meetings thinking about the bathroom. He avoids long drives. He pushes to urinate. He starts to accept that his stream is slow. His doctor refills the medication. Everyone moves on. But the bladder may not be moving on.

The bladder may be working harder every day. It may be pushing against resistance. It may be leaving urine behind. It may be becoming more irritable. It may be stretching. It may be losing strength slowly enough that the patient does not notice until the situation becomes serious.

This is one of the most frustrating patterns in BPH care. The patient and doctor wait because the problem is "not that bad," and then suddenly the patient is in the emergency room unable to urinate.

But urinary retention is often not as sudden as it feels. The final event may be sudden, but the process may have been building for years. That is why waiting should be a decision, not a default.

If the bladder is emptying well, symptoms are tolerable, the stream is acceptable, and the prostate is not creating a dangerous pattern, monitoring may be appropriate. But if the patient is leaving urine behind, urinating slowly, waking all night, or showing signs that the bladder is under stress, waiting becomes a risk.

Doing nothing is still doing something. Sometimes it means allowing the prostate to keep winning.

"I'M BETTER" IS NOT THE SAME AS "I'M SAFE"

Medication often creates a gray zone. The patient is not terrible. He is not in retention. He is not demanding surgery. But he is also not well. He still wakes up. He still has urgency. The stream is still weak. He still feels that urination takes too long. He still cannot travel comfortably. He still lives with a background concern that his bladder is not reliable.

This is where the phrase "better is not fixed" matters. Better is real. If medication improves symptoms, that counts. But improvement is not the same as resolution, and symptom relief is not the same as bladder protection.

A man may feel somewhat better while still leaving too much urine behind after he urinates. He may wake less often but still have a dangerously slow stream. He may be less bothered but still have prostate tissue bulging into the bladder opening and blocking the exit like a ball valve.

The bladder does not care that the symptom score improved a little. The bladder cares whether it can empty.

That is why every medication plan needs an endpoint. The endpoint cannot be merely "the patient says he is a little better." The endpoint should be meaningful improvement in symptoms, sleep, stream, emptying, and quality of life. If the bladder is still unsafe, the medication has not done enough.

THE CLUES THAT MEDICATION IS REACHING ITS LIMIT

There is rarely one single sign that medication has failed. More often, the picture becomes clear when several clues appear together.

The patient remains bothered despite medication. He still wakes up repeatedly at night. He still has a slow stream. He still waits for urination to start. He still strains. He still has urgency. He still feels he does not empty. He may have side effects from the medication. He may need more than one medication and still not feel right.

Then the measurements confirm the concern. The urine stream is slow. Urine is left behind after he finishes. The prostate is large. Part of the prostate is growing into the bladder opening. The bladder may show signs of working too hard. The PSA may require separate evaluation. There may be recurrent infections, bladder stones, or episodes of retention.

At that point, the conversation has to change. The question is no longer simply, "Should we continue the medication?" The question becomes, "What is the medication failing to fix?"

If the medication cannot overcome the anatomy, the anatomy needs to be addressed. If the bladder is not emptying, the bladder needs to be protected. If the patient's life is still controlled by the bathroom, quality of life has to matter. A man does not need to wait until he is miserable to deserve a better plan.

WHEN THE PROSTATE IS PHYSICALLY BLOCKING THE EXIT

Some prostate problems are mainly functional. The muscle around the prostate and bladder opening is tight, and medication helps relax it.

Other prostate problems are more structural. The gland is larger. The channel is narrowed. The middle part of the prostate may be pushing upward into the bladder opening. The outlet is being physically distorted. In those cases, medication may not be powerful enough.

This is easiest to understand with the ball-valve concept. If prostate tissue is bulging into the bladder opening, the bladder may try to empty, but the tissue interferes with the exit. A relaxing pill may reduce some muscle tension, but it does not make the tissue disappear. It does not change the fact that something is sitting at the doorway.

That is why some men say medication helped at first but never fully solved the problem. The pill treated the part it could treat. The anatomy remained.

This is where modern prostate care has to be honest. If the problem is mechanical, the solution may need to be mechanical or anatomical. That does not automatically mean traditional surgery. It means the treatment has to match the problem. Medication cannot be expected to do what it was never designed to do.

WHEN THE BLADDER IS LEAVING URINE BEHIND

A man can urinate every day and still not empty his bladder. This is one of the most important points in the book.

If a significant amount of urine remains after urination, the system is not working properly. The cause may be prostate blockage, bladder weakness, or both. But whatever the cause, the finding matters.

Leftover urine can increase the risk of infections. It can contribute to bladder stones. It can worsen frequency because the bladder never truly starts from empty. It can signal that the bladder is struggling to push through the outlet. If it continues to rise, the patient may be moving toward retention.

Medication may be enough if the amount left behind improves and the bladder remains safe. But if the leftover urine stays high or keeps increasing, the plan has to be reconsidered. A man should not be told he is fine because he can still urinate if he is leaving a large amount behind every time.

That is not fine. That is a warning.

WHEN NIGHTTIME URINATION IS DESTROYING SLEEP

Some men do not think of nighttime urination as a serious medical issue because they have lived with it for so long. They say, "I only get up three times."

Only three times every night is not a small problem. It is chronic sleep interruption. It affects energy, mood, focus, metabolism, testosterone, cardiovascular health, and sexual function. It can make a man feel older than he is.

Medication may reduce nighttime urination in some patients. But if the man remains sleep-deprived despite treatment, the issue deserves a deeper look.

Is he waking because the bladder does not empty? Is the prostate blocking? Is the bladder irritated? Is sleep apnea causing nighttime urine production? Is alcohol involved? Are evening fluids, diabetes, leg swelling, heart function, or kidney issues contributing?

Not all nighttime urination is from the prostate. But when prostate obstruction is part of the problem, continued sleep destruction is a sign that the current plan may not be enough.

Quality of life is not cosmetic. Sleep is medicine. If the prostate-bladder system is destroying sleep, the treatment plan should be taken seriously.

WHEN SIDE EFFECTS BECOME THE PROBLEM

Sometimes medication fails because the patient cannot tolerate it. A man may have dizziness, lightheadedness, low blood pressure symptoms, fatigue, reduced ejaculation, sexual side effects, decreased libido, or erectile changes depending on the medication. Some men tolerate these side effects easily. Others find them unacceptable. This is personal.

A side effect that one man considers minor may be a major problem for another. A man who is sexually active may care deeply about ejaculation changes. A man prone to falls may not tolerate dizziness. A man already struggling with libido may not want a medication that could make it worse.

Patients should not be expected to accept side effects indefinitely if the benefit is modest. If a medication gives partial urinary relief but creates unacceptable sexual or systemic side effects, it may not be the right long-term plan. In some cases, a different medication may help.

In other cases, the better approach is to address the prostate anatomy more directly.

The goal is not just to avoid procedures. The goal is to preserve the man's function and quality of life.

WHEN INFECTIONS OR STONES APPEAR

Recurrent urinary infections in a man should not be brushed off. Men do not get repeated urinary infections for no reason. There may be an underlying source. One common contributor is poor bladder emptying. If urine remains in the bladder after urination, bacteria have a better environment to persist. If bladder stones form, those stones can become a hiding place for bacteria. Antibiotics may help temporarily, but the infection may return because the underlying problem remains.

Bladder stones are also important. They can cause irritation, blood in the urine, urgency, pain, and infection. They often point to a bladder that is not emptying well.

If a man with BPH develops recurrent infections or bladder stones, medication alone may no longer be a reasonable plan. The doctor has to ask why the infections or stones are happening. Is the prostate blocking? Is urine being left behind? Does the bladder need help? Does a stone need to be removed? Does the prostate need to be treated to prevent recurrence?

Antibiotics do not fix obstruction. A pill for prostate relaxation may not remove the reason stones formed. This is why complications change the conversation.

WHEN RETENTION HAPPENS

Urinary retention is the event many men fear. Retention means the bladder cannot empty. In acute retention, the man cannot urinate despite a full bladder. The pain and pressure can be severe. The usual emergency solution is a catheter to drain the urine.

For some men, retention is the first time they realize how serious the prostate problem has become. They may have had symptoms for years, but because they could still urinate, they thought they were managing. Retention changes everything.

After retention, the question is not only how to get the catheter out. The question is why retention happened, whether the bladder can recover, whether the prostate is blocking, and what treatment is needed to prevent recurrence.

Some men pass a voiding trial after medication. Others fail. Some need additional testing to see whether the bladder is strong enough. Some need a procedure. Some may need a catheter longer than expected because the bladder has been stretched or weakened.

This is why I do not like waiting for retention. It is far better to recognize danger before the emergency. A catheter should not be the first serious prostate evaluation.

PROCEDURES ARE NOT ALL THE SAME

One reason men stay on medication too long is fear. They hear the word procedure and think of the most invasive surgery they can imagine. They picture hospitalization, bleeding, sexual dysfunction, incontinence, long recovery, and loss of control. Modern prostate treatment is broader than that.

Some procedures heat or shrink tissue. Some open the urine channel by removing tissue. Some use lasers. Some use waterjet technology. Some pull tissue aside. Some treat the prostate through its blood supply. Some are office-based or outpatient. Some preserve ejaculation better than others. Some are better for smaller glands. Some are better for larger glands. Some are better when the prostate grows into the bladder opening. Some are better when future options need to be preserved.

The point is not that one procedure is best for everyone. The point is that moving beyond medication does not automatically mean traditional surgery.

A man should not reject the entire category of procedures because he has an outdated image in his mind. He should ask which option matches his prostate anatomy, bladder function, sexual priorities, medical condition, and goals. The modern conversation is not medication versus surgery. It is: what is the least destructive effective way to solve this specific problem?

THE GOAL IS NOT TO DO MORE

When I talk about moving beyond medication, I am not arguing that every man should have a procedure early. That would be just as wrong as keeping every man on pills forever. The goal is not to do more.

The goal is to do the right thing at the right time. Some men should be monitored. Some should take medication. Some should adjust lifestyle factors. Some should address constipation, sleep apnea, diabetes, or bladder irritation. Some should have a prostate procedure. Some should have bladder testing first. Some should have cancer-risk evaluation before anything else.

Modern medicine is not aggressive because it measures. It is aggressive when it acts without understanding. It is also careless when it refuses to act despite clear evidence that the bladder is suffering.

The best care is neither passive nor reckless. It is measured.

MATCHING TREATMENT TO ANATOMY

When medication is not enough, the next step should be based on anatomy and function. A smaller prostate with certain types of obstruction may be treated differently than a very large prostate. A prostate that grows into the bladder opening may require a different strategy than one that grows outward. A man with a strong bladder and clear blockage is different from a man with a weak bladder and unclear obstruction. A man who strongly wants to preserve ejaculation may choose differently than a man whose main priority is maximum opening of the channel. A man with multiple medical issues may need an approach with lower anesthesia or recovery burden. This is where modern prostate care becomes individualized.

The wrong question is, "What procedure do you do?" The better question is, "What procedure fits this prostate and this man?" If the doctor cannot explain why a particular treatment matches the patient's anatomy, the patient should ask more questions. A procedure should not be chosen because it is convenient, heavily marketed, or familiar. It should be chosen because its mechanism matches the problem.

THE PSYCHOLOGICAL BARRIER

Many men delay because crossing from medication to procedure feels psychologically significant. Taking a pill feels easy. It feels reversible. It feels private. It does not require admitting the problem has progressed.

A procedure feels like a bigger step. It requires planning. It forces the man to acknowledge that the issue is real. It may bring up fears about sexuality, recovery, catheter time, complications, anesthesia, and aging. Those fears are understandable. But fear should not be allowed to make the decision alone.

A man should be given a clear explanation of what is happening, what the risk of waiting is, what the realistic benefits of treatment are, and what side effects or recovery to expect. When men understand the anatomy and the bladder risk, the decision often becomes clearer.

The goal is not to pressure the patient. The goal is to remove the fog.

WHAT MEN SHOULD ASK WHEN MEDICATION IS NOT ENOUGH

When medication is no longer working well enough, a man should ask the doctor to explain the reason in plain language. Is the prostate too large for medication alone? Is part of it growing into the bladder opening? Is urine being left behind? Is the stream too slow? Is the bladder overactive because of obstruction? Is the bladder becoming weak? Are infections or stones related to poor emptying? Is the current medication causing side effects? What are the risks of waiting another year? Which options fit the anatomy? Which options preserve ejaculation? Which options preserve future treatment choices?

These are not aggressive questions. They are intelligent questions.

A man should not be made to feel difficult for wanting to understand why a plan is being recommended. The doctor should be able to explain it without hiding behind jargon. The patient does not need to know every technical abbreviation. He needs to know whether the current treatment is enough and what happens if it is not.

MOVING BEYOND REFILLS

There is a point where another refill is not care. It is delay.

If a man is doing well, medication can be continued. If he sleeps well, empties well, urinates well, and has no meaningful side effects, that may be a good plan. But if he is still struggling, if the bladder is not emptying, if the prostate is physically blocking the bladder opening, or if complications are appearing, the plan must evolve.

Medicine should not be static when the disease is progressing. The prostate changes. The bladder changes. The man's life changes. The treatment plan should change when the evidence changes.

That is not aggressive. That is modern.

DR. SHUSTERMAN'S MODERN PROSTATE TAKEAWAY

Medication has an important role in BPH, especially early and in properly selected men. But medication is not enough when it fails to protect the bladder, fails to restore meaningful quality of life, or fails to address a mechanical blockage.

A man should not stay on pills for years because they helped a little. He should know whether the bladder empties, whether urine is left behind, whether the stream is too slow, whether the prostate is growing into the bladder opening, and whether the current plan is truly working.

Procedures are not failure. Sometimes waiting too long is the failure.

The goal is not to rush every man into treatment. The goal is to identify the moment when continued medication becomes passive instead of protective. Modern prostate care should be smarter than endless refills. When medication is not enough, the question should change from "Can I keep living with this?" to "What is the right treatment before the bladder becomes the disease?"

CHAPTER 12

REZŪM: TREATING SMALLER PROSTATES WITHOUT TRADITIONAL SURGERY

WHERE REZŪM FITS IN MY PRACTICE

AFTER PAE, Rezūm is the other BPH procedure I use most often in properly selected men. I see it as a strong second pillar of modern prostate care, especially for smaller or moderately enlarged prostates whose anatomy fits water-vapor treatment.

Rezūm is quick to perform and, in experienced hands, can have a low serious-side-effect profile. The tradeoff is recovery. Because Rezūm is performed through the urinary channel and creates controlled inflammation inside the prostate, most men should expect a temporary catheter afterward, often about seven days in my practice.

Men also need realistic expectations. Depending on prostate size and the amount of tissue treated, there may be a one-to-three-month window where urinary symptoms can temporarily increase before the final improvement becomes clear. That does not mean the treatment failed. It means the prostate is healing and remodeling.

This is why I present Rezūm as a targeted procedure, not a

universal procedure. When the prostate is smaller or moderate and the anatomy fits, Rezūm can be excellent. When the gland is larger, more complex, or significantly growing into the bladder opening, PAE often deserves priority discussion.

For many years, men thought about prostate procedures in only one way. If medication stopped working, they assumed the next step was surgery. Not a small procedure. Not a targeted treatment. Surgery. They imagined a hospital, an operating room, bleeding, a long recovery, sexual side effects, and the fear that treatment would permanently change the way they functioned.

That fear kept many men on medication far longer than they should have stayed. It also shaped the old culture of BPH care. Men were told to tolerate symptoms. Keep taking pills. Wait. Delay. Avoid intervention until the situation became severe. In some cases, men waited until they went into urinary retention and needed a catheter before anyone seriously revisited the plan.

That is not how modern prostate care should work. The development of less invasive treatments changed the conversation. Rezūm is one of those treatments. It is not the answer for every man, and it should not be presented as magic. But in properly selected patients, it offers an important middle ground between indefinite medication and more aggressive tissue-removing surgery.

Rezūm uses water vapor energy to treat enlarged prostate tissue from inside the prostate. The goal is to reduce obstruction without the same level of cutting, resection, or tissue removal associated with traditional operations.

The idea is simple enough for patients to understand: instead of carving out a channel, the procedure delivers controlled steam energy into the obstructing prostate tissue. Over time, the treated tissue shrinks and the channel opens more naturally. That is why patient selection matters so much.

Rezūm is not just "a prostate procedure." It is a tool. And like every tool in medicine, it works best when the mechanism matches the anatomy.

WHY REZŪM EXISTS

To understand Rezūm, you have to understand the gap it was designed to fill. Medication can help many men, especially early. A relaxing pill can reduce muscle tension around the prostate opening. A shrinking pill can slowly reduce prostate size in selected men. Daily tadalafil can help some men with both erectile dysfunction and urinary symptoms. But medication has limits.

If the prostate tissue is physically obstructing the urine channel, a pill may only partially help. If the man still wakes up at night, still strains, still has a slow stream, or still leaves urine behind after urination, then medication may not be enough. At some point, the problem becomes anatomical.

Historically, once medication failed, men were often pushed toward more aggressive surgical options. Those procedures can be effective, but they can also come with more recovery, more bleeding risk, more anesthesia, and greater concern about ejaculation or other sexual side effects.

Rezūm was developed as a less invasive way to treat obstructing prostate tissue in selected men. It is designed to reduce the tissue causing blockage without turning every patient into a traditional surgery case. That is the role I see for Rezūm: not as a miracle and not as a cure-all, but as a targeted option for men whose prostate anatomy fits the treatment.

HOW REZŪM WORKS

Rezūm uses water vapor, or steam, to deliver thermal energy into prostate tissue. The treatment is performed through the urinary channel. A small device is placed into the prostate area, and controlled bursts of water vapor are delivered into the obstructing tissue. When that water vapor enters the tissue, it releases energy. That energy damages selected prostate cells in the treated zone. Over the following weeks and months, the body gradually resorbs some of that treated tissue, and the pressure on the urine channel can decrease.

Patients often want to know whether the prostate opens immediately. The honest answer is no, not in the way some tissue-removing operations open the channel immediately. Rezūm is not a carving procedure. It is a tissue-treatment procedure. The prostate responds over time.

That difference is important because it shapes recovery expectations. Some men feel improvement relatively early. Others take longer. Inflammation and swelling after the procedure can temporarily make urinary symptoms worse before they improve. This is not unusual. The prostate has been treated, and the body needs time to heal.

Patients who understand that process do better emotionally during recovery. They are less likely to panic if the first few weeks are not perfect. Rezūm is a delayed-improvement treatment. The final result should not be judged too early.

WHO IS USUALLY A GOOD CANDIDATE?

FIGURE 12.1

Where Rezum Fits

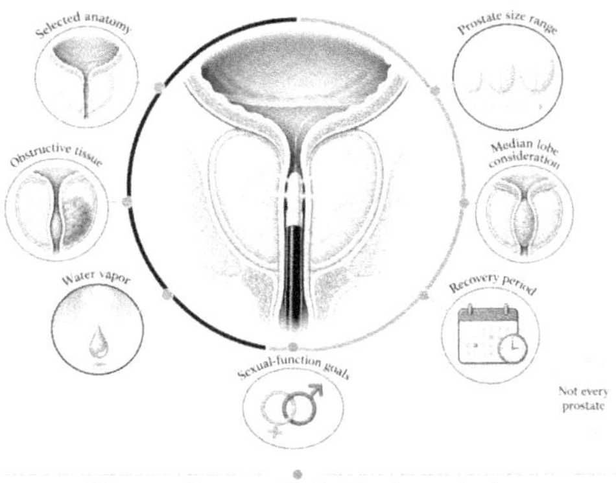

Water-vapor therapy may fit selected anatomy and goals, but it is not a universal BPH solution.

Figure 12.1 - Where Rezum Fits. Water-vapor therapy is a selected option, not a universal solution.

In my practice, Rezūm is generally most attractive for men with smaller or moderately enlarged prostates, especially when the anatomy can be treated efficiently. A common practical range is under about sixty grams, although the decision is not based on size alone. A prostate under sixty grams may be a good candidate if the symptoms are bothersome, medication is not enough, the bladder still has reasonable function, and the internal anatomy fits the procedure.

That does not mean Rezūm can never be used in larger prostates. In experienced hands, it can be applied more broadly. I have treated much larger glands. But as the prostate becomes larger, the procedure may require more treatment sites, the healing period may become more demanding, and symptom worsening during recovery may last longer.

Patients need to understand this honestly. A larger prostate can sometimes be treated with Rezūm, but the patient should not expect the same recovery profile as a smaller gland. Once a man needs many treatment injections, the amount of treated tissue increases, and the inflammatory recovery can become more significant. The procedure is still minimally invasive compared with major surgery, but the recovery may not feel "minimal" to the patient in the first weeks.

That is why I do not choose Rezūm by size alone. I look at the picture: prostate size, shape, whether tissue is growing into the bladder opening, how much urine is left behind, how slow the stream is, how strong the bladder seems, what the patient wants to preserve, and what other options remain. Treatment should follow anatomy.

THE MIDDLE PART OF THE PROSTATE

One important question before Rezūm is whether the middle part of the prostate is pushing upward into the bladder opening. Patients may hear doctors call this a median lobe or intravesical protrusion.

The plain-English idea is that part of the prostate is bulging into the bladder outlet and can act like a ball valve. When the bladder tries to empty, that tissue can interfere with the exit.

Rezūm can treat selected middle-lobe tissue, and this is one of its advantages compared with some approaches that do not handle this anatomy well. But the details matter. A small or moderate middle-lobe problem may be different from a large amount of tissue sitting inside the bladder opening.

When prostate tissue grows into the bladder, the healing process may also be slower. The treated tissue is close to the bladder lining, and the patient may have more urgency, irritation, or delayed improvement. In some men, especially with significant tissue protruding into the bladder, the recovery can take several months before the final benefit becomes clear.

This is not a reason to avoid Rezūm automatically. It is a reason to set expectations correctly. The patient should know what kind of anatomy he has before treatment.

WHY I LIKE REZŪM FOR THE RIGHT PATIENT

Rezūm fits an important philosophy in modern prostate care: treat the obstruction while preserving options. It does not remove large amounts of tissue the way more aggressive operations do. It does not require the same kind of resection through the prostate channel. It can be done in an outpatient setting. It can reduce symptoms in properly selected men while generally preserving future treatment choices. That last point matters.

A man's first procedure should not burn every bridge. Prostate enlargement is an aging condition. A man treated in his fifties or sixties may need more prostate care later in life. The future matters. A treatment that improves symptoms while preserving anatomy and future options is valuable.

Rezūm also fits men who want to move beyond medication but are not ready for or do not need a more aggressive operation. These patients may be tired of pills, bothered by side effects, still waking up at night, or still urinating poorly, but they do not necessarily need major tissue removal. For that kind of patient, Rezūm may offer a reasonable middle path.

WHAT REZŪM IS NOT

Rezūm should not be oversold. It is not instant. It is not painless recovery for everyone. It is not the best choice for every prostate. It is not a guarantee that no other treatment will ever be needed. It is not a substitute for proper evaluation.

The patient should not be told, "This is quick and easy," without understanding the recovery. The procedure itself may be brief, but recovery is a process. Urgency, burning, frequency, temporary worsening of symptoms, catheter time, urinary discomfort, and delayed improvement can occur. Most patients tolerate the process, but they should be prepared.

I do not like marketing language that makes prostate procedures sound like spa treatments. These are real medical procedures. Even when they are minimally invasive, the patient deserves a serious explanation. Rezūm can be excellent for the right man. But the right man has to be selected carefully.

ANESTHESIA AND COMFORT

Patients often ask whether Rezūm hurts. The answer depends on how it is performed. In some settings, Rezūm may be done with local anesthesia, oral sedation, or office-based comfort measures. In my own practice, I prefer a more comfortable approach using monitored anesthesia, often with propofol-based sedation. The patient is asleep or deeply comfortable for a brief period while the procedure is performed, with appropriate monitoring.

This matters because men should not be made to suffer through a prostate procedure unnecessarily. Anxiety and discomfort are real. A patient who has a bad experience may avoid future care, and that can be harmful.

Comfort is not a luxury in prostate care. It is part of doing the procedure properly.

At the same time, anesthesia should be appropriate to the patient's health, age, medical risk, and setting. The goal is not to overdo anesthesia. The goal is to make the treatment safe, controlled, and tolerable. A man should ask his doctor how the procedure is performed, what type of anesthesia is used, how long he will be monitored, and what he should expect afterward.

THE CATHETER QUESTION

Many men are more afraid of the catheter than the procedure. That is understandable.

After Rezūm, many patients need a temporary catheter while swelling settles and the prostate begins the healing process. The length of catheter time varies depending on prostate size, the number of treatment areas, how much swelling is expected, whether the patient was retaining urine before the procedure, and the doctor's protocol.

A catheter after Rezūm does not mean the procedure failed. In many patients, it is part of the planned recovery.

The key is expectation. If a man is told he may need a catheter for several days, he can prepare. If he is told nothing and wakes up with one, he may feel blindsided.

Patients also need to know that urination may feel worse before it feels better. The prostate has been treated. Swelling and irritation are expected. The body needs time to clear treated tissue and calm down. A good recovery plan is part of the procedure.

RECOVERY IS NOT THE SAME FOR EVERY MAN

Recovery after Rezūm varies. Some men improve steadily. Some have burning, urgency, frequency, or a temporary worsening of urinary symptoms. Some need catheter support longer than expected. Some feel frustrated in the first few weeks because they expected immediate improvement.

This is why I explain the mechanism before the procedure. Rezūm works by treating tissue and allowing the body to remodel that tissue over time. That is different from cutting a wide-open channel immediately. The improvement curve may be gradual.

A patient should not judge the final result in the first few days. He should also not be ignored if recovery symptoms are severe, persistent, or unusual. Follow-up matters. Urine testing may be needed if infection is suspected. Medications may be used temporarily to help with irritation. The catheter plan may need adjustment. The doctor should guide the patient through recovery, not simply perform the procedure and disappear.

SEXUAL FUNCTION AND EJACULATION

One reason many men consider Rezūm is the possibility of improving urinary symptoms while preserving sexual function. Any prostate treatment can have sexual implications, and no honest doctor should promise zero risk. But compared with more aggressive tissue-removing operations, Rezūm is generally considered more favorable for preserving erections and ejaculation in properly selected patients. This matters because men care about sexual function.

They may not always say it directly, but they care. They want to urinate better, but they do not want to trade urinary improvement for a sexual side effect they were not prepared for. Ejaculation changes, erection concerns, orgasm changes, and confidence all deserve discussion before treatment.

In my experience, Rezūm does not typically cause erectile

dysfunction. Many men feel more confident sexually once they are urinating better, sleeping better, and less worried about urinary control. But every patient should have an individualized discussion. The goal is not only to open the channel. The goal is to treat the man.

WHY SOME REZŪM TREATMENTS FAIL

No procedure works perfectly for every patient. When Rezūm does not produce the expected improvement, the first step is to understand why. Sometimes the prostate was too large for the degree of treatment performed. Sometimes the middle part of the prostate was under-treated. Sometimes one side of the gland remains obstructive. Sometimes the bladder was already weak before the procedure. Sometimes urgency persists because the bladder had been irritated for years. Sometimes the diagnosis was incomplete from the beginning. This is why follow-up evaluation matters.

If a patient does not improve, the answer is not simply, "Rezūm failed." The question is what part of the system remains abnormal. Is the channel still blocked? Is there untreated tissue? Is the bladder emptying? Is the stream improved? Is the bladder overactive? Is the bladder weak?

In selected cases, a small targeted repeat treatment may help if the issue is residual obstructing tissue. In other cases, a different procedure may be needed. In still others, the prostate may be open enough, but the bladder needs treatment. The failure analysis should be anatomical and functional, not emotional.

REZŪM AFTER OTHER TREATMENTS

Rezūm can also have a role after other prostate treatments in selected patients. For example, some men may undergo prostate artery embolization, which treats the prostate through its blood supply, and later still have a smaller amount of residual obstructing tissue. In that setting, Rezūm may be useful as a targeted follow-up treatment. The prostate may be less vascular and smaller after embolization, which can make a secondary tissue treatment more focused.

This is not a universal pathway, and it should not be presented as a formula. But it reflects a broader modern principle: prostate care can be staged and individualized. Not every man needs one massive intervention. Sometimes the best plan is to reduce the gland, preserve anatomy, reassess, and then treat any remaining obstruction if needed. That is different from the old one-size-fits-all surgical mindset.

HOW REZŪM FITS WITH PAE

Rezūm and prostate artery embolization are different tools. Rezūm treats tissue from inside the prostate using water vapor energy. PAE treats the prostate through the blood supply, reducing blood flow to the gland so it can shrink and soften over time. These treatments are not interchangeable. They fit different patients and different anatomies.

In broad terms, I tend to think of Rezūm as a strong option for selected smaller and moderate prostates, especially when the anatomy is suitable. I think of PAE as especially important for larger prostates, significant prostate tissue growing into the bladder, and men who want an anatomy-preserving, image-guided approach.

There is overlap. Medicine is not rigid. A man with a moderate prostate may be considered for either depending on anatomy, bladder function, goals, and physician expertise. But the philosophy remains the same: choose the treatment whose mechanism matches the problem. The best procedure is not the one with the best advertisement. The best procedure is the one that fits the anatomy.

REZŪM VERSUS TRADITIONAL SURGERY

Traditional prostate surgeries remove or carve out tissue to open the urine channel. They can be effective, especially in certain patients.

Procedures such as TURP or laser enucleation have a real role in urology.

But they are more anatomy-altering than Rezūm. They may carry greater concerns about bleeding, ejaculation changes, catheter time, recovery, and other risks depending on the patient and procedure.

Rezūm does not try to compete with every surgical operation in every situation. It occupies a different space. It is designed for selected men who need more than medication but may not need or want a more aggressive operation. That distinction is important.

A man should not be offered Rezūm if his anatomy is poorly suited for it. He also should not be pushed toward major surgery if a less invasive option is appropriate. Modern care is not about loyalty to one procedure. It is about matching the patient to the right tool.

THE PATIENT WHO SHOULD PAUSE

There are men who should pause before choosing Rezūm. A man with a very large prostate may need a broader discussion. A man already in severe retention may need careful bladder evaluation. A man with a very weak bladder may need pressure testing. A man with a large amount of prostate tissue inside the bladder opening may need to understand the possibility of slower healing or a different treatment strategy. A man expecting immediate improvement may be disappointed if he does not understand the recovery curve.

This does not mean Rezūm is wrong in all of those situations. It means the doctor should not oversimplify.

If the patient hears only, "It is a quick procedure," the explanation is incomplete. He should understand why Rezūm fits him, what it is expected to improve, how long recovery may take, what side effects are possible, whether a catheter is expected, and what the backup plan is if symptoms persist.

The best patients are not necessarily the least anxious. They are the best informed.

WHAT A MAN SHOULD ASK BEFORE REZŪM

Before choosing Rezūm, a man should be able to understand the answer to several questions in plain English. How large is my prostate? Is the prostate growing into the bladder opening? How much urine is left behind after I urinate? How fast does my urine come out? Does my bladder still seem strong? Am I a good candidate for Rezūm, or am I being offered it because it is simply available? How many treatment areas do you expect? Will I need a catheter? How long might recovery take? What urinary symptoms may temporarily worsen? What sexual side effects are possible? What happens if the treatment does not work well enough? What future options remain?

The patient does not need to memorize technical terms. He needs to understand the plan. A good doctor should be able to explain why Rezūm makes sense for that specific prostate. If the answer is vague, the patient should ask again.

DR. SHUSTERMAN'S MODERN PROSTATE TAKEAWAY

Rezūm is an important modern option for selected men with BPH. It uses water vapor energy to treat obstructing prostate tissue and can help men move beyond medication without immediately jumping to more aggressive tissue-removing surgery.

But Rezūm is not magic. It is not instant. It is not right for every prostate.

It works best when the anatomy fits the mechanism. In my practice, I think of Rezūm primarily for smaller and moderately enlarged prostates, though selected larger glands can be considered with careful counseling. If the prostate is very large, if a large amount of tissue is growing into the bladder opening, or if the bladder may already be weak, the conversation must be more detailed.

The value of Rezūm is not only that it can improve urinary symptoms. Its value is that, in the right patient, it can treat obstruction while preserving options. Modern prostate care should not force men to choose between endless medication and traditional surgery. Rezūm belongs in the middle of that conversation: targeted, less invasive, anatomy-based, and useful when the patient is selected properly.

CHAPTER 13

PAE AND THE LARGE-PROSTATE OPTION

WHERE PAE FITS IN MY PRACTICE

IN MY PRACTICE, prostate artery embolization is not a side note in the BPH discussion. For many properly selected men with prostate enlargement, PAE is the option I evaluate first. That is my position, not a consensus guideline, and the reasoning is anatomical. I set it out below so you can weigh it for yourself and raise it with your own urologist.

The reason is practical. PAE treats the prostate through the blood vessels rather than through the penis and urinary channel. Most other prostate procedures approach the gland through the same channel a man uses to urinate. That difference matters to patients because direct urinary-channel manipulation can mean more burning, urgency, frequency, catheter time, and postoperative irritation.

PAE is image-guided and vascular. It reduces the blood supply feeding the enlarged prostate so the gland can shrink and soften over time. In properly selected men, especially men with larger glands or prostate tissue growing into the bladder opening, this can address the obstruction while avoiding unnecessary disruption of the urinary channel.

This does not mean every man is a PAE candidate. The anatomy must fit. The bladder still has to be evaluated. The operator must be experienced. But when the case fits, PAE is often the most elegant option because it treats the prostate from the outside in rather than through the urine channel.

For a long time, men with large prostates were given a limited story. They were told to take medication for as long as possible. If the medication stopped working, they were told they might eventually need surgery. If the prostate was very large, the conversation often became even more intimidating. Bigger gland, bigger procedure, more anesthesia, more recovery, more fear. That old story made many men wait.

They waited because they feared surgery. They waited because the medication helped a little. They waited because they were told they were stable. They waited because they thought a procedure meant cutting through the prostate channel. They waited because nobody clearly explained that the bladder might be paying the price while they delayed.

Prostate artery embolization changed that conversation. PAE is not just another BPH procedure. It represents a different way of thinking about the prostate. Instead of approaching the prostate only through the urine channel, PAE treats the prostate through its blood supply. Instead of cutting, shaving, carving, or removing tissue from inside the urethra, the procedure uses imaging to guide tiny particles into selected arteries feeding the prostate. By reducing blood flow to targeted prostate tissue, the gland can shrink and soften over time.

The concept is elegant. The prostate is an organ that depends on blood supply. If the blood supply is reduced in a controlled, targeted way, the prostate can decrease in size and pressure. As it shrinks, the blockage may improve. The bladder may empty more easily. The stream may improve. Nighttime urination may decrease. The man may get relief without the same kind of direct tissue removal used in traditional surgery. That is why PAE matters. It gives men, especially men with larger glands or prostate tissue growing into the bladder opening, a modern option that did not exist in the old prostate playbook.

HOW PAE WORKS

FIGURE 13.1

How PAE Works

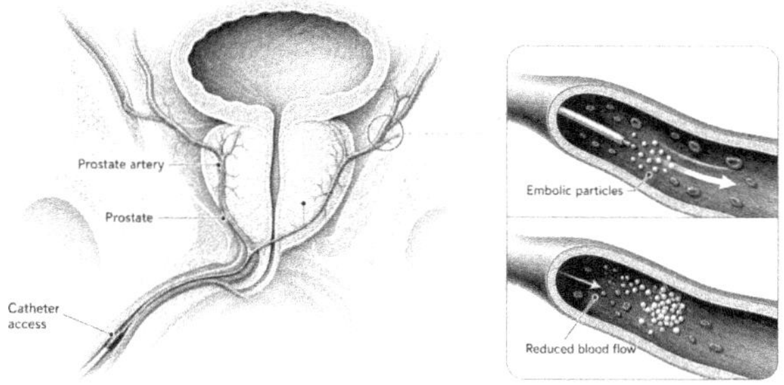

Prostate artery embolization reduces blood flow to prostate tissue through an image-guided vascular approach.

Figure 13.1 - How PAE Works. PAE treats the prostate through its blood supply.

PAE stands for prostate artery embolization. The word embolization may sound intimidating, but the principle is straightforward. An interventional radiologist places a small catheter into the arteries, usually through the wrist or groin, and uses imaging to navigate to the small blood vessels supplying the prostate. Once the correct vessels are identified, tiny particles are released to reduce blood flow to selected parts of the prostate.

The prostate tissue does not disappear immediately. This is not a procedure where a channel is carved open in real time. Instead, the prostate gradually responds after its blood supply is reduced. Over weeks and months, the gland may shrink, soften, and create less pressure around the urine channel and bladder opening.

Patients sometimes ask, "So you are killing the prostate?" That is not the way I explain it. The goal is not to destroy the entire prostate. The goal is to reduce blood flow to the enlarged obstructing tissue so the gland becomes less bulky and less obstructive.

A better patient explanation is this: the prostate has grown too large and is squeezing or blocking the urinary exit. PAE reduces the blood supply that feeds that enlargement, allowing the gland to shrink and the obstruction to improve.

It is a vascular solution to a prostate obstruction problem. That is what makes it different.

WHY THE BLOOD SUPPLY MATTERS

Doctors have known for a long time that the prostate is a vascular organ. It has a blood supply, and that blood supply can be important in symptoms, growth, and bleeding.

Historically, embolization was used in some patients to control severe prostate bleeding. Men with enlarged prostates can develop bleeding from fragile blood vessels inside the gland. In those cases, reducing the blood supply helped control bleeding. Over time, doctors recognized that men treated this way were not only bleeding less. Some were also urinating better.

That observation helped open the door to PAE as a BPH treatment. The logic makes sense. If an enlarged prostate depends on blood supply, then reducing that blood supply can reduce the size and pressure of the gland. The treatment does not need to cut through the urinary channel to affect the prostate. It can treat the gland from the inside of the vascular system.

That idea is important because many traditional prostate procedures focus on the urethra. They treat the obstruction by going through the same channel the man urinates through. PAE approaches the problem from a different direction. For the right patient, that difference can matter a lot.

THE LARGE-PROSTATE PROBLEM

Large prostates create a special challenge. Medication may help some men with large glands, but it often does not do enough. A relaxing pill may reduce muscle tone around the prostate opening, but it cannot make a large gland small. A shrinking pill may reduce prostate volume slowly in selected men, but it can take months, may cause side effects, and may not be enough when the bladder is already struggling.

Traditional procedures can be effective, but as the gland becomes larger, the treatment conversation often becomes more complex. The patient may need a more involved operation. Recovery may be more significant. Catheter time, bleeding risk, sexual side effects, and anesthesia concerns may become more important. Men who are older, medically complex, sexually active, or strongly interested in preserving function may hesitate.

PAE fills an important gap in this setting. It is particularly attractive for men with larger prostates because the mechanism fits the problem. If the prostate is large because it is well supplied by blood vessels and has grown over time, reducing that blood supply can help reduce the bulk of the gland.

This is why I think of PAE as a major option for many larger prostates. It is not the only option. It is not right for every man. But it should be part of the modern conversation far more often than it has been historically.

WHEN THE PROSTATE GROWS INTO THE BLADDER

PAE is also important when the prostate grows upward into the bladder opening. Patients may hear this described as a median lobe or intravesical protrusion. The phrase is less important than the image. Part of the prostate is bulging into the bladder outlet. When the bladder tries to empty, that tissue can block the exit like a ball valve.

This type of anatomy can be frustrating because medication often does not work well enough. A pill can relax the prostate opening, but it cannot remove a piece of tissue sitting at the bladder exit. The patient may improve slightly and still remain obstructed.

PAE can be useful in this setting because it treats the prostate globally through the blood supply. Instead of focusing only on the channel, it can reduce the bulk and vascularity of the gland, including tissue contributing to the blockage.

In my own thinking, once prostate tissue is growing meaningfully into the bladder opening, the treatment conversation changes. The prostate does not have to be enormous for PAE to enter the discussion. A moderately enlarged prostate with significant ball-valve growth into the bladder may be more clinically important than a larger prostate growing outward.

That is why I do not look only at total size. I look at behavior. What is the prostate doing to the bladder? If the prostate is growing into the bladder opening and the bladder is struggling, medication alone becomes a weaker argument.

PAE IS NOT JUST FOR THE GIANT PROSTATE

Many patients and even physicians think of PAE only as a treatment for extremely large glands. That is too narrow.

PAE is certainly important for very large prostates. But in my view, the size threshold should not be rigid. A forty- or fifty-gram prostate with significant tissue bulging into the bladder opening may deserve a PAE discussion if symptoms, urine flow, and bladder emptying support it.

The issue is not simply whether the prostate crosses an arbitrary number. The issue is whether the anatomy is creating a problem that medication is unlikely to solve well.

A man with a modest-sized prostate and no major obstruction may not need PAE. A man with a similar-sized prostate but clear ball-valve blockage, slow stream, persistent symptoms, and urine left behind may be different. The treatment should match the anatomy, not just the number.

This is one of the most important shifts in modern BPH care. We are moving away from a simplistic size-only model and toward a functional model. How large is the prostate? Where is it growing? What is it doing to the bladder? Is the bladder emptying? Is the stream slow? Is the patient suffering? What future options should be preserved? Those questions matter more than any single number.

WHY PAE IS UNDERDISCUSSED

PAE is still underdiscussed in many prostate conversations. There are several reasons for that.

First, PAE is often performed by interventional radiologists, not traditional urologists. That means it sits between specialties. Some urologists may not offer it, may not be familiar with it, or may not have a strong referral pathway. When a treatment is outside a doctor's usual toolkit, it may not be discussed enough.

Second, PAE is not marketed in the same way as some branded procedures. Certain BPH treatments have major device-company branding behind them. Patients hear about them. Doctors see advertising. The procedure becomes part of the public conversation. PAE is less of a simple consumer brand, even though the concept is powerful.

Third, medicine changes slowly. Urology, like many fields, can be conservative. A treatment may make sense mechanistically and still take years to become widely adopted. Training patterns, referral habits, reimbursement, institutional preferences, and specialty boundaries all affect how quickly newer approaches spread.

That does not mean PAE is right for everyone. But it does mean many patients never hear about it when they should. A modern prostate discussion should include every reasonable option that fits the patient, not only the options available in one office or one surgical lane.

THE PATIENT EXPERIENCE

Patients often want to know what PAE feels like compared with traditional prostate procedures. The experience is different because the procedure is performed through the blood vessels rather than through the urinary channel. There is no device cutting through the prostate channel. There is no resection from inside the urethra. There is typically no direct injury to the bladder lining from a cutting prostate instrument.

The interventional radiologist uses imaging to guide the catheter to the prostate arteries. The patient may receive sedation or anesthesia depending on the center and patient factors. The procedure requires detailed vascular mapping because the prostate blood supply can vary, and precision matters.

Afterward, patients may have pelvic discomfort, burning, urinary frequency, temporary worsening of symptoms, fatigue, or a post-procedure inflammatory response. Some men improve quickly. Others improve gradually over weeks to months as the prostate shrinks and softens.

The recovery experience varies. That should be explained honestly.

PAE is often easier for many men than more invasive prostate surgery, but it is still a real medical procedure. It should not be sold as nothing. It should be presented as a serious, image-guided treatment with potential benefits, limitations, and risks.

IMPROVEMENT CAN BE GRADUAL

PAE does not work like opening a clogged pipe with a tool. It works by changing the prostate's blood supply and allowing the tissue to respond over time. Some men notice improvement fairly quickly, sometimes even within days or weeks. Others improve more gradually over several months. This delayed improvement should be expected.

Patients who understand the mechanism are less likely to panic if the first week is not perfect. The prostate may swell or become irritated temporarily before it shrinks. Urinary symptoms may fluctuate. Some men need supportive medication during recovery. Follow-up is important.

The key is that PAE is a remodeling procedure. It changes the biology of the gland rather than mechanically cutting an immediate channel.

That is both an advantage and a limitation. The advantage is that it preserves the urinary channel and avoids direct tissue removal. The limitation is that the final effect may take time, and not every patient gets enough improvement. As with every treatment in this book, patient selection matters.

PRESERVING ANATOMY AND FUTURE OPTIONS

One of the major reasons I like PAE is that it preserves anatomy. It does not cut out the prostate channel. It does not remove large amounts of tissue through the urethra. It does not burn or resect the bladder neck. It does not create the same internal surgical field as traditional tissue-removing procedures. That preservation can matter.

A man treated with PAE may still have future options if symptoms persist or recur. He may later have Rezūm, TURP, HoLEP, Aquablation, or another treatment if needed, depending on the anatomy and clinical situation. In some cases, reducing the size and blood supply of the prostate first may make later procedures easier or less bloody.

This is a key modern principle: the first treatment should not burn every bridge. Prostate enlargement is a long-term condition.

Men are living longer. A man treated in his fifties, sixties, or seventies may need additional prostate care later. Preserving options is valuable.

That does not mean PAE always avoids future treatment. It means PAE often fits a strategy that respects the future.

SEXUAL FUNCTION

Sexual function is a major concern for men considering prostate treatment. Many patients are afraid to ask directly. They may worry about erections, ejaculation, orgasm, libido, and confidence. A doctor should bring these issues into the open.

In general, one of the advantages of PAE is that it tends to be favorable from a sexual-function standpoint compared with more aggressive tissue-removing procedures. Because PAE does not cut through the prostate channel or remove tissue around the bladder neck, the risk of certain ejaculation changes may be lower than with some traditional operations.

No honest physician should promise zero risk. Men vary. Anatomy varies. Procedures vary. But PAE is often attractive to men who want to preserve sexual function while treating urinary obstruction.

This matters because urinary improvement should not be viewed in isolation. The goal is not just to make the stream better. The goal is to treat the man. A treatment that improves urination but damages sexual identity, confidence, or quality of life may not feel like success to the patient.

PAE AND THE BLADDER

The central question in BPH is always bladder safety. PAE may help by reducing the prostate obstruction and allowing the bladder to empty with less resistance. In men whose bladder is still strong enough, this can improve flow, reduce leftover urine, decrease urgency, improve nighttime urination, and reduce the sense of incomplete emptying.

But if the bladder has already become very weak, PAE may not fully solve the problem. This is not unique to PAE. Any prostate treatment can disappoint if the bladder has lost too much strength before the obstruction is relieved. That is why evaluation before treatment matters.

If a man has very high leftover urine, retention, failed catheter removal attempts, or concern for bladder weakness, additional testing may be needed to understand whether the bladder can recover. The patient should know whether the treatment goal is symptom relief, bladder protection, catheter removal, reduction of prostate size, or avoiding more aggressive surgery.

PAE can be powerful. But it still depends on the bladder's ability to respond.

RISKS AND LIMITATIONS

Every procedure has risks and limitations. PAE requires vascular expertise. The prostate arteries can be small and variable. The physician must avoid blocking blood flow to unintended areas. Imaging, anatomy, experience, and technique matter.

Potential issues can include pelvic discomfort, urinary irritation, temporary symptom worsening, urinary infection, blood in the urine or semen, groin or wrist access-site issues, contrast exposure, radiation exposure, and rare non-target embolization. Some men may not be ideal candidates because of arterial anatomy, severe atherosclerosis, kidney issues, contrast allergy, or other medical factors.

PAE may also fail to provide enough relief in some patients. The prostate may not shrink enough. The obstruction may persist. The bladder may be too weak. The patient may eventually need another procedure.

None of that makes PAE a bad treatment. It makes it real medicine.

Every good treatment has indications, limitations, and risks. The goal is to choose wisely and explain honestly.

PAE VERSUS TRADITIONAL SURGERY

Traditional prostate surgeries often work by removing or cutting tissue to open the urine channel. These procedures can be effective, especially when the anatomy requires more immediate or definitive opening.

PAE works differently. It treats the gland through the blood supply and allows shrinkage over time. It does not immediately carve an open channel. It may have a different recovery profile, different sexual side-effect profile, and different role in treatment planning. The choice is not simply "PAE is better" or "surgery is better." That is too simplistic.

For the right man, PAE may be the better option. For another man, HoLEP, TURP, Aquablation, Rezūm, or another approach may be more appropriate. A man with a certain prostate size, shape, symptom pattern, bladder function, catheter status, bleeding risk, anesthesia risk, and sexual priorities needs an individualized recommendation.

Modern prostate care should not be procedure loyalty. It should be patient selection.

PAE AND REZŪM TOGETHER

In some men, PAE and Rezūm can be thought of as complementary rather than competing. PAE can reduce prostate size and blood supply. Rezūm can later treat selected residual obstructing tissue from inside the prostate. In my experience, this staged approach can make sense in certain patients who have a larger prostate initially, improve after embolization, but still have a focal area causing obstruction.

This is not a formula for every man. It is a strategy.

It reflects a larger point: modern prostate care does not always need one massive intervention. It can be staged, measured, reassessed, and adjusted. Treat the big component first. See how the bladder and symptoms respond. Then address what remains if needed. That is a different philosophy from the old model of waiting until things are severe and then doing the most aggressive option all at once.

WHO SHOULD CONSIDER PAE?

FIGURE 13.2

PAE Candidate Profile

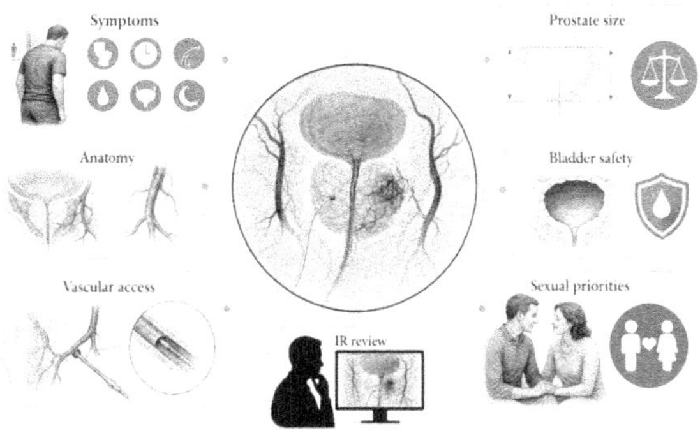

PAE is a selective-use option that depends on anatomy, symptom burden, prostate size, vascular access, and patient goals.

Figure 13.2 - PAE Candidate Profile. PAE depends on anatomy, symptoms, vascular access, and goals.

A man should consider asking about PAE if he has a larger prostate, significant prostate tissue growing into the bladder opening, persistent symptoms despite medication, slow urine flow, urine left behind after urination, side effects from medication, bleeding from an enlarged prostate, or a desire to preserve anatomy and sexual function. That does not mean he automatically needs PAE. It means the option deserves discussion.

The decision should be based on prostate size, shape, bladder function, symptoms, PSA evaluation, medical history, vascular anatomy, and patient goals. The patient should also ask who is performing the procedure. Experience matters. PAE is technically demanding. It should be performed by a physician with appropriate expertise in pelvic embolization and prostate arterial anatomy. The right procedure in the wrong hands is not the right procedure.

WHAT A MAN SHOULD ASK BEFORE PAE

Before choosing PAE, a man should understand the plan in plain language. How large is my prostate? Is part of it growing into the bladder opening? How much urine is left behind after I urinate? How slow is my stream? Does my bladder still seem strong? Why do you think PAE fits my anatomy? What improvement should I realistically expect? How long may it take? What are the risks? What happens if it does not work enough? What future options remain?

He should also ask about the team. Who is the interventional radiologist? How often do they perform PAE? How will follow-up be handled between the urologist and interventional radiologist? How will success be measured? These questions are not excessive. They are how a man makes an informed decision.

A DIFFERENT APPROACH

The reason PAE matters is not only that it is another treatment option. It changes the way men and doctors think about BPH.

For decades, the prostate was often treated from inside the urinary channel. That approach is sometimes necessary and effective. But PAE shows that the prostate can also be treated through its blood supply. It expands the map.

This is especially important in men with large prostates. The old thinking often made these men wait until the problem was severe or pushed them toward more aggressive surgery. PAE offers another path: image-guided, anatomy-preserving, vascular-based treatment.

That does not eliminate the need for surgery in all men. It does not replace every other procedure. But it changes the conversation. And that is what modern prostate care needs.

More options. Better selection. Less fear. Earlier treatment when the bladder is at risk. Less destructive approaches when they fit.

The future is not simply more procedures. The future is smarter procedures.

DR. SHUSTERMAN'S MODERN PROSTATE TAKEAWAY

PAE is one of the most important modern options in BPH care, especially for men with larger prostates, prostate tissue growing into the bladder opening, persistent symptoms despite medication, or a desire to preserve anatomy and future options. It treats the prostate through its blood supply rather than cutting through the urinary channel. Over time, the prostate can shrink and soften, reducing obstruction and helping the bladder empty more easily.

PAE is not magic. It is not instant for every patient. It requires the right anatomy, the right evaluation, and an experienced operator. Some men may still need additional treatment. Some may be better served by another procedure. But PAE changed the prostate conversation.

It showed that the prostate does not always have to be treated by cutting through the channel men urinate through. It can be treated in a more image-guided, vascular, anatomy-preserving way. For the right patient, that changes what is possible.

CHAPTER 14

UROLIFT, AQUABLATION, TURP, HOLEP, AND THE REST OF THE BPH LANDSCAPE

ONE OF THE most confusing parts of modern prostate care is that men now have more options than ever, but more options do not always make the decision easier. A man goes online and searches for BPH treatment. Suddenly he sees a long list of procedures. UroLift. Rezūm. PAE. Aquablation. TURP. GreenLight laser. HoLEP. Simple prostatectomy. Robotic surgery. Office procedures. Hospital procedures. "Minimally invasive" procedures. "Robotic" procedures. "Gold standard" procedures. "Preserve ejaculation" procedures. "No cutting" procedures.

Every option sounds impressive when it is marketed well. That is the problem.

The question is not which procedure has the best advertisement. The question is which procedure fits the man's prostate, bladder, symptoms, sexual priorities, and long-term plan.

This chapter is not meant to convince every man to choose one procedure. It is meant to help him understand the landscape. Each BPH treatment has a mechanism. Each mechanism has strengths and limits. A treatment that works well in one man may be the wrong choice in another. Modern prostate care is not procedure loyalty.

HOW I WEIGH THE OPTIONS

Although this chapter reviews the broader BPH landscape, my own treatment hierarchy is not neutral. In my model, PAE and Rezūm are the core modern BPH procedures I favor most often. PAE usually comes first when the prostate is large, complex, or growing into the bladder opening. Rezūm is the next major option when the prostate is smaller or moderate and the anatomy fits.

The other procedures in this chapter—UroLift, Aquablation, TURP, HoLEP, GreenLight laser, and simple prostatectomy—still have roles. Some men need tissue removal. Some men have anatomy that requires a more aggressive channel-opening operation. But I use those procedures much more selectively because they are generally more disruptive to the urinary channel or less convincing for the kind of anatomy I frequently see.

The point is not to attack every other procedure. The point is to avoid pretending all procedures are equal. They are not. The route of treatment matters. The recovery matters. Catheter time matters. Sexual function matters. The bladder matters. Future options matter. It is anatomy-based decision-making.

THE WRONG QUESTION

Patients often ask, "Doctor, what is the best procedure?" It is a natural question, but it is the wrong question. There is no single best BPH procedure for every man. A small prostate with mild obstruction is not the same as a very large prostate. A prostate growing outward is not the same as one bulging into the bladder opening. A man with a strong bladder is not the same as a man whose bladder has been weakened by years of obstruction. A man who desperately wants to preserve ejaculation may choose differently than a man whose main goal is maximum opening of the channel. A man in urinary retention may need a different strategy than a man who is bothered but still empties well.

The better question is, "Which treatment mechanism fits my problem?" That question changes everything. If the prostate tissue is mainly squeezing the urine channel from the sides, one set of options may make sense. If the prostate is very large, another set may make sense. If prostate tissue is growing into the bladder opening like a ball valve, the discussion changes again. If the bladder is already weak, the doctor may need to test bladder strength before promising that any prostate procedure will solve the problem.

The prostate is not one shape. BPH is not one pattern. Procedures are not interchangeable. Treatment should follow anatomy.

PULLING TISSUE ASIDE: UROLIFT

UroLift is one of the best-known minimally invasive prostate procedures because it has been heavily marketed to patients. The idea is simple. Small implants are placed to pull prostate tissue away from the urine channel. The goal is to open the channel without cutting, burning, or removing tissue. For selected men, especially those with smaller glands and favorable anatomy, that concept can be attractive.

The appeal is obvious. It is usually quick. It is less destructive than tissue-removing surgery. It is often discussed as having a favorable sexual side-effect profile, especially for ejaculation. Men who fear more invasive procedures may find the idea appealing. But the mechanism also explains the limitation.

UroLift does not shrink the prostate. It does not remove tissue. It does not treat the blood supply. It does not make a large gland small. It does not melt or vaporize the obstruction. It pulls tissue aside.

That may work when the prostate is small enough and the obstruction pattern is favorable. It may work best when the side lobes of the prostate are pushing inward and can be mechanically held open. But if the gland is larger, if the obstruction is more complex, or if the middle part of the prostate is growing into the bladder opening, the mechanism may not be strong enough. This is where patient selection becomes everything.

A procedure that pulls tissue aside can be useful when the problem is tissue that can be pulled aside. It becomes less convincing when the problem is too much tissue, tissue in the wrong place, or anatomy that cannot be opened well with implants.

THE UROLIFT FAILURE PATTERN

I have performed many UroLift procedures, and I understand why the procedure became popular. In the right patient, it can help. But I have also seen the failure patterns.

Some men improve for a period of time and then symptoms return. The prostate continues to grow. The tissue eventually overwhelms the implants. The channel that looked more open after the procedure becomes obstructed again.

In other men, the anatomy is distorted. When implants pull tissue from specific points, the prostate channel may not open in a smooth, natural way. On cystoscopy, where we look inside the urinary channel with a small camera, some failed cases can look puckered or narrowed. The channel may appear pulled in certain directions rather than truly opened.

Patients do not need to understand every technical detail. They need to understand the practical lesson: pulling tissue aside is not the same as treating the underlying growth.

That does not mean UroLift is always bad. It means it has a role. I think of it as a selected-patient procedure, often more reasonable in smaller prostates with favorable anatomy and a strong desire to preserve ejaculation. It should not be used as if every prostate is a UroLift prostate.

THE MARKETING PROBLEM

UroLift also illustrates a larger issue in BPH care: marketing can run ahead of nuance. Patients may see commercials or online promotions and think they have found the answer. The promise sounds clean.

No cutting. No heating. Quick recovery. Preserve sexual function. Back to normal fast. Those are attractive claims.

But no procedure should be chosen from a slogan. The doctor still needs to know the prostate size, the shape of the gland, whether tissue is growing into the bladder opening, how much urine is left behind, how fast the urine comes out, and whether the bladder is strong.

If that evaluation is skipped, the procedure becomes a guess. A man should not ask, "Can I have the procedure I saw advertised?" He should ask, "Does that procedure match my anatomy?" That is the difference between consumer medicine and real medicine.

ROBOTIC WATERJET TREATMENT: AQUABLATION

Aquablation is another newer BPH treatment that has received significant attention. The concept is technologically impressive. It uses robotic guidance and a high-velocity waterjet to remove prostate tissue. Imaging helps map the treatment area, and the waterjet removes tissue without the same type of heat used in some other procedures.

On paper, it sounds very modern. Robotic. Image-guided. Precise. Less heat. Effective tissue removal.

For selected patients, Aquablation can improve urinary flow and symptoms. Published studies have shown meaningful improvement in many men, including men with larger glands and certain median-lobe anatomy. It is not a fringe procedure. It has a real place in the BPH landscape.

But here is the issue: a procedure can be technologically advanced and still not be the best choice for every patient. Technology should never replace judgment.

Aquablation removes tissue. That is its strength. It is also why the treatment has to be understood carefully. Removing tissue near the bladder opening, especially when prostate tissue extends into the bladder, can improve obstruction, but it may also create irritation in some men. Some patients may have persistent urgency, frequency, burning, or overactive bladder-type symptoms after the obstruction is relieved.

This is one of the most important distinctions in prostate care. Unblocked is not the same as comfortable.

FLOW IMPROVEMENT IS NOT THE WHOLE STORY

Many BPH studies focus on numbers such as symptom scores, urine flow, prostate volume, retreatment rates, and safety outcomes. Those numbers are important. If a procedure improves the speed of urination and reduces obstruction, that matters.

But a man does not live inside a flow-rate graph. He lives inside his bladder.

If the stream is better but the bladder remains irritated, the patient may still be unhappy. If he urinates faster but has urgency all day, he may not feel cured. If the outlet is open but nighttime urination persists, quality of life may remain poor.

This is not unique to Aquablation. It can happen after many prostate treatments, especially when the bladder has been irritated by years of obstruction. But with any tissue-removing procedure, especially one treating tissue near the bladder opening, doctors and patients should discuss the possibility of persistent storage symptoms.

Storage symptoms are the urgency, frequency, and nighttime urination symptoms that come from the bladder side of the system. Patients usually care about them deeply because they control daily life. A better stream is good. But a better stream is not the only goal.

A CAUTION ABOUT AQUABLATION

My concern with Aquablation is not that it cannot work. It can work.

My concern is that in some patients, especially those with significant prostate tissue growing into the bladder opening, the procedure may trade one problem for another. The obstruction may improve, but the bladder may remain irritated or become more symptomatic. Some men may continue to need overactive bladder medications or additional bladder treatments afterward.

In my practice, I have seen men several years after Aquablation who were told the procedure opened the channel but who still struggled with urgency, frequency, nighttime urination, and bladder irritation. Some were more bothered by the bladder symptoms than they had been by the original slow stream.

This does not prove the procedure is wrong for everyone. It means the patient should be counseled carefully. If a man's main symptoms are urgency and nighttime urination, not just weak stream, the doctor should think hard about whether the bladder has already become part of the disease. Opening the outlet may be necessary, but it may not solve everything.

That is why pre-treatment evaluation matters. A man should know whether his bladder is overactive, whether urine is being left behind, whether the prostate is truly the driver, and what symptoms may persist even after the channel is opened. A procedure that treats obstruction should not be sold as guaranteed comfort.

TURP: THE CLASSIC OPERATION

TURP stands for transurethral resection of the prostate. For decades, TURP was considered the classic surgical treatment for BPH. The procedure is performed through the urinary channel. The surgeon removes obstructing prostate tissue from inside the channel to improve flow.

TURP has helped many men. It can be effective. It remains an important option in the right setting.

But TURP also represents the older paradigm of prostate treatment. It is a tissue-removing operation. It can involve bleeding, anesthesia, catheter time, recovery, and sexual side effects such as retrograde ejaculation. In some men, it can also be followed by urgency or bladder irritation during recovery.

This does not mean TURP is obsolete. It means TURP should be selected thoughtfully.

For a man with the right anatomy, symptoms, and goals, TURP may still be an excellent option. But it should not be the automatic default for every man who fails medication, especially now that less invasive and more anatomy-preserving approaches exist for selected patients.

The question is not whether TURP works. The question is whether TURP is the best match for that specific man.

HOLEP: THE LARGE-GLAND WORKHORSE

HoLEP stands for holmium laser enucleation of the prostate. Patients do not need to remember the full name. The concept is that a laser is used to shell out the obstructing inner portion of the prostate. HoLEP can be especially useful for large glands because it removes a significant amount of tissue and can create a widely open channel.

In experienced hands, HoLEP can be effective. It has become an important option for men with large prostates who need definitive tissue removal.

But HoLEP is still an anatomy-altering operation. It requires specialized skill. Recovery, catheter time, bleeding risk, urinary leakage during recovery, and ejaculation changes need to be discussed. Many men will have retrograde ejaculation or dry ejaculation afterward. That may be acceptable to some patients and unacceptable to others.

HoLEP is powerful. That is both its advantage and its tradeoff.

A man with a very large obstructing prostate and good bladder function may do extremely well with HoLEP. Another man who strongly wants to preserve ejaculation and has a different anatomy may prefer another strategy. Again, the principle is the same: mechanism must match the patient.

GREENLIGHT AND OTHER LASER PROCEDURES

Laser procedures, including GreenLight laser vaporization, are also part of the BPH landscape. These treatments use laser energy to vaporize or remove obstructing prostate tissue. They may reduce bleeding compared with some traditional approaches in selected patients and can be useful in certain settings.

As with all procedures, the details matter. Prostate size, anatomy, bleeding risk, surgeon experience, anticoagulation status, bladder function, and sexual priorities all affect whether a laser procedure makes sense. A patient should not choose a laser procedure because the word laser sounds modern.

Laser is an energy source. It is not a diagnosis. The correct question remains: what is the prostate doing, what is the bladder doing, and does this procedure's mechanism fit?

SIMPLE PROSTATECTOMY

For extremely large prostates, some men may be offered simple prostatectomy. This is not the same as radical prostatectomy for prostate cancer. In a simple prostatectomy, the goal is to remove the enlarged inner portion of the prostate causing obstruction while leaving the outer prostate capsule behind.

This may be done through open, laparoscopic, or robotic approaches depending on the surgeon and setting. Simple prostatectomy can be effective for very large glands, but it is more invasive than many other BPH treatments. It may involve hospitalization, more anesthesia, more recovery, and more surgical risk. For some men, it is appropriate. For others, modern alternatives such as HoLEP or PAE may be considered depending on anatomy, patient priorities, and local expertise.

The important point is that "prostatectomy" can mean different things. A simple prostatectomy for BPH is not the same as radical prostatectomy for cancer. Patients often hear the word and panic. The doctor should explain exactly what is being removed, why, and what the expected effects are. Clear language matters.

OFFICE PROCEDURE VERSUS HOSPITAL PROCEDURE

Another practical issue is where the procedure is performed. Some BPH treatments can be done in an office or outpatient setting. Others require a hospital or operating room. This affects cost, anesthesia, recovery, scheduling, facility fees, and sometimes physician incentives.

This is an uncomfortable but important part of modern medicine. Hospitals and surgical centers invest in equipment. Practices develop expertise in certain procedures. Doctors tend to recommend what they know and what they can offer.

That does not mean recommendations are dishonest. It means patients should understand that availability can influence what gets discussed.

A man should ask whether he is hearing about all reasonable options or only the options available in that specific setting. He should ask why one procedure is being recommended over another. He should ask whether the recommendation is based on his anatomy or on the doctor's usual pathway.

The best procedure is not the one the hospital invested in. The best procedure is the one that fits the patient.

RECOVERY EXPECTATIONS

Every BPH procedure has a recovery profile. Some treatments have more irritation early and gradual improvement. Some open the channel more quickly but involve more tissue removal. Some require a catheter for several days. Some may cause temporary burning, urgency, frequency, blood in the urine, or discomfort. Some may affect ejaculation. Some may require time for the bladder to calm down after years of obstruction.

Patients often ask, "How long until I am better?" The honest answer depends on the procedure, the prostate, the bladder, and the patient's baseline condition. A man treated early with a still-healthy bladder may recover differently from a man treated after years of obstruction and high leftover urine. A smaller prostate may recover differently from a very large gland. A bladder that has been irritated for years may not become calm overnight. This is why expectations are part of treatment. A good doctor should explain not only what the procedure does, but how recovery usually feels, what symptoms may temporarily worsen, and when improvement should be expected.

EJACULATION AND SEXUAL FUNCTION

BPH treatment is not just about urine. Men care about sexual function. They care about erections. They care about ejaculation. They care about orgasm. They care about confidence.

Some procedures have higher risk of retrograde ejaculation, where semen goes backward into the bladder. Some may reduce semen volume. Some may carry risk of erectile changes, although many BPH procedures are not primarily erectile-function procedures. Some preserve ejaculation better in selected men. This discussion should happen before treatment, not after.

A doctor should never assume that ejaculation does not matter because a man is older. Men in their sixties, seventies, and eighties may still be sexually active and may care deeply about preserving function. Even men who are not currently sexually active deserve to know what a procedure may change.

Preserving function is not cosmetic. It is part of treating the man.

RETREATMENT AND FUTURE OPTIONS

Another important issue is retreatment. Some procedures are less invasive but may have a higher chance of needing additional treatment later. Some procedures are more aggressive but may be more durable. Some preserve anatomy and future options better. Some make future procedures more complex.

There is no free lunch in medicine. A man may choose a less invasive treatment because he values recovery and preservation, accepting that future treatment may be possible. Another man may choose a more definitive tissue-removing operation because he wants the strongest chance of durable opening. Both decisions can be reasonable if the patient understands the tradeoffs.

The key is honesty. Patients should not be told only the benefits. They should understand what may happen if the treatment does not work well enough or if symptoms return. A modern prostate plan should think not only about the next three months but also about the next ten years.

THE BLADDER AFTER THE PROSTATE IS TREATED

One of the most important things men need to understand is that prostate treatment does not always immediately normalize bladder behavior. If the bladder has spent years pushing against obstruction, it may remain irritated even after the outlet is opened. Urgency and frequency can persist. Nighttime urination may improve slowly or only partially. Some men need bladder-directed medication, pelvic floor therapy, constipation management, sleep evaluation, or bladder treatments after the prostate is addressed. This does not always mean the procedure failed.

It may mean the bladder became part of the disease. That is why earlier treatment can matter. If obstruction is addressed before the bladder is severely irritated or weakened, recovery may be better. If the patient waits until the bladder is damaged, opening the outlet may not restore everything. A man should not wait until the bladder becomes the problem.

HOW TO THINK ABOUT THE LANDSCAPE

FIGURE 14.1

The BPH Treatment Landscape

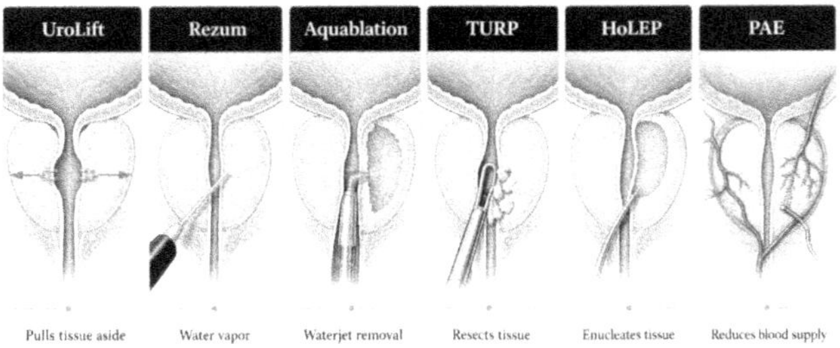

Modern BPH options differ by mechanism, invasiveness, recovery, and the outcomes that matter to each patient.

Figure 14.1 - The BPH Treatment Landscape. Procedures differ by mechanism, invasiveness, recovery, and tradeoffs.

The BPH landscape can be understood in terms of mechanism. Some treatments relax the outlet. Some pull tissue aside. Some shrink tissue with heat or water vapor. Some reduce blood supply. Some remove tissue. Some shell out tissue. Some are more preserving. Some are more definitive. Some are better for certain sizes and shapes.

This is why it is misleading to ask which procedure is best in general. A man should ask which mechanism solves his problem with the least unnecessary damage.

If the problem is early and mild, medication may be enough. If the prostate is smaller or moderate and the anatomy fits, Rezūm may be reasonable. If the prostate is larger or growing into the bladder opening, PAE may be a strong consideration. If major tissue removal is needed, TURP, HoLEP, Aquablation, or another surgical option may be appropriate depending on the patient. If the bladder is weak, pressure testing may be needed before choosing anything.

The correct answer comes from the diagnosis. Not from the brochure.

QUESTIONS PATIENTS SHOULD ASK

A patient does not need to become an expert in every BPH procedure, but he should understand why one is being recommended. He should ask what the procedure actually does. Does it pull tissue aside, shrink tissue, reduce blood supply, or remove tissue? He should ask whether the prostate is small, moderate, large, or very large. He should ask whether the prostate is growing into the bladder opening. He should ask how much urine is left behind after urination and whether the bladder seems strong. He should ask how the procedure may affect ejaculation. He should ask what recovery is usually like and what symptoms may persist. He should ask what future options remain if the treatment does not work well enough.

These questions are not excessive. They are the minimum standard for informed decision-making.

DR. SHUSTERMAN'S MODERN PROSTATE TAKEAWAY

The BPH treatment landscape is crowded, and that can confuse patients. UroLift, Aquablation, TURP, HoLEP, laser procedures, simple prostatectomy, Rezūm, and PAE all have roles, but they are not interchangeable.

UroLift pulls tissue aside. Aquablation removes tissue with a robotic waterjet. TURP shaves out obstructing tissue. HoLEP shells out tissue with a laser. Other laser procedures vaporize or remove tissue. PAE treats the prostate through its blood supply. Rezūm treats selected tissue with water vapor energy.

Each mechanism has strengths. Each has limits.

The best procedure is not the newest, loudest, most advertised, or most technologically impressive procedure. The best procedure is the one that fits the prostate, protects the bladder, respects the patient's sexual priorities, and preserves quality of life.

Modern BPH care should not be procedure-driven. It should be anatomy-driven.

Unblocked is not the same as comfortable. A better stream is not the same as a better life unless the bladder, symptoms, and patient goals are all considered. The prostate is only one part of the decision. The man is the other.

CHAPTER 15

MATCHING THE TREATMENT TO THE ANATOMY

FIGURE 15.1

Match Treatment to Anatomy

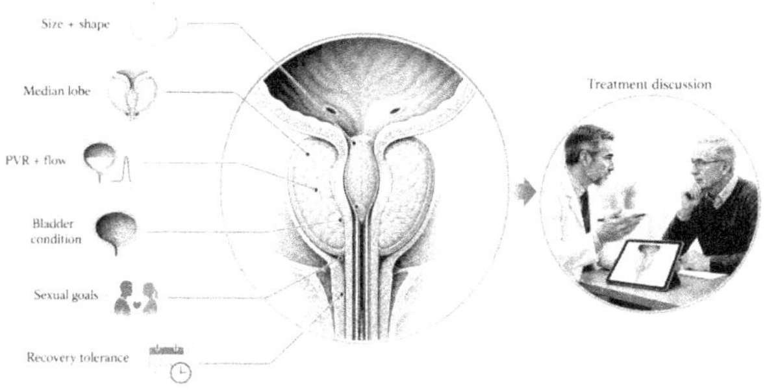

The right BPH treatment depends on prostate anatomy, bladder condition, sexual priorities, recovery tolerance, and future options.

FIGURE 15.1 - MATCH *Treatment to Anatomy. The right treatment depends on anatomy, bladder condition, and goals.*

The most important question in BPH treatment is not, "What is the newest procedure?" It is not, "What procedure does the doctor like?" It is not, "What procedure did my friend have?" It is not,

"What treatment has the best commercial?" The most important question is much simpler: What treatment matches my anatomy?

THE PRACTICAL TREATMENT HIERARCHY

In my practice, the hierarchy usually begins with the least disruptive treatment that can truly solve the anatomical problem. For many enlarged prostates, especially larger glands and prostates that grow into the bladder opening, that means starting the conversation with PAE.

PAE is different because it treats the prostate through the blood vessels. It does not require going through the penis and urinary channel to cut, shave, vaporize, pull, or resect tissue. For properly selected men, that vascular route can mean less urinary-channel irritation, often no postoperative urinary catheter, and a smoother recovery profile than many transurethral procedures.

Rezūm is the next major option I consider. It is quick, targeted, and useful for selected smaller or moderate prostates. But because it is performed through the urinary channel, men should expect catheter time and a healing period during which urinary symptoms may temporarily flare before improving.

The rest of the BPH procedures are more selective tools. They may be right for certain men, but they should not be chosen because they are advertised well or because they are the only thing an office offers. They should be chosen only when their mechanism matches the patient's anatomy and goals.

That is where many men get lost. They think BPH treatment is a menu. Medication, Rezūm, UroLift, PAE, Aquablation, TURP, HoLEP. Pick one. Compare the recovery. Compare the marketing. Compare the side effects. Choose the one that sounds best. That is not how prostate care should work.

The prostate is not the same in every man. Some prostates are only mildly enlarged. Some are massive. Some grow mostly outward. Some squeeze the urine channel from the sides. Some have a middle portion that grows upward into the bladder opening and blocks the exit like a ball valve. Some men have strong bladders that can still push well. Others have bladders that have been struggling for years and may already be weak. Some men are most bothered by slow flow. Others are most bothered by urgency, nighttime urination, or fear of retention. Some men care deeply about preserving ejaculation. Others prioritize the strongest possible opening of the channel.

Those are different patients. They should not all receive the same treatment.

Modern prostate care should not begin with the procedure. It should begin with the anatomy.

THE WRONG WAY TO CHOOSE

A man sees an advertisement for a procedure that promises fast recovery and preserved sexual function. It sounds appealing, so he asks for it. Another man hears from a friend that a certain surgery "fixed everything." Another reads online that one procedure is the "gold standard." Another is told by a doctor that the office offers a certain treatment and that he is a candidate.

Sometimes those recommendations are reasonable. Sometimes they are incomplete.

The problem is that men often hear about procedures before they understand their own prostate. That is backwards.

Before choosing a treatment, a man should know the basic facts. How large is the prostate? Is it mildly enlarged, moderately enlarged, severely enlarged, or very large? Is the prostate growing into the bladder opening? How much urine is left behind after urination? How fast does the urine come out? Does the bladder appear strong, or is it already struggling? Are the symptoms mostly slow stream, urgency, nighttime urination, incomplete emptying, or a combination? Is PSA being evaluated appropriately? Is cancer risk part of the picture? Is sexual function a major priority?

Without those answers, procedure selection becomes guesswork.

A man should not choose a treatment based on the name of the technology. He should choose based on the problem the technology is designed to solve.

SIZE IS ONLY THE FIRST QUESTION

Prostate size matters. A thirty-gram prostate is not the same as a ninety-gram prostate. A prostate over one hundred grams is a different strategic problem than a mildly enlarged gland. Size affects medication choices, procedure selection, expected recovery, and long-term planning. But size is only the first question.

A man can have a moderate-sized prostate that creates major obstruction because it grows in the wrong direction. Another man can have a larger prostate that grows outward and causes fewer symptoms. This is why I care so much about shape and behavior.

The key question is not only how big the prostate is. The key question is what the prostate is doing to the bladder.

If the prostate is simply enlarged but the bladder empties well, the stream is acceptable, and symptoms are mild, a conservative approach may be reasonable. If the prostate is moderately enlarged but bulging into the bladder opening, the situation may be more serious. If the stream is slow and urine is left behind, the treatment discussion should move beyond vague reassurance.

The size tells us how big the gland is. The shape tells us how it behaves. The bladder tells us whether the system is safe.

THE BALL-VALVE PROBLEM

One of the most important anatomical patterns in BPH is when prostate tissue grows upward into the bladder opening. Doctors may call this a median lobe or intravesical prostatic protrusion. Those terms matter medically, but for patients the concept is more important. Part of the prostate is bulging into the bladder outlet. When the bladder tries to empty, that tissue can act like a ball valve and block the exit. This changes the treatment conversation.

A pill that relaxes the prostate opening may help some muscle tightness, but it cannot make that ball-valve tissue disappear. A procedure that works well for side-lobe squeezing may not be enough if the main problem is tissue sitting inside the bladder opening. A treatment designed for smaller, favorable glands may not work as well when the prostate shape is more complex.

This is why a man should not be told only that his prostate is enlarged. He should be told whether the prostate is growing into the bladder opening.

That one detail can explain why medication only helped a little. It can explain why the stream remains slow. It can explain why urine is left behind. It can explain why certain treatments may be better than others. When the prostate acts like a ball valve, the plan must address the ball valve.

THE BLADDER DECIDES THE URGENCY

The prostate may be the visible problem, but the bladder often determines how urgent the situation is. A man can have an enlarged prostate and still empty well. Another man may have a smaller prostate but leave a large amount of urine behind. Those two men are not in the same category.

Urine left behind after urination is one of the clearest signs that the bladder is not emptying normally. The cause may be blockage from the prostate, weakness of the bladder muscle, or both. But the finding matters because it tells us the system is no longer working efficiently.

A man with low leftover urine, a reasonable stream, and tolerable symptoms may have time. He may choose observation, medication, or a less aggressive option.

A man with rising leftover urine, a very slow stream, repeated infections, bladder stones, or retention does not have the same flexibility. The bladder is already showing stress. In that situation, waiting may not be conservative. Waiting may be the thing that allows permanent bladder damage to develop.

That is why I ask a blunt question in BPH care: Is the bladder safe? If the bladder is safe, we have more room to be patient. If the bladder is not safe, the plan must become more serious.

THE STREAM MATTERS, BUT IT DOES NOT EXPLAIN EVERYTHING

A urine flow test tells us how fast the urine comes out. A slow stream is an important clue, but it does not explain everything by itself.

A slow stream can mean the prostate is blocking the outlet. It can also mean the bladder is weak and cannot push strongly. In many older men, both are present. The prostate creates resistance for years, and the bladder eventually loses efficiency.

That distinction matters because treatment expectations depend on it. If the bladder is strong and the prostate is clearly blocking, opening or reducing the obstruction may produce a strong result. If the bladder is weak, the same procedure may not produce the same improvement. The channel may be more open, but the bladder may still not push well.

This is why some men need pressure-based bladder testing before a major treatment decision. If a man has very high urine left behind, retention, failed catheter removal attempts, or symptoms that do not match the prostate size, the doctor may need to know whether the bladder can still generate pressure.

The goal is not to order every test on every patient. The goal is to avoid promising that a prostate procedure will solve a problem that is partly or mainly bladder weakness. The best prostate treatment in the world cannot fully fix a bladder that no longer works well.

MATCHING MEDICATION TO ANATOMY

Medication makes sense when the anatomy fits. If a man has early symptoms, a smaller or moderately enlarged prostate, a bladder that empties well, and no major ball-valve growth into the bladder opening, medication may be a reasonable starting point. A relaxing pill may reduce resistance enough to improve the stream and symptoms. Daily tadalafil may be useful if erectile dysfunction and urinary symptoms overlap. A shrinking medication may be considered in selected men with larger glands who understand the time course and side effects.

But if the anatomy is clearly mechanical, medication becomes less convincing. A very large prostate may not respond enough to a relaxing pill. A ball-valve prostate growth may not respond enough because the issue is tissue in the wrong place. A man leaving a lot of urine behind may not be protected by symptom improvement alone. A man with bladder stones, recurrent infections, or retention has already moved beyond mild disease.

Medication is not wrong. Medication without anatomical logic is wrong. The question is not, "Can we try a pill?" The question is, "Does a pill match the mechanism of this man's problem?"

MATCHING REZŪM TO ANATOMY

Rezūm can be a strong option when the prostate is smaller or moderately enlarged and the obstructing tissue can be treated effectively with water vapor energy. I often think of Rezūm as a useful middle-ground procedure. It can help men who need more than medication but may not need or want a more aggressive tissue-removing operation. It treats prostate tissue without carving out a large channel, and in properly selected patients it can preserve future options. But selection matters.

A smaller or moderate gland with favorable anatomy may respond well. A very large prostate may require many treatment sites, more inflammation, and a longer recovery. A large amount of tissue growing into the bladder opening can be treated in selected cases, but recovery may be slower and symptoms may take longer to improve.

This is where honest counseling matters. Rezūm is not magic. It is a tissue-treatment procedure with a healing curve. It should not be sold as instant or effortless. The right patient is the man whose anatomy fits the tool.

MATCHING PAE TO ANATOMY

Prostate artery embolization fits a different anatomical logic. PAE treats the prostate through its blood supply. It is especially important in men with larger prostates, men with significant prostate tissue growing into the bladder opening, men who want to preserve anatomy, and men who may not be ideal candidates for more aggressive surgery.

In my thinking, PAE should not be reserved only for enormous prostates. A moderately enlarged prostate with a significant ball-valve component at the bladder opening can be a serious problem. If medication is not enough and the bladder is showing stress, PAE may deserve discussion even when the gland is not gigantic.

This is one of the shifts modern prostate care needs. The question is not just the size. It is the behavior.

A prostate that grows into the bladder may behave more dangerously than its volume suggests. PAE can be attractive because it reduces the gland through its blood supply rather than cutting through the urinary channel. It can shrink and soften tissue, preserve the channel, and leave future options open.

PAE is not right for every patient. It requires the right vascular anatomy, an experienced interventional radiologist, and appropriate follow-up. But for the right anatomy, it can be one of the most important tools in the modern BPH landscape.

MATCHING TISSUE-REMOVING SURGERY TO ANATOMY

There are men who need tissue removed. That has to be said clearly.

Modern, less invasive, anatomy-preserving options are important, but they do not eliminate the role of TURP, HoLEP, Aquablation, laser procedures, or other surgical treatments. Some prostates need a more definitive opening. Some men have anatomy that is best handled by tissue removal. Some patients want the strongest possible channel-opening procedure and accept the tradeoffs.

HoLEP can be powerful for large glands in experienced hands. TURP remains effective for selected prostates. Aquablation can improve flow in appropriately selected men. Laser procedures can be useful in certain settings. Simple prostatectomy may still have a role for extremely large glands when other approaches are not appropriate. But tissue-removing procedures should still be selected carefully.

The patient should understand the recovery, catheter time, bleeding risk, irritation, chance of ejaculation changes, and the possibility that bladder symptoms may persist even after the channel is opened. Opening the channel is not the same as curing the bladder. That is one of the most important lessons in the entire BPH discussion.

THE BLADDER SYMPTOM PROBLEM

Many men think the main goal of BPH treatment is to make the stream stronger. That is important, but it is not the only goal.

Some men are more bothered by urgency, frequency, and nighttime urination than by the stream itself. These symptoms come from the bladder side of the system. They may be caused by obstruction, but once the bladder has been irritated for years, it may not calm down immediately after the prostate is treated.

This is why treatment selection has to consider symptoms carefully. If the main complaint is a slow stream and the bladder is otherwise healthy, opening the outlet may produce a clear improvement. If the main complaint is severe urgency and nighttime urination, the doctor must ask whether the bladder has become overactive or damaged. Treating the prostate may still be necessary, but the patient should know that bladder symptoms may need additional time or additional treatment.

This is especially important when evaluating procedures that focus on removing obstruction. A better stream is valuable, but if the patient continues to run to the bathroom all day, he may not feel successful.

The goal is not just flow. The goal is function.

SEXUAL PRIORITIES MATTER

No BPH treatment decision is complete without discussing sexual function. Some men care deeply about ejaculation. Some care mainly about erections. Some are less concerned. Some are not currently sexually active but still want to preserve future possibilities. A doctor should not assume that because a man is older, sexual side effects do not matter.

Different BPH treatments carry different risks. Prostate-relaxing pills can affect ejaculation. Shrinking medications may affect libido or erections in some men. TURP and HoLEP commonly affect ejaculation. Aquablation, Rezūm, UroLift, and PAE may have different sexual side-effect profiles depending on the patient and procedure.

No treatment should be described as having no risk. But the differences matter.

A man should understand the likely effects before treatment, not after. It is not acceptable for a patient to say, "Nobody told me this could happen," after a procedure affects ejaculation or sexual confidence.

Preserving function is not cosmetic. It is part of treating the man.

FUTURE OPTIONS MATTER

BPH is not always a one-time event. A man treated in his fifties or sixties may need more prostate care later. The prostate may continue to change. The bladder may change. Symptoms may return. Cancer-risk evaluation may become relevant. A treatment that works for years may eventually need to be supplemented. That is why future options matter.

Some treatments preserve anatomy better than others. Some may make future procedures more complex. Some are easy to repeat or follow with another treatment. Some are more definitive but more anatomy-altering. Some are best used early; others are best saved for more advanced situations.

A patient should ask not only, "What happens next month?" but also, "What happens if this is not enough?" That question is especially important for younger men, sexually active men, men with large prostates, and men who want to avoid burning bridges. The first procedure should be chosen with the future in mind.

THE PROBLEM WITH ONE-PROCEDURE PRACTICES

Every doctor has training, preferences, and available tools. That is normal.

But patients should be aware that some practices may lean heavily toward the procedures they offer. If a doctor mainly performs one procedure, many patients may be told they are candidates for that procedure. If a hospital has invested in expensive equipment, that technology may become more visible. If a device is heavily marketed, patients may request it before they understand whether it fits.

This does not mean doctors are acting in bad faith. It means systems influence recommendations.

A man should ask whether all reasonable options have been

considered. He should ask why one treatment is preferred over another. He should ask whether the recommendation is based on prostate size, prostate shape, bladder function, sexual priorities, and long-term goals. A good physician should welcome those questions.

If the answer is simply, "This is what we do," that is not enough. The best procedure is not the one that happens to be available. It is the one that fits the patient.

A PRACTICAL WAY TO THINK ABOUT TREATMENT

A man can think of BPH treatment in layers. The first layer is symptoms. How bothered is he? How much is sleep affected? How much does urination control his life?

The second layer is anatomy. How large is the prostate? Is it growing into the bladder opening? Is the channel narrowed from the sides? Is the gland very vascular or very large?

The third layer is bladder function. Is urine being left behind? Is the stream slow? Does the bladder appear strong or weak? Has the patient gone into retention?

The fourth layer is risk. Are there infections, bladder stones, blood in the urine, kidney effects, or cancer-risk questions?

The fifth layer is patient priority. Does he want to preserve ejaculation? Avoid anesthesia? Avoid hospital surgery? Get the strongest possible channel opening? Preserve future options? Minimize medications? When those layers are understood, treatment selection becomes much clearer. Without them, the decision becomes a sales pitch.

THE TREATMENT SHOULD HAVE A REASON

Every treatment should have a reason. If medication is chosen, the reason might be early symptoms, reasonable bladder emptying, and anatomy likely to respond to relaxation. If Rezūm is chosen, the reason might be smaller or moderate obstructing tissue suitable for water vapor treatment. If PAE is chosen, the reason might be a larger gland, prostate tissue growing into the bladder opening, or a desire to preserve anatomy. If HoLEP is chosen, the reason might be a large gland requiring strong tissue removal. If TURP is chosen, the reason might be a prostate size and anatomy well suited to traditional channel-opening surgery. If bladder medication is chosen, the reason should be that the bladder symptoms have been evaluated and emptying is safe.

The reason should be explainable in plain English. If the doctor cannot explain the match, the patient should not be rushed.

Mechanism matters. A treatment without a mechanism is guesswork.

WHAT THE PATIENT SHOULD ASK

A patient does not need to become a prostate expert, but he should ask enough to understand the match. He should ask how large the prostate is, whether it is growing into the bladder opening, how much urine is left behind, how fast the urine comes out, whether the bladder seems strong, and whether the treatment being recommended fits those findings.

He should ask what the treatment actually does. Does it relax muscle, shrink tissue, treat the blood supply, pull tissue aside, heat tissue, or remove tissue? He should ask what symptoms are expected to improve and what symptoms may persist. He should ask about catheter time, recovery, sexual side effects, and future options.

These are not extra questions. They are the core of informed consent. A man should not agree to a prostate procedure because it sounds modern. He should agree because he understands why it matches his anatomy.

DR. SHUSTERMAN'S MODERN PROSTATE TAKEAWAY

The best BPH treatment is not the newest treatment, the most advertised treatment, or the treatment one doctor happens to offer. The best treatment is the one whose mechanism matches the patient's anatomy.

Size matters, but shape matters too. A prostate growing into the bladder opening can behave more seriously than its size suggests. The amount of urine left behind after urination matters. The speed of the stream matters. Bladder strength matters. Sexual priorities matter. Future options matter.

Medication, Rezūm, PAE, UroLift, Aquablation, TURP, HoLEP, laser procedures, and other treatments all have roles. None of them is right for every man.

Modern prostate care should not be procedure-driven. It should be anatomy-driven, bladder-protective, and patient-specific. The real question is not, "What procedure is best?" The real question is, "What treatment makes the most sense for this prostate, this bladder, and this man?"

CHAPTER 16

PSA IS A RISK SIGNAL, NOT A DIAGNOSIS

FEW BLOOD TESTS create as much anxiety in men as PSA. A man goes for routine bloodwork. He feels fine. He is urinating reasonably well. He has no pain. He has no symptoms that feel like cancer. Then the office calls and tells him his PSA is elevated.

Suddenly everything changes. He starts searching online. He reads about prostate cancer, biopsy, surgery, radiation, impotence, incontinence, and death. He remembers a friend who had prostate cancer. He thinks about his father or uncle. He wonders if he has been ignoring something. He may even assume the result already means cancer.

That is the first mistake. PSA is not a cancer diagnosis. PSA is a signal.

It is an important signal, and it should not be ignored. But it is still a signal, not a verdict. An elevated PSA does not automatically mean a man has prostate cancer. A normal PSA does not guarantee that he does not. PSA must be interpreted in context, with the patient's age, prostate size, trend over time, urinary symptoms, inflammation, infection, recent retention, family history, risk factors, and imaging when needed.

This is where modern prostate care needs to be calm and precise. The answer is not panic. The answer is not dismissal. The answer is risk stratification.

WHAT PSA ACTUALLY IS

PSA stands for prostate-specific antigen. It is a protein made by prostate cells.

Most men think of PSA only as a cancer test, but PSA was not created by the body for doctors. It has a biological role. PSA is part of semen. It helps semen liquefy after ejaculation so sperm can move more freely.

That means PSA is a normal prostate product. Every man with a prostate makes some PSA. When doctors measure PSA in the blood, they are measuring a prostate-made protein that has leaked or passed into the bloodstream.

Because prostate cancer cells can produce PSA, the blood test became useful as a cancer-risk tool. But benign prostate cells also produce PSA. An enlarged prostate can raise PSA. Prostate inflammation can raise PSA. Infection can raise PSA. Urinary retention can raise PSA. Recent manipulation or procedures can raise PSA.

This is why PSA is not a simple yes-or-no cancer test. It is a marker of prostate activity. Cancer is one possible cause of that activity. It is not the only cause.

WHY PSA CREATES SO MUCH FEAR

PSA creates fear because it sits between two different dangers. On one side is the danger of missing a serious prostate cancer. Nobody wants to ignore a rising PSA and later discover that an aggressive cancer was present. Early detection can matter, especially for clinically significant cancers that are still treatable.

On the other side is the danger of overreacting. Not every elevated PSA is dangerous. Not every prostate cancer is aggressive.

Some low-risk cancers may never harm the patient. If every PSA elevation is treated like an emergency, men can be exposed to unnecessary anxiety, unnecessary biopsies, overdiagnosis, and overtreatment.

That is why PSA has become controversial in some settings. It is useful, but it must be used intelligently. Modern guidelines emphasize shared decision-making, repeated testing when appropriate, and using PSA as part of a broader risk assessment rather than as a reflex trigger for biopsy. The AUA/SUO guideline describes PSA-based screening as a framework for identifying clinically significant prostate cancer while minimizing harms such as false positives, overdiagnosis, and biopsy-related side effects.

This is the balance every man needs to understand. PSA can save lives when it helps detect important cancer early. PSA can also cause harm when it is interpreted without nuance.

The test is not the problem. The interpretation is the problem.

AN ELEVATED PSA DOES NOT AUTOMATICALLY MEAN CANCER

A high PSA can be caused by many things. The National Cancer Institute explains that a high PSA level can occur from benign prostate conditions, urinary tract infections, prostate disturbance, prostate biopsy, and prostate cancer, among other causes. That is why a single elevated PSA should usually lead to thoughtful evaluation, not immediate panic.

One of the most common benign reasons for PSA elevation is prostate enlargement. If a man has more prostate tissue, he may produce more PSA. That does not make the PSA meaningless. It simply means the number has to be interpreted with prostate size in mind.

Inflammation is another common cause. Prostatitis, urinary infection, and irritation can raise PSA. A man with burning, pelvic discomfort, fever, urinary symptoms, or a positive urine test may need the infection or inflammation addressed before deciding what the PSA truly means.

Urinary retention can also raise PSA. If the bladder has been under pressure or the prostate has been irritated by severe obstruction, the PSA may rise in a way that does not represent cancer. The point is not that elevated PSA is harmless.

The point is that elevated PSA requires explanation. A man should not hear, "Your PSA is high," and assume the diagnosis has already been made. The next step is to understand why it may be high and whether the pattern is concerning enough to justify further testing.

A NORMAL PSA DOES NOT MAKE A MAN BULLETPROOF

The opposite mistake is also common. A man hears that his PSA is normal and assumes he cannot have prostate cancer. That is not quite true.

A lower PSA is generally reassuring, but it is not a guarantee. Some cancers produce less PSA. Some men have risk factors that make a "normal" number less comforting. Some cancers may be found because of MRI, family history, genetic risk, or a concerning trend even before the PSA crosses a traditional cutoff.

This is why the PSA number has to be interpreted with the patient, not just the lab range. Age matters. Family history matters. Prior PSA values matter. Race and ancestry can matter. Genetic mutations can matter. MRI findings matter. The size of the prostate matters. The rate of change matters, although PSA velocity should not be used as the sole reason to move to imaging or biopsy.

Modern prostate care should not reduce cancer risk to one number printed next to a reference range. A man deserves better interpretation than that.

AGE MATTERS

PSA must be interpreted differently depending on age. A PSA that may be acceptable in a seventy-five-year-old man with a very large prostate may be more concerning in a fifty-year-old man with a small prostate. A PSA that appears only mildly elevated on a lab report may deserve attention in a younger man. A PSA that is stable over many years is different from one that is rising steadily.

In my own clinical thinking, I pay close attention when a man under sixty has a PSA around or above 2.5, especially if the number is rising, if the prostate is not large enough to explain it, or if risk factors are present. In men over sixty, a PSA under 4 is often more reassuring, but it is not the story. The trend and context still matter.

The specific number is not the only issue. The pattern is the issue. A man should not ask only, "Is my PSA normal?" He should ask, "Is my PSA appropriate for my age, prostate size, and risk?" That is a much better question.

THE TREND MAY MATTER MORE THAN THE SNAPSHOT

One PSA value is a snapshot. Several PSA values over time create a story.

A PSA that rises slowly over years in a man with a growing benign prostate may be less concerning than a PSA that suddenly jumps. A PSA that fluctuates during infection may settle after treatment. A PSA that continues rising despite no obvious benign explanation deserves more attention. But the trend has to be interpreted carefully.

AUA guidance cautions against using PSA velocity alone as the sole reason for secondary biomarkers, imaging, or biopsy. That does not mean trend is irrelevant. It means trend should be one part of the entire risk picture. A rising PSA should prompt questions.

Was the test repeated? Was there infection? Was there urinary retention? Was the patient recently catheterized or instrumented? Is the prostate enlarged? Is the patient taking medication that lowers PSA? Does he have family history? Does he need a more advanced blood test? Does he need MRI?

The trend tells us where to look. It does not automatically decide everything by itself.

REPEAT THE PSA WHEN IT MAKES SENSE

If a PSA is newly elevated, repeating it can be one of the most practical first steps. PSA can fluctuate. Lab variation, inflammation, infection, ejaculation, vigorous bike riding, urinary retention, recent procedures, and other factors can affect the result. A repeat test does not solve every case, but it can prevent overreacting to a transient elevation.

AUA guidance recommends that clinicians repeat a newly elevated PSA before moving to secondary biomarkers, imaging, or biopsy. This is common sense medicine.

If the PSA normalizes, the conversation changes. If it remains elevated or continues to rise, the concern becomes more real. If it is rising quickly or the clinical picture is concerning, further evaluation may be appropriate.

Repeating the PSA does not mean ignoring it. It means confirming the signal before escalating.

PROSTATE SIZE GIVES PSA CONTEXT

A man's PSA should be interpreted with prostate size in mind. The prostate makes PSA. A larger prostate may produce more PSA because there is more tissue. This is one reason I do not like evaluating PSA without knowing the prostate. A PSA value floating in space is incomplete.

If a man has a very large benign prostate and the PSA is moderately elevated, enlargement may explain part of the number. If a man has a small prostate and the PSA is elevated, the same number may be more concerning.

This does not mean a large prostate protects a man from cancer. A man can have BPH and prostate cancer at the same time. It simply means size helps interpret the signal. That is why prostate ultrasound, MRI volume, or other imaging information can be useful in the PSA discussion.

The patient-friendly idea is simple: if the gland is bigger, it may make more PSA. If the PSA is high for the amount of prostate tissue present, the concern rises.

INFECTION, INFLAMMATION, AND PSA

Prostate inflammation can create confusing PSA results. A man may have urinary burning, pelvic discomfort, urgency, frequency, fever, or abnormal urine testing. His PSA comes back elevated, and he becomes terrified. In that setting, inflammation or infection may be contributing.

If infection is suspected, it should be treated appropriately. If the clinical picture supports prostatitis, the doctor may treat and then repeat PSA after enough time has passed for inflammation to settle. If the PSA falls back toward baseline, that gives useful information. If it remains elevated, continues rising, or does not fit the overall picture, further evaluation is needed.

The key is not to use inflammation as a permanent excuse. I have seen both mistakes. Some men are rushed toward panic without considering infection or retention. Others are told again and again that the PSA is probably inflammation while cancer risk is never properly clarified.

Both approaches are wrong. Inflammation can explain PSA. It should not be allowed to hide cancer indefinitely.

PSA AND PROSTATE MEDICATIONS

Some prostate medications change PSA. Finasteride and dutasteride, medications that can slowly shrink selected enlarged prostates, usually lower PSA. This can be helpful for BPH in certain men, but it complicates PSA interpretation.

A man taking these medications must make sure every doctor reviewing his PSA knows he is on them. The measured number may look lower than it otherwise would. A rising PSA while on these medications can be especially important.

This is another reason medication should not be casual. If a drug affects both prostate size and a cancer-risk marker, the patient needs a monitoring plan. A man should know whether his medication changes PSA interpretation. If he does not know, he should ask.

ISOPSA AND ADVANCED BLOOD TESTING

Traditional PSA testing measures the amount of PSA in the blood. That is useful, but it is not perfect.

Advanced tests can sometimes help refine risk before deciding whether biopsy is needed. IsoPSA is one example. It evaluates structural information related to PSA rather than only the amount of PSA present. The patient does not need to understand the chemistry in detail. The point is that modern risk assessment can be more nuanced than simply looking at one PSA number.

In a man with an elevated PSA where the next step is unclear, advanced blood testing may help decide whether MRI, biopsy, or continued monitoring is appropriate. It can be especially useful when the PSA is abnormal but the story is not straightforward.

This is part of the future of prostate care. The old model was too blunt: PSA high, biopsy. The modern model is smarter: PSA high, confirm it, interpret the context, refine the risk, image when appropriate, biopsy when justified. The goal is to find meaningful cancer while avoiding unnecessary procedures.

MRI BEFORE BIOPSY

FIGURE 17.1

MRI Before Biopsy

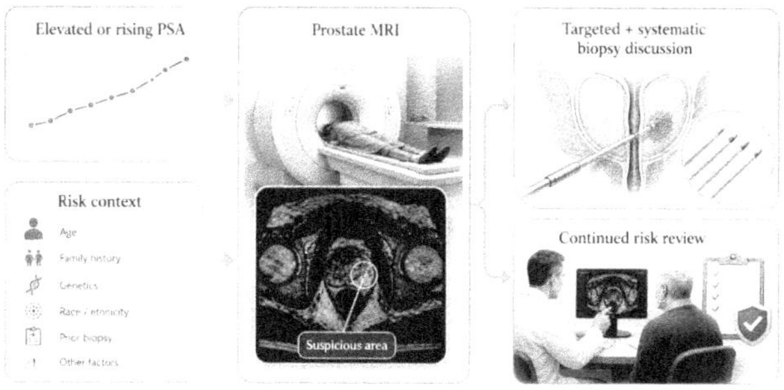

MRI can help locate suspicious areas and refine biopsy decisions in selected men.

Figure 16.1 - MRI Before Biopsy. MRI can refine biopsy decisions in selected men.

MRI has changed prostate cancer evaluation. In the past, many men with elevated PSA were sent directly to biopsy. Biopsy still has a crucial role because tissue diagnosis is how prostate cancer is confirmed. But MRI can help identify suspicious areas, guide biopsy decisions, and reduce blind sampling.

MRI is especially helpful when PSA remains elevated, when prior biopsy was negative but suspicion continues, or when the doctor needs to better understand the prostate before biopsy. A suspicious MRI does not automatically mean cancer, and a negative MRI does not guarantee there is no cancer. But MRI adds important information. It can help distinguish men who need biopsy more urgently from those who may be monitored or evaluated further. This is another example of risk stratification. Modern care should not jump from blood test to biopsy without asking whether additional information would make the decision smarter.

BIOPSY IS THE DIAGNOSIS

PSA does not diagnose prostate cancer. MRI does not diagnose prostate cancer. Advanced blood testing does not diagnose prostate cancer.

Biopsy diagnoses prostate cancer. That distinction matters. PSA and MRI tell us risk. They help decide whether biopsy is necessary and where to sample. But until tissue is examined under the microscope, cancer has not been definitively diagnosed. This is why men should not say, "My PSA says I have cancer." It does not.

A better statement is, "My PSA suggests I need further risk evaluation." That shift in language reduces fear and improves decision-making. A man who understands PSA as a risk signal is less likely to panic and more likely to follow the right pathway.

LOW-RISK CANCER AND THE PSA TRAP

One reason PSA became controversial is that it can lead to the diagnosis of low-risk prostate cancers that may never harm the patient. This is a real issue.

Some prostate cancers are biologically quiet. They may be monitored with active surveillance rather than treated immediately. If every cancer is treated as a life-threatening emergency, men may suffer side effects from treatment they did not need.

But the answer is not to abandon PSA. The answer is to use PSA intelligently.

The goal is to detect clinically significant prostate cancer, not to terrify men over every microscopic low-risk finding. MRI, better biopsy techniques, advanced blood tests, genomic tests, and better active surveillance protocols all help improve that balance. A man should understand that not all prostate cancers behave the same way.

The word cancer creates fear. The risk category creates the plan.

HIGH-RISK MEN NEED EARLIER ATTENTION

Some men should pay attention to PSA earlier. Men with a strong family history of prostate cancer, especially a father or brother affected at a younger age, may need earlier screening. Men with known genetic mutations, such as BRCA2, may be at higher risk. Men of African ancestry have higher risk of prostate cancer and aggressive disease. Men with multiple relatives affected by prostate, breast, ovarian, pancreatic, or related cancers may need a more careful genetic and screening discussion.

These men should not wait until the average age if their risk is above average. Risk should individualize screening.

A man should know his family history. He should know whether relatives had prostate cancer, how old they were at diagnosis, whether the cancer was aggressive, whether anyone had metastatic disease, and whether there are cancers in the family that suggest inherited risk. PSA is not the same test in every man because every man does not start with the same risk.

DO NOT LET FEAR AVOID THE TEST

Some men avoid PSA because they are afraid of what it might show. That is understandable, but it is not wise.

Avoiding a test does not remove the risk. It only removes the opportunity to understand it early. A man who refuses PSA because he fears biopsy or treatment may later face a more advanced cancer that could have been detected earlier.

The answer to PSA anxiety is not avoidance. The answer is better counseling.

A man should know that an elevated PSA does not automatically mean cancer. He should know that a biopsy is not always the immediate next step. He should know that MRI and advanced testing may help refine risk. He should know that low-risk cancer may be monitored. He should know that treatment decisions are more nuanced than they used to be.

When men understand the pathway, PSA becomes less terrifying. Knowledge reduces fear.

DO NOT LET REASSURANCE BECOME NEGLECT

The opposite problem is false reassurance. A man has a PSA that is "only a little high." He is told not to worry. Then it rises again. He is told it is probably age or enlargement. Then it rises again. Years pass. No one measures the prostate. No one orders MRI. No one uses advanced testing. No one discusses biopsy.

Reassurance can be appropriate when it is based on evidence. It is dangerous when it replaces evaluation.

A man with a persistent or rising PSA deserves an explanation. If the explanation is a large benign prostate, inflammation, or recent retention, that should be supported by the clinical picture. If the PSA does not make sense, the risk needs to be clarified. "Probably fine" is not the same as a plan.

WHAT A MAN SHOULD ASK ABOUT PSA

A man does not need to become an expert in prostate cancer screening, but he should ask better questions. He should ask whether his PSA is appropriate for his age. He should ask how it compares with prior values. He should ask whether his prostate size explains part of the number. He should ask whether infection, inflammation, retention, ejaculation, biking, or recent procedures could have affected it. He should ask whether the PSA should be repeated. He should ask whether advanced blood testing or MRI would help. He should ask whether biopsy is truly indicated and why.

These questions do not challenge the doctor. They clarify the plan.

The patient's goal is not to interpret PSA alone. His goal is to make sure the PSA is being interpreted thoughtfully.

DR. SHUSTERMAN'S MODERN PROSTATE TAKEAWAY

PSA is one of the most important tools in men's health, but it is also one of the most misunderstood. PSA is not a cancer diagnosis. It is a prostate-made protein and a cancer-risk signal. It can rise from prostate enlargement, inflammation, infection, retention, procedures, and cancer. It must be interpreted in context.

A man should not panic over one number. He should also not ignore a concerning pattern. Modern PSA care means confirming abnormal results when appropriate, understanding age and risk, considering prostate size, recognizing inflammation and retention, using advanced blood tests or MRI when helpful, and performing biopsy when the risk justifies it.

The goal is not to biopsy every man. The goal is not to miss meaningful cancer.

PSA should not create fear without a plan. It should create a smarter conversation. The right question is not, "Is my PSA high?" The right question is, "What does my PSA mean for me?"

CHAPTER 17

MRI BEFORE BIOPSY

FOR MANY YEARS, the prostate biopsy pathway was too blunt. A man had an elevated PSA. The number worried everyone. The next step was often a biopsy. The doctor sampled the prostate in a systematic pattern, hoping to find whatever might be there. Sometimes cancer was found. Sometimes no cancer was found. Sometimes the biopsy missed a cancer that was present. Sometimes it found a very low-risk cancer that may never have hurt the man but created years of anxiety. That was the old model.

It was understandable for its time, but it was incomplete. Today, prostate MRI has changed the conversation. It allows us to look at the prostate before putting a needle into it. It gives us a map. It can show suspicious areas. It can help decide whether biopsy is necessary, where the biopsy should focus, and how concerned we should be.

MRI does not replace biopsy when biopsy is needed. That is important. A biopsy is still the way prostate cancer is diagnosed. Tissue has to be examined under the microscope.

But MRI can make the biopsy decision smarter. The old model was: PSA is high, biopsy.

The modern model is: PSA is high, understand the risk, look at the prostate, then decide whether biopsy makes sense and where it should be aimed. That is a major improvement.

PSA TELLS US RISK. MRI SHOWS US ANATOMY.

PSA is a blood signal. It tells us that something may be happening in the prostate. It does not show us where. It does not show us whether there is a suspicious area. It does not tell us whether the prostate is large, inflamed, or has a region that looks concerning for cancer.

MRI adds anatomy to the discussion. When a man has an elevated PSA, the first question is not automatically, "How fast can we biopsy?" The better question is, "What is the most intelligent way to understand this risk?"

Sometimes the PSA should be repeated first. Sometimes infection, inflammation, or urinary retention may explain the elevation. Sometimes the prostate is very large, and the PSA may be partly explained by benign enlargement. Sometimes an advanced blood test can help clarify the risk. Sometimes MRI is the next smart step.

A prostate MRI can show whether there are areas that look suspicious. It can show the size of the gland. It can help identify whether a suspicious area is in a location that should be targeted during biopsy. It can also help in men who had a prior negative biopsy but whose PSA remains concerning.

This is why MRI has become one of the most important tools in modern prostate cancer evaluation. It does not diagnose cancer by itself. It helps decide how worried we should be and where to look.

THE PROBLEM WITH BLIND SAMPLING

A traditional prostate biopsy samples tissue in a systematic pattern. The doctor takes cores from different areas of the prostate to look for cancer.

That approach can work, and it has diagnosed many cancers. But the prostate is not a flat surface. It is a three-dimensional gland. Cancer may be small, hidden, anterior, high up, low down, or located in an area that is not easily sampled by a standard pattern.

Without imaging, the biopsy is partly systematic and partly blind. That does not mean it is careless. It means the doctor is sampling based on an anatomic template rather than seeing a specific suspicious target. MRI helps reduce that problem.

If MRI shows a suspicious area, the biopsy can be directed toward that area. Even when a systematic biopsy is also performed, the MRI gives the doctor better information. It changes the biopsy from purely random sampling into a more informed search.

Patients understand this immediately when I use a simple analogy. If a smoke alarm goes off in a house, you can open every door randomly and hope you find the problem. Or you can use a thermal camera and see where the heat is coming from.

PSA is the alarm. MRI helps show where to look.

MRI IS ESPECIALLY USEFUL AFTER A PRIOR NEGATIVE BIOPSY

One of the most frustrating situations in prostate care is the man with a persistently elevated PSA and a prior negative biopsy. He has already gone through the anxiety and discomfort of biopsy. The pathology report did not show cancer. That is reassuring, but the PSA remains elevated or continues to rise. Now everyone is unsure what to do.

Was the biopsy truly negative because there is no cancer? Or did the biopsy miss something?

This is where MRI can be extremely valuable. It can look for suspicious areas that may have been missed by the original sampling. It can show lesions in parts of the prostate that are harder to reach or less likely to be sampled thoroughly in a standard biopsy. It can help decide whether repeat biopsy is necessary and where that repeat biopsy should focus.

A negative biopsy is not always the end of the story. If the PSA pattern still does not make sense, if the risk remains concerning, or if the patient has significant risk factors, MRI can help clarify what was missed or whether continued monitoring is reasonable.

The goal is not to keep biopsying blindly. The goal is to biopsy intelligently when risk remains.

WHAT THE MRI REPORT MEANS

Patients often become confused when they read their MRI report. They see terms like lesion, peripheral zone, transition zone, restricted diffusion, enhancement, capsule, seminal vesicle, and PI-RADS. The language can be intimidating. The most important part for most patients is the suspicion score.

Prostate MRI findings are commonly reported using a system called PI-RADS. The acronym is less important than the concept. It is a score from 1 to 5 that estimates how suspicious an area looks for clinically significant prostate cancer.

A score of 1 or 2 is generally less suspicious. A score of 4 or 5 is more suspicious. A score of 3 is the gray zone.

Patients do not need to memorize the scoring system in detail. They need to understand what the score means for the next decision.

If the MRI shows a clearly suspicious area, especially a 4 or 5, biopsy is often strongly considered if the patient is healthy enough and the result would change management. If the MRI is negative or low suspicion, the next step depends on the PSA pattern, prostate size, family history, overall risk, and clinical judgment. A score of 3 requires the most nuance.

THE GRAY ZONE: MRI SCORE 3

A PI-RADS 3 lesion is neither clearly reassuring nor clearly alarming. That is why I do not treat every score 3 the same way. A score 3 in a man with a mildly elevated but stable PSA, a large prostate that explains the PSA, low-risk history, and reassuring advanced testing may be watched carefully.

A score 3 in a younger man with a rising PSA, small prostate, strong family history, abnormal advanced blood test, or other risk factors may deserve biopsy. The MRI score is not the only decision-maker. The patient is the decision-maker. By that I mean the whole patient: age, health, PSA trend, prostate size, risk factors, family history, prior biopsy history, and personal tolerance for uncertainty.

This is one of the places where medicine cannot be reduced to a simple rule. A score 3 lesion needs judgment. Sometimes the right answer is monitoring. Sometimes the right answer is biopsy. The question is not, "What is the score?" The question is, "What does this score mean in this man?"

MRI CAN HELP AVOID SOME UNNECESSARY BIOPSIES

One of the major benefits of MRI is that it can help reduce unnecessary biopsies in selected patients. If a man has a mildly elevated PSA and MRI is reassuring, especially when the prostate is large and other risk factors are low, the doctor may choose close monitoring rather than immediate biopsy. That may spare the patient discomfort, infection risk, anxiety, and the possibility of diagnosing a very low-risk cancer that may never have mattered.

This is not the same as ignoring the PSA. It is a risk-based decision.

The patient must still be followed. PSA should be monitored. Symptoms and prostate size should be understood. Advanced blood testing may be used when appropriate. If the PSA rises, the MRI changes, or the risk picture worsens, biopsy may still become necessary.

MRI helps us avoid some biopsies. It does not give permission to stop thinking.

MRI CAN HELP FIND CLINICALLY IMPORTANT CANCER

The other benefit of MRI is that it can help find cancers that matter. The goal of prostate cancer detection is not to find every microscopic focus of low-risk disease. The goal is to find clinically significant cancer — the kind that may grow, spread, or require treatment during the man's lifetime.

MRI is useful because suspicious lesions can be targeted. If there is a region that looks concerning, the biopsy can focus on it rather than relying only on systematic sampling. This improves the chance of finding important cancer when it is present.

That is the balance modern prostate care is trying to achieve. Do not biopsy every man reflexively. Do not miss aggressive cancer. MRI helps move us toward that balance.

MRI IS NOT PERFECT

MRI is powerful, but it is not perfect. A negative MRI does not guarantee that there is no cancer. Some cancers are too small to see. Some are not obvious on imaging. Some are in areas that are difficult to interpret. Image quality can vary. Radiologist experience matters. The strength of the MRI magnet, the protocol used, patient movement, inflammation, bleeding from prior biopsy, and prostate size can all affect interpretation.

A suspicious MRI also does not guarantee cancer. Inflammation, scarring, benign nodules, and other changes can sometimes look concerning. That is why biopsy is still needed when the suspicion is high enough. Patients should not treat MRI as a magic answer.

MRI is a tool. A good tool, but still a tool. The best results come when MRI is combined with PSA interpretation, prostate size, advanced blood testing when appropriate, clinical judgment, and high-quality biopsy technique.

THE QUALITY OF THE MRI MATTERS

Not all prostate MRIs are equal. A prostate MRI should be done with a proper prostate protocol and interpreted by radiologists experienced in prostate imaging. The details matter. Poor imaging can create false reassurance or false alarm. A vague MRI report may not help much. A high-quality MRI can provide information that changes the entire plan.

This is why patients should not think of MRI as simply checking a box. Where the MRI is done matters. Who reads it matters. Whether it is a true prostate MRI matters. Whether the images are good enough to guide a biopsy matters.

If the MRI is going to influence whether a man has a biopsy, the quality of the MRI should be taken seriously. A bad map can be worse than no map if everyone trusts it too much.

MRI AND PROSTATE SIZE

MRI can also measure prostate size. That is important because PSA should be interpreted in context. A larger prostate may produce more PSA. A smaller prostate with an elevated PSA may be more concerning. MRI can help show the prostate volume and provide additional anatomic information.

This does not mean a large prostate cannot have cancer. It can. A man can have benign enlargement and prostate cancer at the same time. But size helps interpret the PSA signal.

If a man has a very large prostate, a mildly elevated PSA may be partly explained by volume. If a man has a small prostate and a PSA that seems too high for the amount of tissue present, the concern may rise.

MRI adds this context. Again, the point is not that one number decides everything. The point is that modern prostate evaluation should connect the pieces. PSA, prostate size, MRI findings, symptoms, family history, and risk factors all belong in the same conversation.

MRI BEFORE FIRST BIOPSY

There has been a major shift toward using MRI before biopsy in many men with elevated PSA or concerning risk. This makes sense. If we are going to put a needle into the prostate, we should first ask whether imaging can show us where the most suspicious area is.

This does not mean every man must have MRI before every biopsy in every setting. There may be urgent or unusual situations where biopsy is needed without delay. Access, cost, quality, and clinical context all matter. But as a modern principle, MRI before biopsy is often the smarter pathway.

It respects the patient. It respects the prostate's anatomy. It reduces blind decision-making. It may help avoid unnecessary biopsy in some men and improve targeting in others. A man should feel comfortable asking his doctor, "Should I have a prostate MRI before biopsy?" That is a reasonable question.

MRI AFTER A NEGATIVE BIOPSY

MRI is also important after a negative biopsy when concern remains. If the PSA continues to rise, if the patient has risk factors, or if the doctor remains concerned, a prior negative biopsy should not automatically end the evaluation. The first biopsy may have sampled benign tissue while missing a suspicious area.

MRI can help identify whether there is a lesion that needs targeted sampling. This is especially important because repeating the same type of biopsy over and over without new information is frustrating and may still miss the key area. MRI gives the doctor a new map.

A man with a persistently concerning PSA after a negative biopsy should not accept vague reassurance forever. He should ask whether MRI could help clarify the risk.

MRI AND ACTIVE SURVEILLANCE

MRI is also useful after prostate cancer has already been diagnosed, especially in men on active surveillance. Active surveillance means monitoring a low-risk cancer carefully rather than treating it immediately. The goal is to avoid unnecessary treatment while still catching signs of progression early.

MRI can help monitor the prostate over time. It can show whether a suspicious area is stable or changing. It can help guide repeat biopsy decisions. It can provide another layer of information beyond PSA alone.

But MRI should not create false comfort. Surveillance still requires structure. PSA, examination when appropriate, repeat imaging, biopsy timing, pathology, and the patient's overall risk all matter.

Active surveillance is not doing nothing. It is disciplined monitoring. MRI can be part of that discipline.

MRI AND TREATMENT PLANNING

MRI can help not only with diagnosis but also with treatment planning. If cancer is found, MRI can provide information about where the lesion is, whether it appears confined, whether there is concern near the capsule, whether seminal vesicles are involved, and whether focal therapy may be considered in selected cases. It can help radiation oncologists, urologists, and focal therapy specialists understand the anatomy.

MRI is not the only staging tool. In higher-risk disease, PSMA

PET scans and other imaging may be needed. But MRI remains central to understanding the prostate itself.

This matters because prostate cancer treatment should not be based only on the word cancer. It should be based on grade, risk category, location, volume, patient age, health, sexual function, urinary function, and goals. MRI helps define the battlefield before treatment begins.

WHEN MRI IS NOT ENOUGH

There are situations where MRI cannot answer the question completely. If PSA is strongly concerning despite a negative MRI, biopsy may still be needed. If advanced blood tests are concerning, the doctor may still recommend biopsy. If the patient has high-risk family history or a very concerning PSA pattern, imaging alone may not be enough reassurance.

This is important because patients sometimes want MRI to replace biopsy completely. It cannot always do that.

MRI can reduce unnecessary biopsy. MRI can improve targeting. MRI can help guide risk. But if the risk remains significant, tissue diagnosis may still be necessary.

The patient-friendly line is simple: MRI is the map. Biopsy is the proof.

FEAR OF BIOPSY SHOULD NOT MISUSE MRI

Some men want MRI because they are afraid of biopsy. That is understandable. Biopsy can create anxiety. Men worry about pain, infection, bleeding, sexual side effects, and what the results may show.

MRI can help decide whether biopsy is truly needed, but it should not be used as an excuse to avoid biopsy when the risk is high. A suspicious MRI should not be ignored because the patient prefers not to know. A rising PSA with concerning features should not be dismissed because the first MRI was not alarming.

Fear is real, but fear should not drive the plan. The goal is not to biopsy unnecessarily. The goal is not to avoid biopsy at all costs. The goal is to diagnose meaningful cancer when it matters and avoid unnecessary procedures when risk is low. MRI helps us make that decision more intelligently.

THE PATIENT'S MRI QUESTIONS

A man considering MRI should understand why it is being ordered. He should ask what question the MRI is supposed to answer. Is it being used because PSA is elevated? Because PSA is rising? Because a prior biopsy was negative? Because a biopsy is being planned? Because low-risk cancer is being monitored? Because treatment planning is needed?

He should ask whether the MRI is a dedicated prostate MRI and whether it will be read by someone experienced in prostate imaging. He should ask what the score means if a lesion is found. He should ask whether a negative MRI would change the plan. He should ask whether a suspicious MRI would lead to biopsy.

These questions make MRI part of a strategy rather than just another test. A test is only useful if everyone knows what decision it is meant to guide.

DR. SHUSTERMAN'S MODERN PROSTATE TAKEAWAY

MRI has changed prostate cancer evaluation because it gives us a map before biopsy. PSA is a risk signal. MRI helps show whether there is a suspicious area in the prostate. Biopsy proves whether cancer is present. MRI is especially useful when PSA is elevated, when risk is unclear, when a prior biopsy was negative but suspicion remains, or when active surveillance and treatment planning require better anatomic information.

But MRI is not magic. A negative MRI does not guarantee there is no cancer. A suspicious MRI does not prove cancer. The quality of the MRI and the experience of the radiologist matter. The result must be interpreted with PSA, prostate size, family history, risk factors, advanced blood testing when appropriate, and clinical judgment.

The modern pathway is not PSA panic followed by blind biopsy. The modern pathway is smarter: understand the signal, image the prostate, target what matters, and biopsy when the risk justifies it.

MRI is the map. Biopsy is the proof.

CHAPTER 18

PROSTATE BIOPSY: WHEN IT IS NEEDED AND HOW IT SHOULD BE DONE

FIGURE 18.1

Biopsy Route Comparison

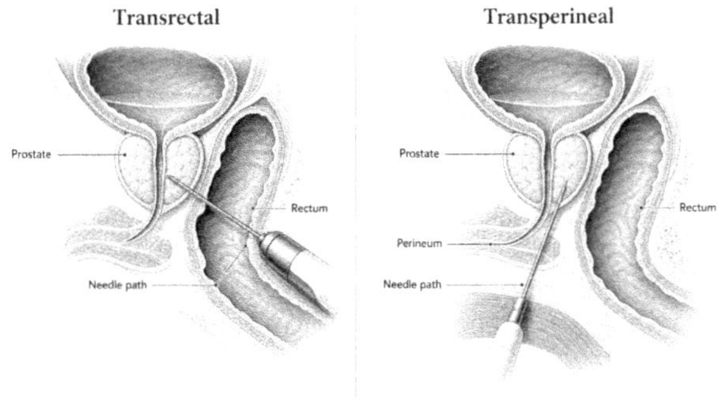

Transrectal and transperineal biopsy routes sample prostate tissue differently and carry different practical considerations.

FIGURE 18.1 - BIOPSY ROUTE COMPARISON. *Transrectal and transperineal routes have different practical considerations.*

Aprostate biopsy is one of the most feared words in men's health. The fear is understandable. A man hears "biopsy" and immediately imagines cancer, pain, infection, bleeding, embarrassment, and bad news. He may not fully understand what the biopsy involves, but he knows enough to be nervous.

That anxiety often begins before the procedure is even recommended. It starts with a PSA result. The number is elevated. The patient is told he may need further evaluation. He searches online. He reads about prostate cancer. He reads about biopsy complications. He reads conflicting opinions about biopsy routes, MRI targeting, infection risk, antibiotics, and whether biopsy is even necessary.

By the time he sees the urologist, he may already be overwhelmed. The first thing he needs to understand is this: a biopsy is not done because the doctor knows cancer is present. A biopsy is done because the risk is high enough that tissue needs to be checked.

PSA is a signal. MRI is a map. Advanced blood tests can refine risk. But biopsy is the proof.

That does not mean every elevated PSA needs a biopsy. It does not mean every MRI finding requires immediate tissue sampling. It does not mean biopsy should be casual. It means that when the risk of clinically meaningful prostate cancer is high enough, the only way to know what is present is to sample tissue and have a pathologist examine it.

A biopsy should answer a real question. It should not be performed reflexively, and it should not be avoided when the risk justifies it.

WHAT A PROSTATE BIOPSY ACTUALLY DOES

A prostate biopsy samples small cores of tissue from the prostate. Those tissue samples are sent to a pathology lab, where they are examined under a microscope. The pathologist looks for cancer cells and, if cancer is found, determines how aggressive the cancer appears. This is a major point for patients.

The biopsy is not just about whether cancer is present. It is also about what kind of cancer is present.

Prostate cancer is not one disease. Some prostate cancers are low risk and may be watched carefully. Others are more aggressive and need treatment. The biopsy helps determine the Grade Group, Gleason pattern, number of involved samples, percentage of involvement, and sometimes other features that influence the plan.

A man should not think of biopsy as a simple yes-or-no test. It is the test that begins risk classification. If cancer is found, the next question is not automatically, "When do we remove the prostate?" The next question is, "What is the risk category, and what does this mean for this man?" That distinction matters because biopsy can diagnose cancers that require different approaches.

WHEN BIOPSY BECOMES NECESSARY

A prostate biopsy should be considered when the risk of clinically significant cancer becomes high enough. That risk may come from several places. A PSA may be elevated for the man's age. The PSA may be rising in a concerning pattern. A prostate MRI may show a suspicious area. An advanced blood test may suggest increased risk. A prior biopsy may have been negative, but the PSA may continue to rise. A man may have a strong family history or inherited risk that lowers the threshold for further evaluation.

Biopsy is not based on fear. It is based on risk.

A man with a mildly elevated PSA, a very large prostate, reassuring MRI, low-risk family history, and stable trend may not need immediate biopsy. Another man with the same PSA but a small prostate, rising trend, suspicious MRI, and strong family history may need biopsy.

The number alone does not decide. The whole picture decides.

This is why modern prostate care should not jump directly from PSA to biopsy without asking whether the risk has been properly clarified. Sometimes the PSA should be repeated. Sometimes infection or retention should be addressed. Sometimes MRI should be obtained. Sometimes an advanced blood test can help. But when those pieces point toward meaningful risk, biopsy should not be delayed indefinitely.

Avoiding biopsy does not make cancer disappear. It only delays knowing.

MRI CHANGES THE BIOPSY CONVERSATION

MRI has changed prostate biopsy because it gives the doctor a map before sampling. In the older model, biopsy was often performed in a systematic pattern without knowing whether a specific suspicious area was present. That approach still has a role, but MRI allows a smarter strategy. If MRI shows a concerning lesion, the biopsy can target that area.

This does not mean systematic sampling is useless. Some cancers may still be found outside the MRI-visible lesion. Depending on the patient and the approach, the doctor may take targeted samples from suspicious areas and systematic samples from the rest of the gland. The goal is to reduce the chance of missing meaningful cancer.

Patients should understand the difference. A systematic biopsy samples the prostate by pattern. A targeted biopsy samples a suspicious area seen on imaging.

In many modern cases, both ideas are combined. The purpose is not to take more tissue for no reason. The purpose is to answer the risk question accurately.

THE MRI SCORE AND BIOPSY DECISION

MRI reports often use a scoring system to describe how suspicious a prostate lesion appears. Patients may see scores from 1 to 5. A score of 1 or 2 is usually less concerning. A score of 4 or 5 is more concerning. A score of 3 is the gray zone.

When MRI shows a clearly suspicious lesion, especially a 4 or 5, biopsy usually becomes a serious discussion, assuming the man is healthy enough that the result would matter. In my practice, a man under eighty with a 4 or 5 lesion generally needs strong consideration for biopsy. In older men, the decision depends more heavily on overall health, life expectancy, and whether diagnosing the cancer would change treatment.

A score of 3 requires judgment. A score of 3 in a low-risk man may be watched. A score of 3 in a man with a rising PSA, strong family history, smaller prostate, abnormal advanced blood test, or other risk factors may deserve biopsy.

The score is not the whole decision. The man is the decision. The point is to avoid both extremes: biopsying every borderline finding and ignoring meaningful risk.

BIOPSY ROUTE: THROUGH THE RECTUM OR THROUGH THE SKIN

There are two main ways to biopsy the prostate. One route is transrectal, meaning the needle passes through the rectal wall into the prostate under ultrasound guidance. This has been the traditional approach for many years.

The other route is transperineal, meaning the needle passes through the skin between the scrotum and anus into the prostate. This approach has become more popular because it may reduce infection risk by avoiding passage through the rectal wall.

There is a major debate in modern urology about which route should be preferred. Many European guidelines increasingly favor the transperineal route because of infection concerns. AUA/SUO guidance recognizes that laboratory biomarkers, MRI, and biopsy techniques can improve detection and safety when biopsy is necessary, while studies continue to compare transrectal and transperineal approaches. Current evidence generally suggests both approaches can detect cancer effectively when performed well, with infection risk being one of the major differentiators.

Patients do not need to become experts in the debate. They need to understand the practical question.

Which route is safest and most accurate in the hands of the doctor performing it? That matters more than ideology.

MY VIEW ON TRANSRECTAL BIOPSY

In my own practice, I continue to favor transrectal ultrasound-guided biopsy when it is done carefully, efficiently, and with a strong infection-prevention protocol. That statement may surprise some readers because transperineal biopsy has gained significant momentum. I understand why. Infection risk after transrectal biopsy is real because the needle passes through the rectal wall. Antibiotic resistance is also a real concern. For many practices, moving toward transperineal biopsy makes sense.

But medicine is not only about route. It is about execution.

A well-performed transrectal biopsy in experienced hands, with appropriate patient selection, careful technique, and strong antibiotic prophylaxis, can be fast, accurate, and well tolerated. In my practice, I have had excellent safety outcomes with my protocol. That experience matters to how I counsel patients, while still recognizing that other physicians may reasonably prefer transperineal biopsy.

The wrong conclusion would be to say one route is always correct for every patient and every doctor. The right conclusion is that biopsy should be performed by someone who can explain their route, technique, infection-prevention strategy, targeting strategy, and safety outcomes. A patient should ask how the doctor does biopsies and why.

INFECTION RISK MUST BE RESPECTED

Infection is one of the complications men fear most after biopsy. The concern is legitimate. Any biopsy route can have complications, but transrectal biopsy specifically introduces the possibility of bacteria from the rectum entering the prostate or bloodstream. This is why antibiotic prophylaxis and patient selection matter.

Some centers perform rectal swabs to check for resistant bacteria. Some use targeted antibiotics. Some use enhanced prophylaxis. Some have shifted toward transperineal biopsy to reduce infection risk. The exact protocol varies by practice. What should not vary is seriousness.

A prostate biopsy should never be casual about infection prevention. A patient should know what antibiotics or preventive measures are being used, what symptoms should prompt a call after the procedure, and what to do if fever develops. Fever after biopsy is not something to watch casually at home. It needs prompt medical attention.

Biopsy is usually safe when done properly, but safe does not mean risk-free. The patient deserves a plan.

PAIN AND COMFORT

Men often fear biopsy pain more than they admit. A prostate biopsy should not be torture. With proper local anesthesia, technique, and patient preparation, most men tolerate it well. Some feel pressure. Some feel brief sharp sensations. Some feel anxiety more than pain. The experience varies, but the procedure should be manageable.

Comfort matters because a bad biopsy experience can affect future care. A man who has a traumatic procedure may avoid follow-up, delay repeat biopsy when needed, or resist prostate care altogether. The doctor should explain what the patient will feel, how numbing is done, how long the procedure takes, and what to expect afterward.

Some men may need additional anxiety control or sedation depending on their situation. Others do fine with local anesthesia. The approach should be individualized. The goal is not only to obtain tissue. The goal is to obtain tissue accurately and humanely.

WHAT HAPPENS AFTER BIOPSY

After a prostate biopsy, some bleeding is common. A man may see blood in the urine, stool, or semen. Blood in the semen can last longer than men expect and may look alarming. In many cases, it is not dangerous, but patients should be warned in advance so they do not panic.

Some men have soreness or urinary irritation. A small amount of discomfort can be normal. Severe pain, inability to urinate, heavy bleeding, chills, or fever are not normal and should be addressed promptly.

Patients should receive clear instructions. What activity should be avoided? When can they resume exercise or sex? What symptoms are expected? What symptoms are urgent? When will results be available? Who will call them? What happens if cancer is found? What happens if the biopsy is negative?

The days after a biopsy are psychologically difficult. Men wait for pathology results, often imagining the worst. Communication matters during that period. A patient should not feel abandoned after the tissue is taken.

IF THE BIOPSY IS NEGATIVE

A negative biopsy is reassuring, but it is not always the end of the story. If the PSA falls, the MRI is reassuring, and the overall risk is low, continued monitoring may be appropriate. But if the PSA remains concerning, continues to rise, or does not match the clinical picture, the evaluation should continue.

A biopsy can miss cancer. That is why MRI, targeted sampling, advanced blood tests, and follow-up trends matter. A prior negative biopsy should reduce concern, but it should not create permanent false reassurance if the risk pattern remains abnormal. The patient should ask: what is the plan now?

Will PSA be repeated? Should MRI be repeated? Was the suspicious area adequately sampled? Do advanced blood tests make sense? When would another biopsy be considered? A negative biopsy without a follow-up plan is incomplete.

IF THE BIOPSY SHOWS LOW-RISK CANCER

If biopsy shows low-risk prostate cancer, the patient's first reaction is usually fear. That is normal. The word cancer is powerful.

But low-risk prostate cancer is often different from the cancers men imagine. Many low-risk prostate cancers can be managed with active surveillance rather than immediate treatment. Active surveillance means careful monitoring with PSA, imaging, repeat biopsy when appropriate, and clinical follow-up. It is not ignoring cancer. It is watching a low-risk cancer closely so treatment can be avoided unless there are signs of progression.

This is why biopsy results must be explained carefully. The patient should know the Grade Group, the Gleason pattern, how many samples were positive, how much cancer was in each sample, whether MRI findings match the biopsy, and whether genomic testing might help. The question after diagnosis is not simply, "Do I have cancer?" The question is, "What kind of cancer is it?" That question determines the plan.

IF THE BIOPSY SHOWS HIGHER-RISK CANCER

If the biopsy shows higher-risk cancer, the conversation changes. Higher grade cancer, more extensive involvement, or concerning features may require staging and treatment planning. MRI, PSMA PET scans, genomic testing, radiation consultation, focal therapy evaluation, hormone therapy discussion, or surgical opinions may all become relevant depending on the risk category.

The biopsy is the doorway into this next level of decision-making. This is also where patients need time and guidance. A man who hears "higher-risk cancer" may feel pressured to act immediately. Timely care is important, but panic should not drive treatment. The patient needs risk classification, staging, functional discussion, and a clear understanding of options. The goal is cancer control while preserving the man's life and function as much as possible.

BIOPSY IN OLDER MEN

Biopsy decisions become more nuanced in older men. A healthy seventy-eight-year-old with a concerning MRI and rising PSA may benefit from diagnosis. A frail eighty-seven-year-old with multiple serious medical conditions and a borderline PSA may not benefit from biopsy because the result may not change management.

Age alone should not decide, but life expectancy and health status matter. In my practice, I generally biopsy clearly suspicious MRI lesions in men under eighty when the clinical picture supports it. Over eighty, I become more selective. I want to know whether the man is healthy enough to benefit from diagnosis and treatment, whether he has at least a meaningful life expectancy, whether the cancer risk is high enough, and whether the result would actually change what we do.

The point is not to deny care based on age. The point is to avoid procedures that do not help the patient. A biopsy should be performed when the result matters.

BIOPSY TECHNIQUE AND EXPERIENCE MATTER

A prostate biopsy is not only a decision. It is a technical procedure.

Experience matters. Ultrasound quality matters. MRI interpretation matters. Targeting matters. Knowledge of prostate anatomy matters. Infection prevention matters. Comfort matters. Sampling strategy matters.

Patients often assume a biopsy is a biopsy. It is not. A rushed biopsy performed without understanding the MRI, prostate size, lesion location, prior history, and patient risk is different from a thoughtful biopsy performed with a clear plan.

The patient should ask whether the suspicious area will be targeted, whether systematic samples will also be taken, how many cores are expected, what route will be used, what infection prevention is planned, and how complications are handled. These are not unreasonable questions. They are the foundation of informed consent.

COGNITIVE TARGETING, FUSION, AND SKILL

When MRI shows a suspicious area, there are different ways to target it. Some practices use MRI-ultrasound fusion systems, where MRI images are digitally fused with real-time ultrasound to guide biopsy. Others use cognitive targeting, where the physician reviews the MRI and uses ultrasound anatomy and experience to sample the corresponding area.

Fusion technology can be useful, especially in many settings. It can help standardize targeting and improve confidence that the MRI-visible lesion is sampled. But technology is not a substitute for skill.

A physician who understands prostate anatomy, MRI location, ultrasound appearance, and biopsy technique can perform high-quality targeted sampling. A fusion system in inexperienced hands is not automatically superior to careful targeting by an experienced operator.

The patient does not need to choose technology blindly. He should ask how the lesion will be targeted and how the doctor ensures the suspicious area is sampled. Again, the principle is the same throughout this book.

Mechanism matters. Execution matters.

THE PATIENT SHOULD NOT BE PASSIVE

A man facing biopsy should be calm, but not passive. He should understand why biopsy is being recommended. He should know what risk signal triggered it. Was it PSA? MRI? Family history? Prior negative biopsy with persistent concern? Advanced blood test? He should know whether the MRI showed a suspicious area and what that means. He should know what route the doctor plans to use. He should know how infection risk is reduced. He should know what to expect after the procedure. He should know when results will come back and how they will be explained.

A patient who asks these questions is not difficult. He is informed.

That matters because biopsy is a turning point. If negative, the patient needs a follow-up plan. If positive, the patient enters the world of prostate cancer risk classification and treatment decisions. Either way, the biopsy should not feel like an isolated event. It should be part of a strategy.

THE GOAL OF BIOPSY

The goal of biopsy is not to find every microscopic abnormality at all costs. The goal is to detect clinically meaningful prostate cancer when the risk is high enough, classify it accurately, and guide the next decision. That is why biopsy should be neither automatic nor avoided out of fear.

If the risk is low, a biopsy may create more harm than benefit. If the risk is high, avoiding biopsy may delay diagnosis of a cancer that should be treated. Modern prostate care is about finding the balance.

PSA gives the signal. MRI gives the map. Biopsy gives the proof. A man needs all three concepts in the right order.

DR. SHUSTERMAN'S MODERN PROSTATE TAKEAWAY

A prostate biopsy is not a punishment for an elevated PSA. It is not something to do casually, and it is not something to avoid when the risk is real.

Biopsy is how prostate cancer is diagnosed and classified. PSA, MRI, and advanced blood tests help decide whether biopsy is needed, but tissue is still the proof.

A modern biopsy decision should be based on risk, not panic. It should consider PSA pattern, age, prostate size, MRI findings, family history, advanced testing when appropriate, prior biopsy history, and whether the result will change care.

The biopsy route should be chosen based on safety, accuracy, physician experience, infection-prevention protocol, patient comfort, and the clinical situation. Transperineal biopsy has gained momentum because of infection-risk advantages in many settings. Transrectal biopsy can still be safe and effective when performed carefully with a strong protocol and experienced hands.

The patient should understand why biopsy is needed, how it will be done, how infection risk is reduced, what side effects to expect, and what the results will mean. PSA is the signal. MRI is the map. Biopsy is the proof.

CHAPTER 19

PROSTATE CANCER GRADES, STAGES, AND RISK GROUPS

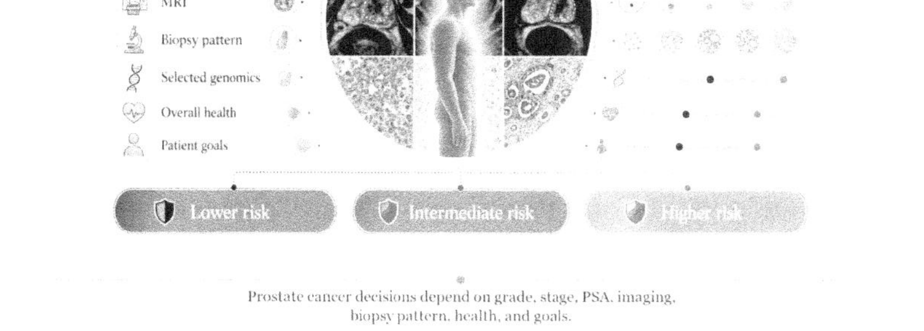

FIGURE 19.1 - RISK GROUP, *Not Just Cancer. Risk groups help determine whether monitoring or treatment is appropriate.*

The word cancer is never small. A man can be calm, successful, logical, and medically sophisticated, but when he hears "prostate cancer," the room changes. He may stop hearing the rest of the sentence. He may immediately picture surgery, radiation, incontinence, impotence, chemotherapy, pain, and death. He may think of someone he knew who had aggressive cancer. He may assume that cancer means immediate treatment. That fear is understandable.

But it is also where many bad decisions begin. Prostate cancer is not one disease. Some prostate cancers are slow-growing and may never threaten the man's life. Others are aggressive and need serious treatment. Some can be monitored carefully. Others need radiation, focal therapy, hormone therapy, surgery, or a combination of treatments. Some are confined to the prostate. Others have already spread outside it.

The word cancer tells us something important has been found. It does not tell us the whole plan. The plan comes from risk.

That is why this chapter matters. A man diagnosed with prostate cancer must understand the language of grade, stage, PSA, biopsy volume, imaging, and risk group. He does not need to become an oncologist, but he does need to understand enough to avoid both panic and neglect. The question is not simply, "Do I have prostate cancer?" The better question is, "What kind of prostate cancer do I have, and what is the real risk?"

THE FIRST SHOCK

When a biopsy comes back positive, many men hear only the word cancer. They may not hear the Grade Group. They may not understand the Gleason score. They may not know how many biopsy samples were positive. They may not know whether the cancer was found in one small area or throughout the gland. They may not understand whether MRI showed a small lesion or a more concerning pattern. They may not know whether the PSA is mildly elevated or highly suspicious. They may not know whether the cancer is likely confined to the prostate.

All of those details matter. A man with one tiny focus of low-grade cancer is not in the same situation as a man with high-grade cancer in multiple biopsy cores. A man with a PSA of 5 is not in the same situation as a man with a PSA of 50. A man with cancer confined to the prostate is not in the same situation as a man with cancer in lymph nodes or bones.

The diagnosis is only the beginning. Risk classification is what turns fear into a plan.

GLEASON SCORE: WHAT THE PATHOLOGIST SEES

After a biopsy, the tissue is examined under a microscope. The pathologist looks at how abnormal the prostate cells appear and how they are arranged. This is where the Gleason score comes from.

Patients often find the Gleason system confusing because the numbers do not behave the way they expect. A man may hear "Gleason 6" and think it sounds high because 6 out of 10 sounds like more than half. In prostate cancer, however, Gleason 6 is generally considered the lowest grade cancer commonly reported on biopsy.

The older Gleason system adds two patterns together. The first number is the most common pattern seen in the cancer, and the second number is the next most common pattern. That is why a man may hear 3+3, 3+4, 4+3, 4+4, or 4+5.

The order matters. A 3+4 cancer is not the same as a 4+3 cancer. In 3+4, the less aggressive pattern is dominant, with some pattern 4 present. In 4+3, the more aggressive pattern is dominant. That difference can change the risk group and the treatment discussion.

This is one of the most important concepts for patients to understand. Not all Gleason 7 cancers are the same. A 3+4 and a 4+3 may both add up to 7, but they do not behave the same way.

GRADE GROUPS: A CLEARER LANGUAGE

Because the Gleason system confused so many patients, modern pathology also uses Grade Groups. Grade Group 1 usually corresponds to Gleason 6. Grade Group 2 usually corresponds to Gleason 3+4. Grade Group 3 usually corresponds to Gleason 4+3. Grade Group 4 usually corresponds to Gleason 8. Grade Group 5 usually corresponds to Gleason 9 or 10.

The National Cancer Institute describes this Grade Group framework in its patient prostate cancer treatment information, and it is now widely used to help communicate risk more clearly. For patients, Grade Group is often easier to understand than the old Gleason language. Grade Group 1 is the lowest-risk category. Grade Group 5 is the highest-grade category. The higher the Grade Group, the more aggressive the cancer appears under the microscope. But even Grade Group is not the story.

A man with Grade Group 2 in one small biopsy sample may not be the same as a man with Grade Group 2 in many samples. A man with Grade Group 3, where pattern 4 dominates, is different from a man with low-volume Grade Group 2. A man with Grade Group 4 or 5 generally needs a much more serious staging and treatment discussion.

The grade tells us how the cancer looks. The volume and stage tell us how much disease we are dealing with and where it may be.

WHY GLEASON 6 IS DIFFERENT

Gleason 6, or Grade Group 1, is the prostate cancer diagnosis that creates the most confusion. The word cancer scares the patient. But many Grade Group 1 prostate cancers behave in a very low-risk way. They may grow slowly. They may never spread. They may never require treatment during the man's lifetime, especially if he is older or has other health issues.

That is why active surveillance has become the preferred approach for many men with low-risk prostate cancer. Active surveillance means careful monitoring rather than immediate treatment. The cancer is not ignored. It is followed with PSA testing,

MRI when appropriate, repeat biopsy when needed, and clinical judgment.

This is not doing nothing. It is structured observation. The goal is to avoid unnecessary treatment and preserve urinary and sexual function while still watching closely for signs that the cancer is changing.

Current AUA/ASTRO localized prostate cancer guidance recommends active surveillance as the preferred management option for low-risk disease, and AUA materials describe favorable intermediate-risk patients as candidates for active surveillance in selected situations when features such as low tumor volume and low percentage of Gleason pattern 4 are present. This is a major shift from the old era when many men with low-risk prostate cancer were treated immediately.

For many men with Grade Group 1 disease, the best treatment may be no immediate treatment. But the word immediate matters. Active surveillance requires discipline.

ACTIVE SURVEILLANCE IS NOT IGNORING CANCER

Some patients hear "active surveillance" and think the doctor is minimizing cancer. That is not the idea.

Active surveillance is not denial. It is not laziness. It is not avoiding care. It is a strategy for low-risk or carefully selected favorable-risk prostate cancer.

The reason active surveillance exists is that treatment has costs. Surgery and radiation can affect erections, ejaculation, urinary control, bowel function, energy, and quality of life. If a cancer is unlikely to harm the man, immediate treatment may create more harm than benefit. But surveillance must be active.

The patient must return for follow-up. PSA must be monitored. MRI may be repeated. Biopsy may be repeated depending on the situation. If the cancer shows signs of progression, treatment may become appropriate. A man on active surveillance should not disappear for five years and assume everything is fine.

That is not surveillance. That is neglect. The modern approach is to separate low-risk cancer from aggressive cancer and treat each appropriately.

FAVORABLE INTERMEDIATE RISK

Intermediate-risk prostate cancer is a broad category. This is where patients can become especially confused because the word intermediate sounds like one group, but it includes different cancers.

A favorable intermediate-risk cancer may include a small amount of Gleason 3+4, meaning Grade Group 2, with other reassuring features. These men may still have options. Some may choose treatment. Some, especially with low-volume disease, low PSA density, limited pattern 4, and reassuring imaging, may be considered for active surveillance after careful counseling.

This is not the same as saying all intermediate-risk cancers should be watched. It means some favorable cases deserve a nuanced discussion.

This is also where genomic testing can help. Tests that evaluate gene-expression patterns in the cancer may provide additional information about whether the cancer behaves more quietly or more aggressively. Oncotype DX Genomic Prostate Score and similar tools can sometimes help when the decision between surveillance and treatment is not obvious.

The patient-friendly idea is simple: sometimes the microscope tells part of the story, but the biology may need further clarification. A man with favorable intermediate-risk prostate cancer should not be rushed blindly, but he also should not be falsely reassured. He needs a careful risk discussion.

UNFAVORABLE INTERMEDIATE RISK

Unfavorable intermediate-risk cancer is different. This may include Gleason 4+3 disease, more extensive cancer, higher PSA, or other features suggesting that the cancer is more likely to behave aggressively. In my mind, the distinction between 3+4 and 4+3 is critical. Both add up to 7, but they are not the same disease.

A 4+3 cancer has pattern 4 as the dominant pattern. That means the more aggressive architecture is the majority. I treat that very differently from a small amount of 3+4.

In many cases, 4+3 behaves much closer to higher-risk disease than patients expect. It is not the type of finding I casually place into the same mental category as low-volume 3+4. This is why men need to see the actual biopsy details, not just the final score.

How much pattern 4 is present? How many samples are positive? How much cancer is in each sample? Is there cribriform pattern? Is there intraductal carcinoma? Are there MRI findings suggesting a larger lesion? Is the PSA rising quickly? These details can move a man from a surveillance conversation into a treatment conversation. The biology matters.

HIGH-RISK PROSTATE CANCER

High-risk prostate cancer is a different category. This may involve a higher PSA, a higher Grade Group, more aggressive Gleason patterns, concerning clinical stage, or imaging findings suggesting more advanced disease. These cancers require serious staging and treatment planning. The first question is whether the cancer is truly localized.

A man with high-risk prostate cancer should not assume the disease is confined to the prostate just because it was found on biopsy. Modern imaging, including PSMA PET scanning in appropriate patients, can help evaluate whether cancer has spread to lymph nodes, bones, or other sites.

This matters because treatment changes if cancer has spread. A high-risk localized cancer may be treated with radiation and hormone therapy, surgery in selected cases, or multimodal therapy. A cancer that has spread may require systemic treatment and a different strategy. The higher the risk, the more important staging becomes. The future of cancer treatment starts with knowing where the cancer actually is.

STAGE: WHERE THE CANCER IS

Grade tells us how aggressive the cancer cells look. Stage tells us where the cancer is.

Is it confined to the prostate? Does it appear to extend outside the prostate capsule? Are the seminal vesicles involved? Are lymph nodes involved? Are bones involved? Is there distant spread? This is the difference between local disease and systemic disease.

Patients often mix up grade and stage. They may think a higher Gleason score automatically means cancer has spread. That is not necessarily true. A cancer can be high grade but still localized. A cancer can also be lower grade but more extensive than expected, although this is less common. Both grade and stage matter.

A man with cancer confined to the prostate may have different options than a man with cancer in the bones. That is why imaging is so important when risk is high enough.

MRI helps evaluate the prostate and nearby anatomy. PSMA PET can help look for spread in higher-risk cases. CT and bone scans may still be used in certain situations, but PSMA PET has become one of the most important modern tools for staging prostate cancer when appropriate. The treatment plan should not be made in the dark.

PSA STILL MATTERS AFTER DIAGNOSIS

After cancer is diagnosed, PSA remains important. The PSA level helps place the patient into a risk group. A very low PSA with low-grade cancer is different from a high PSA with high-grade disease. PSA trend also matters. A rapidly rising PSA can be more concerning than a stable number. But PSA still does not act alone.

A man can have a high PSA because of a large prostate and also have low-volume cancer. Another man can have a modest PSA and a more aggressive cancer. PSA must be interpreted with biopsy grade, cancer volume, MRI findings, prostate size, and overall risk.

This is why patients should not obsess over PSA alone once cancer is found. The question becomes how PSA fits into the entire risk profile.

CANCER VOLUME: HOW MUCH WAS FOUND

The amount of cancer in the biopsy matters. A man with one tiny focus of Grade Group 1 disease is not the same as a man with cancer in many biopsy samples. A man with a small amount of Grade Group 2 is different from a man with extensive Grade Group 2 or 3 disease.

Patients should ask how many biopsy samples were positive and how much cancer was present in each. They should also ask whether the MRI lesion matches the biopsy findings. If MRI showed a large suspicious lesion but the biopsy found only a tiny amount of low-grade cancer, the doctor should make sure the suspicious area was adequately sampled. If the biopsy found more aggressive cancer than expected, staging may become more important.

Cancer volume helps separate a small finding from a more extensive disease process. The word cancer is not enough. How much cancer matters.

CRIBRIFORM AND INTRADUCTAL FEATURES

Some pathology features make prostate cancer more concerning. Two of the important terms patients may hear are cribriform pattern and intraductal carcinoma. These are microscopic patterns seen by the pathologist. Patients do not need to understand every detail, but they should know that these findings can be associated with more aggressive behavior.

If cribriform or intraductal features are present, the patient should ask how they affect the risk category and treatment recommendation. This is especially important in men who otherwise might be considered for active surveillance. Certain adverse pathology features can make surveillance less appropriate.

Again, modern prostate cancer care is not just about the headline Gleason score. The details matter.

GENOMIC TESTING

Genomic testing can help in selected prostate cancer cases. These tests examine gene activity in the tumor tissue to provide additional information about the cancer's behavior. They are not needed for every man, but they can be useful when the decision is uncertain, especially in low-risk or favorable intermediate-risk disease.

A patient may ask, "Do I need treatment now, or can I safely watch this?" Sometimes the biopsy, PSA, MRI, and clinical factors are enough to answer. Sometimes they are not. Genomic testing may help refine the risk. This is part of the move toward personalized prostate cancer care.

Two cancers that look similar under the microscope may not behave exactly the same way biologically. Genomic testing tries to provide another layer of information. The test should not replace clinical judgment, but it can support it.

RISK GROUPS CREATE THE PLAN

The point of all this information is to place the patient into a risk category. Low-risk cancer is often best managed with active surveillance. Favorable intermediate-risk cancer may require a careful discussion between surveillance and treatment depending on volume, pattern, imaging, genomic testing, and patient preference. Unfavorable intermediate-risk cancer usually pushes more strongly toward treatment. High-risk cancer requires staging and a serious treatment plan. Metastatic cancer requires systemic thinking.

This is why men should not make decisions based only on emotion. When the diagnosis is new, the instinct may be to get the cancer out immediately. That instinct is understandable. But immediate treatment is not always the best choice, especially for low-risk disease. In other cases, the instinct may be denial. The man does not want treatment, so he minimizes the cancer. That can be dangerous when the risk group is unfavorable or high.

Risk groups exist to protect men from both overreaction and underreaction. They turn fear into structure.

THE PATIENT'S FIRST QUESTIONS AFTER DIAGNOSIS

After a prostate cancer diagnosis, a man should not leave the office with only the phrase, "You have cancer." He should understand the grade, the volume, the stage information available, and the next step. He should ask: What is my Grade Group? Is this Gleason 3+3, 3+4, 4+3, 8, 9, or 10? How many biopsy samples were positive? How much cancer was in each sample? Was the MRI lesion sampled? Is there pattern 4, and how much? Are there cribriform or intraductal features? What is my PSA, and does it fit the cancer found? Do I need genomic testing? Do I need PSMA PET or other staging? Am I low risk, favorable intermediate risk, unfavorable intermediate risk, high risk, or metastatic? Is active surveillance reasonable, or should treatment be recommended? These questions are not academic.

They determine whether the man watches, treats, images further, tests further, or seeks additional opinions. A prostate cancer diagnosis should begin with explanation, not panic.

DO NOT TREAT THE WORD ALONE

One of the biggest mistakes in prostate cancer care is treating the word cancer rather than the risk. A low-risk cancer may not need immediate treatment. Treating it aggressively may expose the patient to urinary, sexual, and bowel side effects without improving survival. On the other hand, a high-risk cancer should not be casually watched because the patient is afraid of side effects. Both mistakes come from failing to define risk.

A man should not choose surgery, radiation, focal therapy, or surveillance because the word cancer scares him. He should understand what type of cancer he has and what the realistic risk is.

The goal is not to be passive. The goal is to be accurate.

DR. SHUSTERMAN'S MODERN PROSTATE TAKEAWAY

Prostate cancer is not one disease. The word cancer creates fear, but the risk group creates the plan.

A man with Grade Group 1 disease may be a candidate for active surveillance. A man with favorable intermediate-risk disease may need a nuanced discussion. A man with 4+3 disease, high-volume pattern 4, cribriform or intraductal features, high PSA, concerning MRI, or high-risk staging features needs a more serious treatment conversation.

The biopsy diagnosis is only the beginning. The important details are the Grade Group, Gleason pattern, amount of cancer,

PSA, MRI findings, genomic risk when appropriate, and whether imaging shows disease outside the prostate.

Do not treat the word cancer automatically. Treat the biology. A man should not ask only, "Do I have prostate cancer?" He should ask, "What kind of prostate cancer do I have, what is the risk, and what plan matches that risk?"

CHAPTER 20

MODERN PROSTATE CANCER TREATMENT OPTIONS

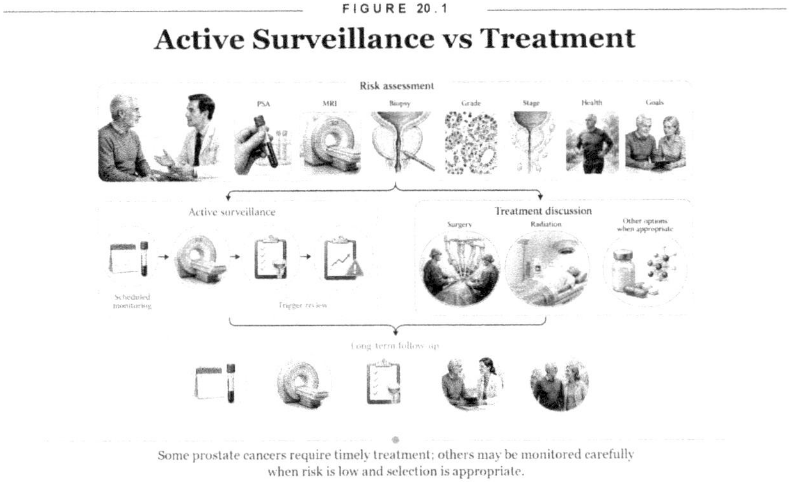

FIGURE 20.1 - *Active Surveillance vs Treatment. Some cancers need treatment; others can be monitored carefully.*

The hardest part of prostate cancer care is not always finding the cancer. Sometimes the hardest part is deciding what to do after it is found.

A man hears that his biopsy shows prostate cancer, and his first instinct is often immediate action. Get it out. Kill it. Treat it. Do something now. That reaction is human. The word cancer creates urgency. It creates fear. It makes men feel that any delay is dangerous.

But prostate cancer is not one disease, and treatment should not be one reaction. Some prostate cancers need treatment. Some need careful monitoring. Some need staging before a decision is made. Some need radiation. Some may be candidates for focal therapy. Some may require hormone therapy with radiation. Some may require systemic treatment if the disease has spread. Some men may be better served by observation rather than aggressive intervention because of age, health, or very low-risk disease.

The most important idea is this: do not treat the word cancer. Treat the risk. That is where modern prostate cancer care begins.

A man should not choose surgery because he panicked. He should not choose radiation because someone told him it was easier. He should not choose focal therapy because it sounds modern. He should not choose surveillance because he wants to avoid the problem. Every option has a role, and every option has tradeoffs.

The right treatment depends on the biology of the cancer, the stage, the man's age and health, urinary function, sexual priorities, life expectancy, imaging, and what the patient values most. The goal is not just to control cancer. The goal is to control cancer while preserving the man.

THE FIRST QUESTION IS RISK

Before discussing treatment, the first question should always be risk. Is this low-risk disease that may be watched carefully? Is it favorable intermediate-risk disease where surveillance or treatment may both be reasonable depending on details? Is it unfavorable intermediate-risk disease that should usually be treated? Is it high-risk disease that needs staging and a serious treatment plan? Has the cancer spread beyond the prostate? Those questions come before choosing a treatment.

A man with one tiny focus of low-grade cancer should not be in the same conversation as a man with high-grade cancer in many biopsy samples. A man with cancer confined to the prostate should not be treated the same way as a man with cancer in lymph nodes or bones. A man who is eighty-eight and medically fragile should not automatically be treated like a healthy fifty-eight-year-old.

Risk creates the plan. Without risk classification, treatment becomes emotional. And prostate cancer treatment should not be driven by emotion alone.

ACTIVE SURVEILLANCE

Active surveillance is one of the most important concepts in modern prostate cancer care. It means carefully monitoring selected prostate cancers instead of treating them immediately. This is most often used for low-risk prostate cancer, and in some selected men with favorable intermediate-risk disease.

Patients sometimes hear surveillance and think, "So we are doing nothing?" That is wrong. Active surveillance is not doing nothing. It is disciplined monitoring. The man is followed with PSA testing, repeat imaging when appropriate, repeat biopsy when needed, and careful reassessment over time. If the cancer remains quiet, the patient avoids or delays treatment and preserves urinary and sexual function. If the cancer shows signs of becoming more aggressive, treatment can be started.

This strategy exists because some prostate cancers are unlikely to harm the patient during his lifetime. Treating every low-risk cancer immediately can expose men to side effects without improving their lives. That is the part many patients struggle to accept.

They hear the word cancer and assume treatment must begin immediately. But the biology matters more than the word. If the cancer is low-grade, low-volume, and carefully monitored, surveillance may be the most intelligent choice. The goal is not to ignore cancer. The goal is to avoid harming the man by overtreating a cancer that may never hurt him.

WATCHFUL WAITING IS DIFFERENT

Active surveillance should not be confused with watchful waiting. Active surveillance is a structured plan for men who may still be candidates for curative treatment if the cancer changes. The goal is to monitor closely and intervene if needed.

Watchful waiting is usually less intensive and is often used in men who are older, frailer, or unlikely to benefit from curative treatment. In that setting, the goal may be to avoid treatment unless symptoms develop. Those are different strategies. A healthy sixty-year-old with low-risk cancer on active surveillance is not the same as an eighty-nine-year-old with multiple serious medical conditions being watched conservatively.

Patients should ask which strategy is being recommended and why. The words matter because the goals are different.

RADIATION THERAPY

Modern radiation therapy is one of the most important treatment options for localized prostate cancer. Radiation treats cancer by damaging the DNA of cancer cells so they cannot continue dividing. The treatment can be delivered from outside the body using external beam radiation, or from inside the prostate using radioactive seed placement or other forms of brachytherapy. Some men receive radiation alone. Others, especially with higher-risk disease, may receive hormone therapy along with radiation to improve cancer control.

Radiation has changed dramatically over time. Modern planning, imaging, dose delivery, and targeting are far more sophisticated than older radiation approaches. The goal is to deliver an effective dose to the prostate and cancer while limiting exposure to the bladder, rectum, and surrounding tissues as much as possible.

For many men, radiation can provide excellent cancer control without removing the prostate. That matters.

I often prefer modern radiation over radical prostate removal for many patients because it can treat the cancer while avoiding the immediate functional trauma of removing the organ. This is especially important for men who are concerned about urinary leakage, erectile function, and quality of life.

That does not mean radiation is free of side effects. No treatment is.

Radiation can cause urinary burning, frequency, urgency, bowel irritation, rectal symptoms, fatigue, erectile changes over time, and, rarely, more serious complications. Some side effects appear during treatment, while others may develop months or years later. The patient must understand these risks.

But radiation deserves to be discussed seriously and fairly. It is not a second-class treatment. It is a major modern prostate cancer treatment option.

HORMONE THERAPY WITH RADIATION

Some prostate cancers grow in response to male hormone signaling. Hormone therapy, often called androgen deprivation therapy, lowers or blocks testosterone signaling to help control the cancer.

Patients often find this emotionally difficult because testosterone is tied to identity, energy, libido, muscle, mood, and sexual function. Hormone therapy can cause hot flashes, fatigue, decreased libido, erectile problems, muscle loss, weight gain, metabolic changes, mood changes, bone thinning, and other effects.

That is why hormone therapy should not be presented casually. In prostate cancer, hormone therapy is often used together with radiation for certain intermediate-risk and high-risk cancers. It can make radiation more effective and reduce the risk of recurrence in selected patients. In more advanced disease, hormone therapy may be part of systemic treatment.

The key is matching the intensity of treatment to the risk of the cancer. A low-risk cancer does not need the same treatment as high-risk disease. A man should understand why hormone therapy is being recommended, how long it is expected to continue, what side effects are likely, and how those side effects will be managed.

Hormone therapy can be powerful. It also has a cost.

RADICAL PROSTATECTOMY

Radical prostatectomy means removing the entire prostate, usually along with the seminal vesicles, for prostate cancer. Today, if surgery is performed, it is commonly done robotically.

Patients often assume that removing the prostate is the most definitive option because the cancer is physically taken out. That is an understandable way to think. Surgery provides the entire prostate for pathology. It gives a final specimen. It allows PSA to be followed after removal, often with the expectation that PSA should become undetectable.

For some men, radical prostatectomy is a reasonable option. But I do not believe it should be treated as the automatic default for most men.

Removing the prostate is a major functional event. The prostate sits at the intersection of urination, ejaculation, erections, and pelvic anatomy. Surgery can affect urinary control. It can affect erections. It eliminates normal ejaculation. It can change orgasm. Recovery can take time. Even with excellent surgeons and robotic technique, the man is not simply having a cancer removed from an isolated part of the body. He is having an organ removed from the center of the male urinary and sexual system.

That does not mean surgery is wrong. It means surgery should be chosen carefully.

A man should understand why surgery is being recommended

over radiation, focal therapy, or surveillance. He should understand the likelihood of urinary leakage, erectile dysfunction, ejaculation loss, penile length changes, need for rehabilitation, and the possibility of additional treatment if pathology shows more aggressive disease.

Robotic surgery is a technique. It is not a guarantee of perfect functional outcome.

WHY I AM CAUTIOUS ABOUT RADICAL PROSTATECTOMY

I am cautious about radical prostatectomy because I have seen the functional consequences. I have seen men whose cancer may have been controlled but whose urinary and sexual function changed dramatically. I have seen men struggle with leakage. I have seen men lose erections. I have seen men deal with dry orgasm or no ejaculation. I have seen men who felt that the treatment changed their identity.

For high-risk cancer in a properly selected patient, surgery may be part of a reasonable plan. For certain younger men who strongly prefer surgery and understand the tradeoffs, it may be appropriate. For some patients, surgery provides staging and pathologic information that helps guide next steps.

But for many localized prostate cancers, especially when modern radiation or other options are available, I do not automatically recommend removing the prostate. This is an opinion shaped by patient experience, functional priorities, and the fact that prostate cancer care should not be reduced to "cut it out."

The cancer must be treated. But the man must be preserved whenever possible.

FOCAL THERAPY

Focal therapy is one of the most interesting areas in prostate cancer treatment. The idea is simple: instead of treating the entire prostate, treat the cancerous area while leaving the rest of the prostate alone.

This approach is attractive because many prostate cancers are found in a specific region of the gland. With modern MRI and targeted biopsy, we can often identify the dominant lesion more clearly than in the past. Focal therapy attempts to destroy the cancer focus while reducing damage to surrounding structures involved in erections, urinary control, ejaculation, and bowel function.

Different technologies can be used for focal therapy, including high-intensity focused ultrasound, cryotherapy, laser ablation, irreversible electroporation, and other approaches depending on the center. The promise is appealing: cancer control with fewer side effects.

But focal therapy must be chosen carefully. It is not right for every man. Prostate cancer can be multifocal, meaning more than one area of cancer may exist in the gland. A focal treatment may miss disease elsewhere if mapping is incomplete. Long-term comparative data are still evolving. Follow-up after focal therapy is essential, including PSA, MRI, and repeat biopsy when appropriate.

Focal therapy is not a shortcut. It is a precision strategy.

For the right patient, it can make a lot of sense. For the wrong patient, it can undertreat disease.

WHO MAY BE A CANDIDATE FOR FOCAL THERAPY

A good focal therapy candidate usually has cancer that appears localized, visible, and targetable. The cancer should be in a region that can be treated safely. The rest of the prostate should be reasonably evaluated so that important disease elsewhere is not being ignored. The patient should understand that follow-up is not optional.

Focal therapy is often most attractive in selected men with intermediate-risk disease that is localized and well mapped, or in certain men who want to avoid or delay whole-gland treatment and accept the need for close monitoring. It may also be considered in some recurrence settings after prior treatment, depending on the situation.

But a man with aggressive, widespread, high-volume, or poorly mapped disease is usually not an ideal focal therapy candidate. The patient-friendly explanation is this: focal therapy works best when the target is clear, the rest of the prostate has been adequately checked, and the cancer risk is appropriate. The treatment is only as good as the map.

THE NEED FOR HONEST FOLLOW-UP

Every prostate cancer treatment requires follow-up, but focal therapy especially demands it. Because the entire prostate remains in place, PSA does not usually drop to zero. The untreated prostate tissue can still make PSA. That means PSA interpretation after focal therapy is more nuanced than after radical prostatectomy.

MRI may be used to monitor the treated area and the rest of the gland. Repeat biopsy may be needed to confirm the treated cancer is controlled and to check for cancer elsewhere. The patient must understand that focal therapy is not "treat it and forget it."

The benefit is preserving more of the prostate and surrounding function. The tradeoff is that monitoring remains important.

That is not a weakness if the patient understands it. It is part of the strategy.

TREATMENT SHOULD MATCH THE MAN'S PRIORITIES

A prostate cancer treatment plan should not be made only from the doctor's perspective. The patient's priorities matter.

Some men value maximum cancer control even if side effects are more likely. Others are terrified of urinary leakage. Some care most about erections. Some care deeply about ejaculation. Some want to avoid hormone therapy if possible. Some want the least invasive reasonable option. Some want the option with the longest track record. Some want to avoid surgery. Some want the cancer physically removed because psychologically they cannot live with it inside them.

These priorities are not irrational. They are part of decision-making.

The doctor's job is to make sure the patient understands the risk and tradeoffs clearly. The patient's job is to be honest about what matters most to him. A treatment that is perfect on paper but unacceptable to the man's values is not the right treatment.

LOW-RISK DISEASE: OFTEN SURVEILLANCE

For many men with low-risk prostate cancer, the best initial treatment is active surveillance. This is one of the most important messages in modern prostate cancer care. A low-risk cancer should not automatically lead to surgery or radiation. If the cancer is small, low-grade, and well characterized, immediate treatment may do more harm than good.

This is not the same as ignoring cancer. The patient must be monitored. If the cancer changes, treatment can be offered. But many men can avoid treatment for years, and some may never need it. This is where patients must resist panic.

The word cancer is not enough reason to rush. The biology decides.

FAVORABLE INTERMEDIATE-RISK DISEASE: THE GRAY ZONE

Favorable intermediate-risk prostate cancer requires nuance. Some men in this category may still be considered for surveillance, especially if the cancer volume is low, the more aggressive pattern is limited, MRI is reassuring, genomic testing is favorable, and the patient understands the risk. Other men may be better served by treatment. This is where shared decision-making becomes important.

A man may reasonably choose radiation. Another may consider focal therapy. Another may choose surveillance with strict monitoring. The decision depends on details, not slogans. If the doctor presents only one option, the patient should ask why. Favorable intermediate-risk disease is often where modern prostate cancer care becomes individualized.

UNFAVORABLE INTERMEDIATE-RISK AND HIGH-RISK DISEASE

Unfavorable intermediate-risk and high-risk prostate cancer usually require more active treatment. These cancers are more likely to progress and may have a higher risk of spread. The treatment plan may include radiation with hormone therapy, surgery in selected cases, focal therapy only in very selected circumstances, or combination approaches. Higher-risk disease also deserves careful staging, often with advanced imaging such as PSMA PET when appropriate. This is not the setting for casual surveillance.

A man with higher-risk disease should not delay because he is afraid. He should get staged properly, understand the options, and move toward a treatment plan.

The goal is not panic. The goal is timely, intelligent action.

PSMA PET AND STAGING

For higher-risk prostate cancer, one of the most important modern tools is PSMA PET imaging. PSMA PET is a scan that can help detect prostate cancer outside the prostate, including lymph nodes or bones, more sensitively than older imaging in many cases. It is not needed for every low-risk patient. But when the cancer is higher-risk, knowing whether disease has spread is crucial.

If the cancer is truly localized, local treatment may be curative. If it has spread, the plan changes. This is why staging matters before committing to treatment.

A man should not undergo a major local treatment for higher-risk disease without asking whether appropriate staging has been done. The future of cancer treatment starts with knowing where the cancer actually is.

WHEN CANCER HAS SPREAD

If prostate cancer has spread beyond the prostate, treatment becomes systemic as well as local. Hormone therapy is often central. Additional medications may be added depending on the extent of disease, whether the cancer is sensitive or resistant to hormone therapy, the patient's health, genetic testing, symptoms, and prior treatment. Radiation may still be used in selected cases for prostate control, bone pain, or specific metastatic sites. Chemotherapy, targeted therapy, immunotherapy, radiopharmaceuticals, and clinical trials may become relevant depending on the disease.

This is a different conversation from low-risk localized cancer. The point for patients is that staging changes the map.

A man should understand whether his cancer is localized, locally advanced, node-positive, or metastatic. Those words are not just labels. They determine treatment strategy.

SIDE EFFECTS ARE NOT SECONDARY

In prostate cancer care, side effects are not a minor afterthought. They are central to the decision.

Surgery, radiation, focal therapy, hormone therapy, and systemic treatments all have different side-effect profiles. Some effects are urinary. Some are sexual. Some involve bowel function. Some involve energy, muscle, metabolism, mood, hot flashes, bone density, or cardiovascular risk.

A man may live many years after prostate cancer treatment. That means the quality of those years matters.

Doctors sometimes focus on cancer control, and of course cancer control is essential. But patients live with the consequences of treatment every day. Urinary leakage matters.

Erectile function matters. Ejaculation matters. Bowel symptoms matter.

Fatigue matters. Body composition matters. A treatment plan that ignores function is incomplete.

THE SECOND OPINION

Prostate cancer is one of the diagnoses where a second opinion can be helpful. The reason is not that the first doctor is wrong. It is that treatment choice often depends on perspective. A surgeon may emphasize surgery. A radiation oncologist may emphasize radiation. A focal therapy specialist may emphasize focal treatment. A medical oncologist may emphasize systemic therapy for advanced disease. Each specialist sees the cancer through the lens of their tools.

The patient benefits from hearing more than one perspective when the decision is significant. A man should not feel guilty for seeking a second opinion. A good doctor should welcome it, especially when the choice is complex. The patient should gather his PSA history, MRI report, biopsy pathology, imaging, genomic test results, and treatment recommendations so that the second opinion is informed.

The goal is not to collect endless opinions until one says what the patient wants to hear. The goal is to understand the options clearly.

DO NOT RUSH FROM FEAR

Some prostate cancers require timely treatment. But many decisions do not need to be made in panic.

A man newly diagnosed with localized prostate cancer should

usually take enough time to understand the grade, stage, risk group, imaging, and options. He should not disappear for months. But he also should not schedule a life-changing treatment before he understands the tradeoffs.

Fear pushes men toward immediate action. Modern care pushes men toward informed action. Those are not the same. The right decision should still make sense after the fear settles.

DR. SHUSTERMAN'S MODERN PROSTATE TAKEAWAY

Modern prostate cancer treatment is not one-size-fits-all. Low-risk prostate cancer is often best managed with active surveillance. Favorable intermediate-risk disease requires a nuanced discussion. Unfavorable intermediate-risk and high-risk disease usually require treatment and appropriate staging. Metastatic disease requires systemic thinking.

Radiation is a major modern treatment option and, in many men, may preserve function better than removing the prostate. Radical prostatectomy has a role, but it should not be the automatic default. Focal therapy is an exciting option for selected men when the cancer is visible, localized, and properly mapped. Hormone therapy can be important, especially with higher-risk disease, but it has real side effects and should be explained honestly.

The treatment should match the cancer risk and the man's priorities. Do not treat the word cancer. Treat the biology, the stage, the patient's function, and the life he wants after treatment.

CHAPTER 21

PROSTATITIS: THE CONFUSING PROSTATE DIAGNOSIS

FIGURE 21.1

Prostatitis Is Not One Thing

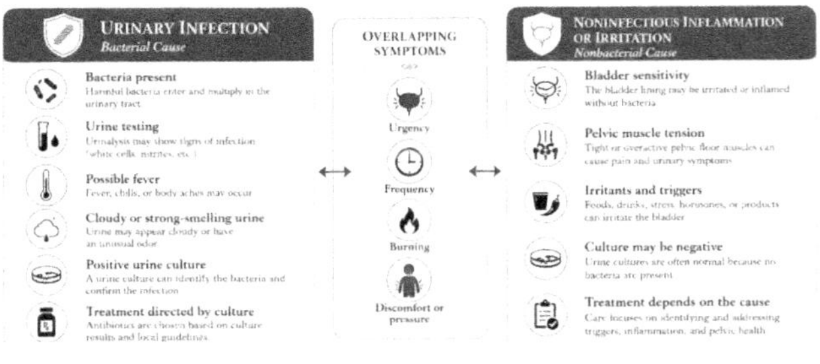

Pelvic pain, urinary symptoms, inflammation, infection, and pelvic-floor dysfunction can overlap under the word prostatitis.

FIGURE 21.1 - PROSTATITIS *Is Not One Thing. Infection, inflammation, pelvic floor, bladder, and bowel factors may overlap.*

Prostatitis may be one of the most confusing words in urology. A man hears it and usually assumes he has an infection. Sometimes that is true. Sometimes it is not. Sometimes the prostate is inflamed.

Sometimes bacteria are involved. Sometimes the symptoms feel like they are coming from the prostate, but the real problem is the bladder, pelvic floor, bowel, urinary blockage, a stone, or a mixture of several things at once. That is why prostatitis frustrates patients.

It can cause burning, pressure, pelvic discomfort, urinary frequency, urgency, pain with ejaculation, testicular discomfort, rectal pressure, fever in severe cases, or a general feeling that something is wrong deep in the pelvis. The symptoms can be frightening because they are difficult to localize. Men often cannot tell whether the pain is in the prostate, bladder, penis, testicles, rectum, lower back, or pelvis. Everything feels connected because anatomically, it is connected.

The prostate sits in a crowded neighborhood. The bladder is above it. The rectum is behind it. The urine channel passes through it. The pelvic floor muscles surround the area. Nerves run through the region. The bowel, bladder, prostate, and pelvic muscles all live close together. When one part of that system becomes irritated, the entire area can feel involved.

This is why a man with prostatitis-like symptoms can feel miserable even when testing does not show a simple infection. The key is not to throw the word prostatitis at every pelvic symptom and move on. The key is to ask what kind of prostatitis we are dealing with, whether bacteria are truly present, whether the bladder is emptying, whether the prostate is obstructing, whether a stone or infection source is being missed, and whether the pelvic floor or bowel is part of the problem.

Prostatitis is not one simple diagnosis. It is a category that needs careful thinking.

THE WORD CREATES CONFUSION

The word prostatitis literally means inflammation of the prostate. That sounds straightforward. In practice, it is not.

Inflammation can come from infection, but it does not always. A man can have bacteria in the urine and a true prostate infection. Another man can have pelvic pain and urinary symptoms without clear bacteria. Another may have recurrent urinary infections because urine is being left behind in the bladder. Another may have a bladder stone acting like a hiding place for bacteria. Another may have constipation and pelvic floor muscle tension creating symptoms that feel like prostate pain.

All of these men may be told they have prostatitis. That is the problem.

A label that includes too many different mechanisms becomes less useful. The patient hears one word, but the causes and treatments may be different.

A bacterial infection needs a different plan than pelvic floor dysfunction. A bladder stone needs a different plan than inflammation. A man retaining urine because of prostate blockage needs a different plan than a man with chronic pelvic pain and normal emptying.

The diagnosis should not stop at the word prostatitis. It should begin there.

ACUTE BACTERIAL PROSTATITIS

The clearest version of prostatitis is acute bacterial prostatitis. This is a true infection of the prostate. The patient may feel very sick. He may have fever, chills, burning with urination, pelvic pain, urinary urgency, difficulty urinating, and sometimes trouble emptying the bladder. The urine test may show signs of infection. A urine culture may grow bacteria.

This is not a vague condition. It is a real infection and should be treated seriously.

Acute bacterial prostatitis can make men very uncomfortable and sometimes quite ill. In more severe cases, a patient may require urgent care, antibiotics, and close monitoring. If he cannot urinate, that becomes even more serious and must be managed carefully.

This is one area where antibiotics absolutely matter. When bacterial infection is suspected, treatment should not be delayed casually. The prostate can be difficult for some antibiotics to penetrate, and treatment may need to be longer than a simple bladder infection.

The important point is that acute bacterial prostatitis has a clinical picture. The patient is usually more acutely ill. The urine findings may support infection. The timing is often faster. The symptoms are not just vague discomfort for years. When infection is real, treat it.

CHRONIC BACTERIAL PROSTATITIS

Chronic bacterial prostatitis is different. The man may not be severely ill, but he may have recurrent urinary infections, urinary symptoms, pelvic discomfort, or episodes that improve with antibiotics and then return. Sometimes the prostate acts as a reservoir where bacteria can persist. Sometimes the urine culture repeatedly grows the same organism. Sometimes symptoms flare after periods of feeling better.

This condition can be frustrating because the patient may feel that the infection never fully goes away. The key is to prove, as much as possible, whether bacteria are part of the problem. A urine test and culture matter. The pattern matters. Has the same bacteria returned? Does the patient have fever or systemic symptoms? Is there burning? Is there urine left behind after urination that may be increasing infection risk? Is there a bladder stone? Is the prostate obstructing the bladder outlet? Is there another source of infection?

If bacteria are present or strongly suspected, antibiotics may be appropriate. But if the patient keeps receiving antibiotics without cultures, without reassessment, and without a search for why infections recur, the plan is incomplete. Repeated infections in a man should raise the question: why is this happening?

WHEN ANTIBIOTICS HELP

I do not believe in pretending bacterial prostatitis does not exist. It does.

There are men who need antibiotics. If a patient has bacteria in the urine, a positive culture, signs of infection, fever, burning, acute worsening, or a clinical picture that strongly suggests bacterial prostatitis, antibiotics can be the right treatment.

A reasonable antibiotic trial can also provide information. If a man has symptoms consistent with infection and improves clearly with treatment, that response matters. It does not prove everything forever, but it is useful evidence. The problem is not antibiotics when they are used for the right reason.

The problem is endless antibiotics when the diagnosis does not fit or the patient does not improve. If the symptoms return repeatedly, if cultures are negative, if the urine does not support infection, if the patient never gets real relief, or if antibiotics only create temporary partial improvement, the doctor has to step back and ask what else is going on.

Antibiotics are a tool. They are not a personality. A good urologist should know when to use them and when to stop repeating the same failed plan.

WHEN ANTIBIOTICS DO NOT SOLVE THE PROBLEM

Many men with prostatitis-like symptoms do not have a clear bacterial infection. They may have pelvic pressure, urinary frequency, discomfort after ejaculation, testicular aching, rectal pressure, or burning sensations, but the urine culture is negative and there is no clear evidence of infection. They may be given antibiotics anyway because both patient and doctor want to do something. Sometimes the patient feels a little better. Sometimes he does not. Sometimes he improves while taking the medication and then relapses.

This is the point where the diagnosis must be reconsidered. Maybe the pelvic floor muscles are tight. Maybe constipation is increasing pressure in the pelvis. Maybe the bladder is irritated. Maybe there is hidden obstruction from the prostate. Maybe urine is left behind after urination. Maybe there is a stone. Maybe the patient has nerve-related pelvic pain. Maybe stress physiology is amplifying the symptoms. Maybe there is more than one cause.

If the patient has taken several antibiotic courses and still has the same problem, the answer is not automatically another course. The answer is a better diagnosis. This is where prostatitis becomes less about one organ and more about the entire male pelvis.

THE PROSTATE-BLADDER LINK IN PROSTATITIS SYMPTOMS

Men with prostate inflammation often have urinary symptoms. They may urinate frequently. They may feel urgency. They may have burning. They may feel they cannot empty. They may have pressure in the pelvis or discomfort near the bladder outlet. But those symptoms overlap with BPH and bladder dysfunction.

A man with benign prostate enlargement may develop urinary retention or incomplete emptying. Urine left behind can increase infection risk. The bladder may become irritated. The symptoms may be labeled prostatitis when the deeper issue is obstruction.

This is why a man with recurrent prostatitis symptoms should not be evaluated only with a urine test and antibiotics. He should also be evaluated as a prostate-bladder patient.

How much urine is left behind after he finishes? How fast does the urine come out? Is the prostate enlarged? Is part of the prostate growing into the bladder opening? Has he had bladder stones? Has he had recurrent infections? Has anyone looked inside the bladder?

These questions matter because the infection or inflammation may be downstream from another problem. If the bladder is not emptying, the prostate problem is not only inflammation. It may be obstruction.

BLADDER STONES AND THE HIDDEN SOURCE

A bladder stone can make prostatitis and urinary infection confusing. A man may be treated over and over with antibiotics. He feels better temporarily. Then the symptoms return. Everyone calls it another infection or another prostatitis flare.

But if a stone is sitting in the bladder, it can act like a hiding place for bacteria and irritation. Antibiotics may reduce the bacterial load, but they do not remove the stone. The symptoms return because the source remains. The question then becomes: why did the stone form?

Often, bladder stones in men are related to incomplete emptying. The bladder is not draining well. Urine sits behind. Crystals form. Stones develop. Infection becomes more likely. The man is treated for infection, but the underlying emptying problem remains. This is why cystoscopy, a small camera test that looks inside the urinary channel and bladder, can be so important in selected men.

Cystoscopy answers questions antibiotics cannot. If there is a stone, remove the stone. If there is obstruction, evaluate and treat the obstruction. If the bladder is not emptying, protect the bladder. Do not keep treating the symptom while missing the source.

PAIN WITH EJACULATION

Pain with ejaculation is one of the symptoms that can make men very anxious. It can occur with inflammation of the prostate, pelvic floor muscle tension, infection, seminal vesicle irritation, or other pelvic pain conditions. It can also occur after periods of sexual inactivity, during pelvic stress, or when the surrounding muscles are tight and irritated.

Men often worry that pain with ejaculation means something dangerous. Sometimes it needs evaluation, especially if it is new, severe, persistent, associated with blood in the semen, fever, urinary symptoms, or elevated PSA. But in many cases, it is part of a broader prostatitis or pelvic pain syndrome.

The key is not to panic and not to ignore it. A doctor should ask when it started, whether there is blood in the semen, whether urination burns, whether urine testing suggests infection, whether the patient has pelvic floor symptoms, constipation, or prostate enlargement. PSA may need to be interpreted carefully if inflammation is present.

Sexual symptoms should not be dismissed. They affect confidence, relationships, and quality of life. Men may not volunteer them unless asked directly. A modern urologist should ask.

BLOOD IN THE SEMEN

Blood in the semen is another symptom that frightens men. The medical term is hematospermia. The patient-friendly explanation is simple: the man sees blood or a rusty discoloration in the semen.

In many men, especially younger men, blood in the semen is often benign and related to inflammation, irritation, infection, recent sexual activity, or a recent procedure. But age and context matter. In an older man, especially if blood in the semen is persistent, recurrent, associated with elevated PSA, blood in the urine, pain, or other symptoms, further evaluation may be appropriate.

The prostate and seminal vesicles contribute fluid to semen, so inflammation in this region can create visible changes. That does not automatically mean cancer, but it does deserve thoughtful evaluation in the right context. Again, the principle is the same.

Do not panic. Do not ignore. Understand the signal.

PELVIC FLOOR DYSFUNCTION

The pelvic floor is one of the most underappreciated parts of the male pelvis. These muscles help coordinate urination, bowel movements, ejaculation, pelvic support, and pain signaling. When they are too tight, irritated, or poorly coordinated, they can create symptoms that feel like prostate disease.

A man may have urinary frequency, urgency, pelvic pressure, testicular discomfort, pain after ejaculation, rectal pressure, or difficulty starting urination. He may be told he has prostatitis, but repeated urine cultures are negative and antibiotics do not solve the problem. In that situation, pelvic floor dysfunction should be considered.

This does not mean every man with pelvic pain has a pelvic floor problem. It also does not mean every man should be sent to pelvic floor therapy while real obstruction is ignored. A man with a large prostate, slow stream, and urine left behind needs evaluation for blockage.

But when obstruction, infection, stones, and other causes do not explain the symptoms, the pelvic floor may be a major part of the problem. Pelvic floor physical therapy can be helpful for selected men. The goal is not bodybuilding. It is relaxation, coordination, trigger point work, breathing, posture, and retraining muscles that may be stuck in a guarded, irritated state. The prostate may be blamed, but the muscles may be driving the pain.

CONSTIPATION AND PELVIC PRESSURE

Constipation can worsen prostatitis-like symptoms. This is not a side issue. It is common and important.

The rectum sits directly behind the prostate and bladder area. When a man is constipated, straining, or carrying a large stool burden, the entire pelvis can feel more crowded and irritated. Pressure increases. Pelvic floor muscles may tighten. Urinary urgency and frequency can worsen. Prostate discomfort may flare. The patient may feel incomplete emptying from both the bowel and the bladder.

Men often do not connect bowel habits with urinary symptoms, but they should. A man with chronic pelvic discomfort should be asked about constipation. How often does he move his bowels? Does he strain? Is the stool hard? Does pelvic pressure worsen when he is constipated? Does urinary frequency improve after a bowel movement?

Constipation may not be the whole diagnosis. But it can be the amplifier. Ignoring it can make prostatitis treatment fail.

STRESS, PAIN, AND THE PELVIS

Chronic pelvic pain can become a cycle. Pain creates anxiety. Anxiety increases muscle tension. Muscle tension worsens pain. The patient becomes hyperaware of every sensation in the pelvis. Urination, ejaculation, sitting, bowel movements, and sexual activity all become mentally loaded. The nervous system becomes sensitized. This does not mean the pain is imaginary.

It means pain is biological, muscular, neurologic, and emotional at the same time. Men sometimes resist this explanation because they think it means the doctor is saying it is "all in their head." That is not the point. Pelvic pain is real. The question is whether the pain is coming from bacteria, inflammation, muscle tension, nerve sensitivity, obstruction, bladder irritation, bowel dysfunction, or a combination.

A modern explanation should validate the symptoms without reducing everything to infection. The patient is not crazy. The system is irritated.

PSA DURING PROSTATITIS

Prostatitis can raise PSA. This creates a difficult situation. A man has pelvic pain or urinary symptoms, gets a PSA test, and the number is elevated. He becomes afraid of cancer. The doctor may suspect inflammation. Antibiotics may be given. The PSA may be repeated.

This can be appropriate, but it must be handled carefully. If PSA rises during a clear infection or inflammatory episode, it may make sense to treat the clinical problem and repeat the PSA after things calm down. If the PSA returns to baseline, that is reassuring. If it remains elevated, rises again, or does not fit the clinical picture, further evaluation may be needed.

The danger is using prostatitis as an endless explanation for PSA elevation. Inflammation can raise PSA. But inflammation should not be used to ignore cancer risk forever.

If the PSA remains abnormal, the doctor should consider prostate size, risk factors, repeat testing, advanced blood tests, MRI, and biopsy when appropriate. A man should not be terrified by one PSA during inflammation, but he should also not let it disappear without follow-up.

WHEN TO LOOK DEEPER

A man with prostatitis symptoms should be evaluated more deeply when the story does not behave like a simple infection. If symptoms keep returning, if antibiotics do not work, if urine cultures are negative, if infections recur, if urine is left behind after urination, if there is blood in the urine, if there are bladder stones, if the stream is slow, if PSA remains elevated, or if the pain pattern suggests pelvic floor involvement, the plan should broaden.

That may mean imaging. It may mean checking how much urine remains after urination. It may mean measuring the urine stream. It may mean cystoscopy. It may mean pelvic floor evaluation. It may mean constipation treatment. It may mean MRI or cancer-risk evaluation. It may mean referral to a specialist with experience in male pelvic pain.

The point is not to overtest every man. The point is to stop repeating failed treatment. If the diagnosis is not behaving as expected, reassess it.

SEX AND PROSTATITIS

Men often ask whether sex makes prostatitis worse or better. The answer depends on the patient.

For some men, ejaculation temporarily relieves pressure. For others, ejaculation triggers pain or a flare of symptoms. Some men notice symptoms after prolonged abstinence. Others notice symptoms after frequent sex or intense pelvic muscle contraction. There is no single rule that fits every man.

In general, I do not like fear-based sexual restriction unless there is a clear reason. A normal sex life is part of male health. If a man notices that ejaculation causes pain, the pattern should be evaluated. If he has infection, treatment may be needed. If he has pelvic floor tightness, therapy may help. If symptoms are severe, temporary adjustment may be reasonable.

The goal is not to make men afraid of sex. The goal is to understand why sex is painful when it is painful. Sexual function is part of prostate care.

THE PATIENT WHO HAS BEEN EVERYWHERE

Many men with chronic prostatitis-like symptoms have already seen several doctors. They have taken antibiotics. They have tried anti-inflammatories. They have changed diets. They have searched online. They have worried about cancer. They have been told it is prostatitis, then not prostatitis, then pelvic floor, then stress, then nothing serious. Some feel dismissed. Some feel embarrassed. Some become obsessed with symptoms because no one has given them a coherent explanation. These patients need structure.

They need a doctor to slow down and separate the possibilities. Is there infection? Is there obstruction? Is the bladder emptying? Is there a stone? Is PSA being followed? Is constipation present? Is the pelvic floor tight? Is there nerve-related pain? What has been tried, and what actually helped?

The goal is not to promise a one-visit cure. The goal is to create a rational plan. Chronic pelvic symptoms can be difficult, but difficult does not mean hopeless.

AVOIDING THE TWO EXTREMES

There are two mistakes in prostatitis care. The first is treating every pelvic symptom as infection and giving antibiotics repeatedly without proof or reassessment.

The second is dismissing infection entirely and telling every man it is stress, pelvic floor, or chronic pain. Both are wrong.

Bacterial prostatitis exists. It should be recognized and treated.

Nonbacterial pelvic pain also exists. It should not be treated forever with antibiotics. The skill is knowing when the story fits infection and when it does not.

That requires history, urine testing, cultures when appropriate, prostate and bladder evaluation, and the humility to change course when the treatment is not working. Prostatitis care should not be automatic. It should be thoughtful.

WHAT A MAN SHOULD ASK

A man told he has prostatitis should ask what evidence supports the diagnosis. Is there bacteria in the urine? Was a culture done? Is this acute infection, recurrent infection, inflammation, or chronic pelvic pain? Is the bladder emptying properly? Is there urine left behind after urination? Is the stream slow? Could the prostate be blocking the bladder opening? Could there be a stone? Could constipation or pelvic floor tightness be involved? If antibiotics are prescribed, what is the endpoint? What happens if symptoms do not improve?

These questions help prevent the diagnosis from becoming vague. A man should not accept years of symptoms under one label without a plan.

DR. SHUSTERMAN'S MODERN PROSTATE TAKEAWAY

Prostatitis is one of the most confusing prostate diagnoses because it can mean several different things. Sometimes it is a true bacterial infection, and antibiotics are appropriate. Sometimes it is inflammation without clear infection. Sometimes the symptoms are coming from the bladder, pelvic floor, bowel, prostate blockage, stones, or chronic pelvic pain pathways. Sometimes several problems overlap.

The key is to avoid lazy diagnosis. If bacteria are present or strongly suspected, treat them. If antibiotics fail, reassess. If infections recur, look for the source. If urine is left behind, evaluate emptying. If bladder stones are present, remove them. If pelvic floor tightness or constipation is driving symptoms, address those directly. If PSA is elevated, follow it intelligently and do not let "prostatitis" become a permanent excuse.

Prostatitis should not be a label that ends the conversation. It should be the beginning of a better one.

CHAPTER 22

CONSTIPATION, PELVIC FLOOR, AND THE CROWDED MALE PELVIS

FIGURE 22.1

The Crowded Male Pelvis

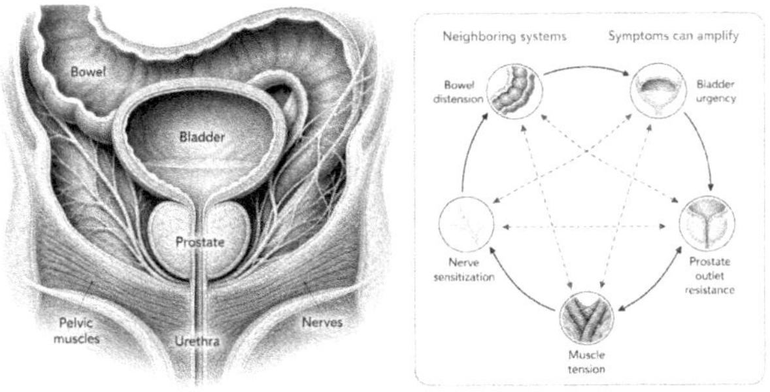

Bowel function, pelvic-floor tension, bladder behavior, and prostate symptoms can amplify one another.

FIGURE 22.1 - *The Crowded Male Pelvis. Bowel, bladder, prostate, and pelvic floor symptoms can amplify one another.*

Men often want every urinary symptom to have one clean explanation. If the stream is weak, it must be the prostate. If there is urgency, it must be the bladder. If there is pelvic pain, it must be prostatitis. If there is nighttime urination, it must be aging.

Real life is usually more complicated. The male pelvis is crowded. The bladder, prostate, rectum, urine channel, pelvic floor muscles, nerves, blood vessels, and bowel all sit close together. They do not function in isolation. When one part becomes irritated, blocked, stretched, inflamed, constipated, tense, or painful, the other parts may react.

This is why some men continue to have symptoms even after they have been treated for the prostate. It is also why some men are told they have prostatitis when the real problem is pelvic floor tension. It is why constipation can make urinary symptoms worse. It is why a man with urgency may need more than a bladder pill. It is why a man with pelvic pain may need more than antibiotics.

The prostate is important, but it is not the only structure in the pelvis. A modern urologist has to think beyond the prostate without ignoring the prostate. That balance is the entire chapter.

THE PELVIS IS A CROWDED NEIGHBORHOOD

The bladder sits in the front of the pelvis. The rectum sits behind it. The prostate sits between them, directly under the bladder and around the urine channel. The pelvic floor muscles form a muscular support system at the bottom of the pelvis. Nerves pass through the region. Blood vessels run nearby. The bowel and urinary system are neighbors. That word matters: neighbors.

If your neighbor is quiet, life is easy. If your neighbor is loud every night, eventually you feel it. The same thing happens in the pelvis. A full rectum can press into the pelvic space. Tight pelvic floor muscles can irritate the bladder and prostate region. A bladder that is struggling to empty can create urgency and pressure. A prostate that is blocking the outlet can make the bladder work harder. Pain in one structure can make surrounding muscles tighten, which then creates more pain.

The organs and muscles talk to each other. Not literally, but functionally. Pressure, inflammation, nerve sensitivity, muscle tension, and mechanical crowding can create symptoms that overlap. That is why the diagnosis must be careful.

When a man says he has pressure, urgency, frequency, pelvic discomfort, constipation, weak stream, pain after ejaculation, or a sensation that he never empties, the prostate may be involved. But the prostate may not be acting alone.

CONSTIPATION IS NOT A MINOR DETAIL

Constipation is one of the most underappreciated contributors to male urinary symptoms. Many men do not bring it up because they do not think it matters. They come to the urologist to talk about urination, not bowel movements. They may be embarrassed. They may assume constipation is a gastrointestinal issue and has nothing to do with the prostate or bladder. That assumption is wrong.

The rectum sits directly behind the prostate and bladder area. When the rectum is full, when stool is hard, when a man strains, or when bowel movements are incomplete, the pelvis becomes more crowded and irritated. That pressure can worsen urinary urgency, frequency, pelvic discomfort, and the feeling that the bladder is not emptying normally.

Constipation can also tighten the pelvic floor. A man who strains every day trains the pelvic muscles into a pattern of tension. Those muscles may then have trouble relaxing during urination, bowel movements, or ejaculation. This is why I ask about bowel habits in men with urinary and pelvic symptoms.

Not because constipation explains everything. Because it often makes everything worse.

THE STRAINING CONNECTION

Straining is a problem whether it happens at the toilet for urine or stool. A man who strains to move his bowels may also strain to urinate. He may not even notice the pattern. The pelvic floor becomes tense. The abdomen bears down. The rectum, bladder, prostate, and pelvic muscles are placed under repeated pressure.

Over time, this can create a cycle. The man is constipated, so he strains. Straining tightens the pelvic floor. A tight pelvic floor makes urination less coordinated. Poor urination increases anxiety and pelvic awareness. Pelvic discomfort makes the muscles guard even more. The next bowel movement becomes more difficult. The cycle continues.

Patients often want the problem to be either prostate or bowel. In many cases, the better answer is that the bowel is amplifying the prostate-bladder problem.

A man may truly have prostate enlargement. He may also have constipation making the symptoms worse. Treating the prostate while ignoring the bowel may produce incomplete improvement. Treating constipation may reduce pressure, urgency, and pelvic discomfort, but it may not solve a true prostate blockage. Both can be true. That is why the evaluation should not be narrow.

THE PELVIC FLOOR IS NOT JUST A WOMEN'S ISSUE

Many men are surprised to learn that they have pelvic floor muscles. They may associate pelvic floor therapy with women after childbirth. They may think the subject has nothing to do with them. But men have pelvic floor muscles too, and those muscles matter.

The pelvic floor helps coordinate urination, bowel movements, ejaculation, pelvic support, and continence. These muscles need to contract when support is needed and relax when urine or stool needs to pass. When the muscles are too tight, poorly coordinated, irritated, or weak, symptoms can develop.

In men, pelvic floor dysfunction can cause urinary frequency, urgency, hesitancy, pelvic pain, testicular discomfort, rectal pressure, pain with ejaculation, bowel symptoms, and sexual dysfunction. Chronic male pelvic pain is often associated with urinary symptoms and sexual symptoms, and modern guidelines increasingly emphasize multidisciplinary evaluation rather than assuming every case is simple infection. The AUA guideline on male chronic pelvic pain covers men with chronic pelvic pain complaints, and the EAU pelvic pain guidance emphasizes that learning to relax and retrain pelvic floor muscles can be useful in pelvic floor pain syndromes.

This does not mean every man with urinary symptoms needs pelvic floor therapy. It means the pelvic floor should be considered when the symptom pattern fits.

A man with a tight pelvic floor may feel like he has prostatitis even when cultures are negative. He may feel burning, pressure, testicular aching, or urinary urgency. He may feel worse after sitting, stress, constipation, or ejaculation. If no one thinks about the pelvic floor, he may receive antibiotics repeatedly without real improvement. That is not modern care.

TIGHT VERSUS WEAK

When people hear "pelvic floor," they often think of strengthening exercises. That can be misleading.

Some men have weak pelvic floor muscles, especially after prostate surgery or other pelvic treatments. These men may need strengthening, coordination, and continence work.

Other men have the opposite problem. Their pelvic floor is too tight. The muscles are guarded, tense, irritated, and unable to relax properly. These men do not need aggressive strengthening as the first step. They often need relaxation, down-training, stretching, breathing, manual therapy, posture work, and coordination. This distinction matters.

Telling every man to do Kegels is not the answer. If a man already has a tight pelvic floor and pelvic pain, strengthening exercises may worsen symptoms. The goal may be to teach the muscles how to relax, not how to contract harder.

That is why pelvic floor therapy should be guided by someone who understands male pelvic pain and male urinary function. The right therapy depends on the muscle problem.

THE PROSTATE STILL MUST BE EVALUATED

There is a danger on the other side of the argument. Some men are told their symptoms are pelvic floor dysfunction when they actually have a prostate blockage. That is also wrong.

A man with a very slow stream, urine left behind after urination, a prostate that is enlarged and growing into the bladder opening, recurrent infections, or retention should not be reassured that everything is pelvic tension. In that man, the prostate-bladder system must be evaluated seriously.

Pelvic floor dysfunction can mimic prostate disease. But it should not be used to ignore obvious obstruction.

This is one of the key principles in this chapter. Do not blame everything on the prostate. Do not blame everything on the pelvic floor. Measure the system. If the bladder empties well, the stream is reasonable, the prostate is not significantly blocking, cultures are negative, and the patient has pelvic pain with muscle tension, then the pelvic floor may be a major part of the diagnosis.

If the stream is very slow, urine is left behind, and the prostate is blocking the outlet, the prostate has to be addressed. Modern care requires both openness and discipline.

WHY PELVIC PAIN FEELS SO CONFUSING

Pelvic pain is difficult because the brain does not always localize it precisely. A man may say the pain is in the prostate, but he may feel it in the testicles, penis, rectum, bladder, lower abdomen, groin, or lower back. He may have pain after ejaculation. He may feel pressure when sitting. He may feel urgency even when the bladder is not full. He may have burning without infection.

This confusion happens because the pelvis shares nerves, muscles, and reflex pathways. Pain in one area can be perceived in another. A tight muscle can create pain that feels like an organ problem. Bladder irritation can feel like prostate pain. Constipation can create urinary pressure. Anxiety can amplify pelvic guarding, and guarding can amplify pain.

This does not mean the pain is imaginary. It means the system is interconnected.

Men sometimes resist pelvic floor or pain explanations because they think the doctor is saying, "It is all in your head." That is not what this means. Pelvic pain is real. The question is whether the pain is coming from infection, obstruction, muscle tension, nerve sensitivity, bowel dysfunction, bladder irritation, or several of these at once. A real symptom deserves a real explanation.

CONSTIPATION AND NIGHTTIME URINATION

Constipation can also contribute to nighttime urinary symptoms in some men. If the rectum is full and the pelvic floor is irritated, the bladder may feel more sensitive. A man may wake more easily to bladder signals. He may feel pressure even when the bladder is not truly full. If he also has prostate enlargement, the combination can be especially frustrating.

This does not mean constipation is the only cause of waking at night. Nighttime urination can come from prostate obstruction, overactive bladder, sleep apnea, diabetes, leg swelling, heart or kidney issues, fluid habits, alcohol, and medications. But constipation is easy to miss.

A man may undergo prostate treatment and still wake at night if the bladder remains irritated by other factors. He may be given bladder medication when the bowel is a major amplifier. He may keep chasing the prostate while ignoring daily straining.

The modern approach should ask the simple question: are the bowels working normally? If the answer is no, fix that too.

THE BOWEL-BLADDER REFLEX

The bowel and bladder are linked by nerve pathways and pelvic mechanics. When the bowel is distended, irritated, or difficult to empty, bladder symptoms can worsen. This is especially obvious in children, but it also matters in adults. A full rectum can affect bladder sensation and emptying. Straining can affect pelvic floor coordination. Chronic constipation can keep the pelvis in a state of tension.

Patients often want to separate specialties. "That is GI." "This is urology." But the body does not care about specialty boundaries. A urologist who ignores bowel habits may miss a major driver of urinary symptoms. A gastroenterologist who ignores urinary symptoms may miss the impact of pelvic floor dysfunction. A pelvic floor therapist who ignores prostate obstruction may miss the root mechanical issue.

The patient needs a coordinated explanation. Not a specialty turf war.

WHEN PELVIC FLOOR THERAPY HELPS

Pelvic floor therapy can be helpful for selected men. A comprehensive therapy program may include education, relaxation training, breathing, stretching, manual therapy, trigger point work, posture changes, biofeedback, and coordination exercises. The exact plan depends on the patient. Studies of comprehensive pelvic floor physical therapy in men with chronic pelvic pain syndrome have shown symptom improvement in many patients, though the evidence base is still developing and the field needs more high-quality research.

The key is selecting the right patient. Pelvic floor therapy is especially reasonable when a man has pelvic pain, pain with ejaculation, testicular discomfort, rectal pressure, urinary urgency or frequency with negative cultures, symptoms worsened by sitting or stress, constipation, or evidence of pelvic muscle tension.

It is also useful after certain prostate treatments, especially after prostate cancer surgery, where men may need help with urinary control and pelvic coordination. But therapy should be individualized. The man with a tight, painful pelvic floor does not need the same plan as the man with leakage after prostate surgery. Again, mechanism matters.

THE ROLE OF STRESS

Stress does not "cause" every pelvic symptom, but it can amplify them. When a man is under stress, muscles tighten. Breathing changes. Sleep worsens. Pain sensitivity increases. The nervous system becomes more reactive. If the pelvis is already irritated, stress can keep the muscles guarded and the symptoms active.

This is particularly common in chronic pelvic pain. The patient feels pain, worries about it, monitors every sensation, tightens the muscles, sleeps poorly, and becomes more sensitive to symptoms. The cycle becomes self-sustaining.

This does not mean the patient is making it up. It means pain, muscles, nerves, and psychology interact.

A modern physician should be able to say that without dismissing the patient. The pain is real. The pelvic tension is real. The urinary symptoms are real. Stress may be one of the factors keeping the system activated. That explanation often helps men more than another antibiotic course they do not need.

SITTING, EXERCISE, AND PELVIC SYMPTOMS

Some men notice pelvic symptoms after prolonged sitting. Others notice symptoms after cycling, heavy lifting, intense core work, or long drives. Some flare after ejaculation. Some worsen during constipation. Some worsen during periods of anxiety or poor sleep. These patterns are clues.

A man with prostate obstruction may not have symptoms that change dramatically with sitting position. A man with pelvic floor tension may feel much worse after sitting for hours. A cyclist may irritate the perineal region and pelvic floor. A man who clenches during stress may worsen pain without realizing it.

The doctor should ask about these triggers. The patient should track them. Patterns help separate obstruction, bladder irritation, infection, muscle tension, bowel dysfunction, and nerve sensitivity. The pelvis is not mysterious when someone takes the time to listen.

AFTER PROSTATE TREATMENT

Some men continue to have urinary symptoms after prostate treatment. This is frustrating, but it does not always mean the prostate treatment failed.

If the prostate blockage is relieved but urgency and frequency persist, the bladder may need time to calm down. If the bladder was overworked for years, recovery may be gradual. If constipation, pelvic floor tension, or sleep apnea is still present, those factors may keep symptoms active. If the bladder is weak, emptying may remain incomplete. If there is residual obstruction, the prostate channel may need re-evaluation.

This is why post-treatment symptoms should be evaluated carefully. Do not assume the procedure failed. Do not assume everything is normal. Ask what part of the system still needs attention.

Sometimes the answer is time. Sometimes bladder medication. Sometimes pelvic floor therapy. Sometimes constipation treatment.

Sometimes repeat testing. Sometimes cystoscopy. Sometimes bladder pressure testing. The right answer depends on the mechanism.

THE PELVIC FLOOR AFTER CANCER TREATMENT

Pelvic floor issues also matter after prostate cancer treatment. After radical prostatectomy, many men need pelvic floor rehabilitation to recover urinary control. The anatomy has changed, and the muscles have to compensate. Pelvic floor therapy can help with continence, coordination, and recovery.

After radiation, some men develop urinary urgency, frequency, pelvic discomfort, bowel irritation, or pelvic floor tension. The treatment may affect tissues in the pelvis, and symptoms can evolve over time. After focal therapy, men may also have urinary or pelvic symptoms depending on the treatment zone, swelling, inflammation, and baseline function.

The point is that prostate cancer treatment is not only about cancer control. It is also about preserving and rehabilitating pelvic function.

Men should be prepared for that. A good treatment plan includes the recovery plan.

THE PATIENT WHO HAS BOTH PROBLEMS

One of the most common real-world situations is the patient who has both prostate obstruction and pelvic/bowel contributors. He may have an enlarged prostate and a slow stream. He may also be constipated. He may have urgency from bladder irritation. He may have pelvic floor tension because he has been straining to urinate and move his bowels for years. He may have pain after ejaculation and wake up at night.

If the doctor treats only one piece, the patient improves only partially. Treat the prostate and ignore constipation, and symptoms may persist. Treat constipation and ignore prostate obstruction, and the bladder may remain at risk. Send the patient to pelvic floor therapy while ignoring urine left behind, and you may miss a dangerous urinary problem. Give bladder medication without checking emptying, and you may worsen retention.

This is why I keep returning to the same principle. Identify the mechanism. If there are multiple mechanisms, treat the major ones in the right order.

THE ORDER MATTERS

When symptoms overlap, the order of treatment matters. If a man has dangerous urine retention, that must be addressed. If he has infection, that may need treatment. If he has a bladder stone, it may need removal. If the prostate is clearly blocking the bladder opening, that has to be part of the plan. If constipation is severe, it should be treated because it may be worsening everything. If pelvic floor tension is prominent, therapy may be important.

The doctor has to decide what is driving the risk and what is amplifying the symptoms. Bladder safety comes first. Infection source matters. Obstruction matters. Then the secondary contributors must be treated so the patient actually feels better. This is how modern prostate care becomes more sophisticated than "take this pill" or "it is just your prostate."

The pelvis is a system. Treat it like one.

WHAT MEN SHOULD NOTICE

A man can help his doctor by paying attention to patterns. Do urinary symptoms worsen when he is constipated? Does pelvic pain worsen after sitting? Does ejaculation trigger discomfort? Does exercise help or hurt? Does stress make symptoms worse? Does he strain to move his bowels? Does he strain to urinate? Does he feel rectal pressure? Does he wake up to urinate even when evening fluids are low? Does he feel better after a bowel movement? These details matter.

They help the doctor determine whether the problem is mainly prostate blockage, bladder irritation, pelvic floor tension, constipation, infection, or a mixed picture. Patients often think these details are too embarrassing or too unrelated to mention.

They are not. In pelvic medicine, the details are the diagnosis.

WHAT A MODERN EVALUATION SHOULD INCLUDE

A modern evaluation of pelvic and urinary symptoms should begin with the story, but it should not stop there. The doctor may need to check urine for infection or blood. The prostate may need to be measured. The bladder may need to be scanned after urination to see how much urine remains. The urine stream may need to be measured. PSA may need to be interpreted in context. Cystoscopy may be needed if there are infections, stones, blood, obstruction concerns, or persistent symptoms. Pelvic floor examination or referral may be appropriate. Constipation should be addressed directly.

Not every man needs every test. But every man deserves a diagnosis that makes sense. A vague label like prostatitis, overactive bladder, or enlarged prostate may not be enough when symptoms persist.

DR. SHUSTERMAN'S MODERN PROSTATE TAKEAWAY

The male pelvis is crowded. The prostate, bladder, bowel, pelvic floor muscles, nerves, and urine channel all live close together. When one part of the system is irritated, the others may react.

Constipation can worsen urinary symptoms and pelvic pressure. A tight pelvic floor can mimic prostatitis or bladder problems. A weak pelvic floor can contribute to leakage, especially after prostate treatment. Prostate obstruction can irritate the bladder and lead to urine being left behind. More than one problem can exist at the same time.

The key is balance. Do not blame every symptom on the prostate. Do not blame every symptom on the pelvic floor. Do not ignore constipation. Do not use pelvic floor therapy as an excuse to miss obstruction. Do not treat the bladder without knowing whether it empties.

The prostate is important, but it lives in a neighborhood. Modern urology has to treat the whole neighborhood.

CHAPTER 23

OVERACTIVE BLADDER, BLADDER FAILURE, AND PERSISTENT SYMPTOMS AFTER PROSTATE TREATMENT

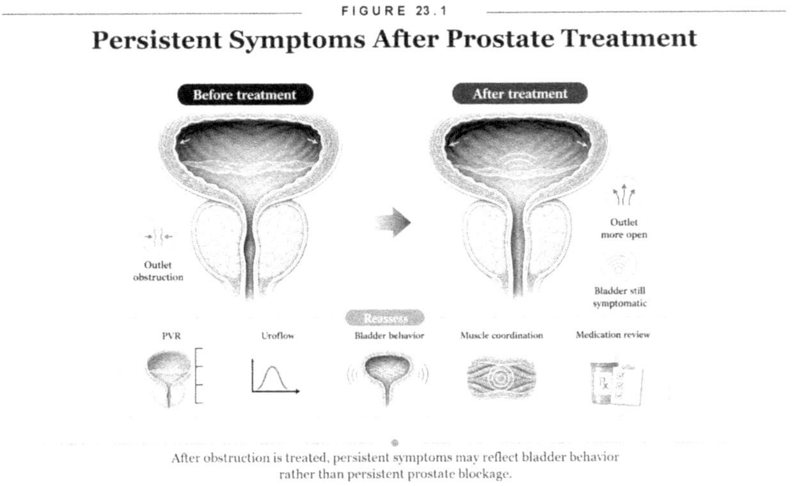

FIGURE 23.1 - *Persistent Symptoms After Prostate Treatment. Persistent symptoms may reflect bladder behavior after obstruction is treated.*

One of the most frustrating moments in prostate care happens after the prostate has been treated. The man expected everything to become normal.

The stream is better. The channel is more open. The prostate obstruction has improved. Maybe the procedure went well. Maybe the doctor says the anatomy looks good.

But the patient is still waking up at night. He still has urgency. He still urinates often. He still feels pressure. He may still feel like the bladder is not behaving normally. He becomes confused. He asks, "If the prostate was the problem and the prostate was treated, why am I still having bladder symptoms?"

That question is important, and it deserves an honest answer. Sometimes the answer is that healing takes time. Sometimes the bladder was irritated for years and does not calm down immediately. Sometimes obstruction remains and needs to be rechecked. Sometimes the bladder muscle became weak from years of pushing against resistance. Sometimes the bladder has become overactive. Sometimes constipation, pelvic floor tension, sleep apnea, diabetes, or medications are still contributing. Sometimes the patient had two problems from the beginning: a prostate problem and a bladder problem. This is where prostate care becomes more complex.

Opening the outlet is not always the same as restoring a normal bladder. The prostate may have started the problem, but after years of obstruction, the bladder can become its own disease.

THE BLADDER IS A MUSCLE, NOT A BAG

Many men think of the bladder as a storage container. That image is only partly correct.

The bladder stores urine, but it is not just a passive bag. It is a muscular organ. It has to relax while it fills, stay quiet while urine is stored, and then contract strongly enough to empty when the time is right. It has to coordinate with the bladder opening, the prostate, the urine channel, and the pelvic floor muscles.

A normal bladder does two opposite jobs well. It stores without complaining, and it empties without struggling. Prostate obstruction disrupts both jobs.

When the prostate narrows the exit, the bladder has to push harder to empty. At first, it may compensate. Later, it may become irritated. It may begin sending urgency signals too early. It may make the man urinate frequently. It may wake him at night. Over time, if the obstruction persists, the bladder may stretch, weaken, and stop emptying completely.

This is why BPH is not only a prostate condition. It is a prostate-bladder condition.

The prostate creates resistance. The bladder adapts. Sometimes that adaptation becomes damage.

OVERACTIVE BLADDER

Overactive bladder is a term used when the bladder sends sudden or frequent signals to urinate. Patients experience it as urgency, frequency, nighttime urination, and sometimes leakage before reaching the bathroom. It can be one of the most disruptive urinary problems because it makes the bladder feel unpredictable.

A slow stream is annoying. Urgency is controlling.

A man with urgency may plan every activity around bathrooms. He may avoid long drives, meetings, theaters, golf, travel, and social events. He may not leak, but he still lives as if he might. That anxiety changes behavior.

The confusing part is that overactive bladder can exist by itself, but it can also develop as a reaction to prostate obstruction. A bladder that has been pushing against a blocked exit may become irritated and unstable. It starts firing signals before it is truly full. The patient feels urgency, but the underlying reason may still be the prostate. That distinction matters.

If the bladder is overactive because the prostate is blocking the exit, simply calming the bladder may not fix the root problem. It may reduce the alarm while the obstruction continues. Before treating overactive bladder in a man, especially an older man, the doctor should ask: is the bladder emptying safely?

DO NOT QUIET THE BLADDER BEFORE CHECKING THE EXIT

Bladder-calming medications can be useful. Some medications relax bladder activity. Others help the bladder store urine more comfortably. These drugs can reduce urgency, frequency, and leakage in properly selected patients. But they can be risky if used without understanding bladder emptying.

If a man already leaves a significant amount of urine behind after urination, calming the bladder may make emptying worse. That does not mean these medications are bad. It means patient selection matters.

A man with urgency should not automatically be treated as if the bladder is the only problem. He should be evaluated for prostate obstruction, urine left behind, slow stream, infection, stones, diabetes, sleep problems, constipation, and other causes.

This is a common mistake. A man says he has urgency. He is given bladder medication. But no one checks how much urine remains after he urinates. No one measures the stream. No one checks whether the prostate is blocking the bladder opening. That is not modern care. Before quieting the bladder, make sure the bladder is not screaming because the exit is blocked.

THE BLADDER CAN BE DAMAGED BY TIME

A bladder can only fight obstruction for so long. In the early stages, the bladder muscle may become stronger or thicker as it works harder to push urine through a narrowed outlet. That may sound beneficial, but it is not necessarily healthy. A bladder that has to generate high pressure every day is under stress.

Over time, the bladder may become more irritable. The man

develops urgency, frequency, and nighttime urination. He may be told he has overactive bladder, but the bladder may be reacting to years of prostate resistance.

If obstruction continues even longer, the bladder may begin to weaken. It may stretch. It may lose its ability to contract effectively. The man may start leaving urine behind. Eventually, he may go into retention or require a catheter. This is what I mean when I talk about bladder failure in the context of prostate obstruction.

The bladder muscle has been pushing against resistance for so long that it can no longer empty properly. That is the stage we want to prevent.

BLADDER FAILURE

The phrase bladder failure sounds dramatic, but patients understand it. It does not mean the bladder suddenly died. It means the bladder is no longer doing its job effectively. It may not contract strongly enough. It may not empty fully. It may leave large amounts of urine behind. The patient may urinate but still retain urine. In more severe cases, he may not be able to urinate at all. This can happen after years of obstruction.

The prostate blocks. The bladder pushes. The man adapts. The bladder compensates. Then the compensation fails.

Once the bladder becomes weak, treating the prostate may still help, but the outcome becomes less predictable. Opening the exit is important, but the bladder still has to push. If the bladder muscle cannot contract well, the patient may continue to retain urine even after the prostate is treated. This is why timing matters.

Treat the prostate before the bladder becomes the disease. That line is not just a slogan. It is the logic of modern BPH care.

RETENTION IS NOT ALWAYS SUDDEN

When a man cannot urinate, it feels sudden. He was urinating yesterday. Today he cannot. He goes to the emergency room. A catheter is placed. The bladder drains. The event feels like a surprise.

But many episodes of urinary retention are not truly sudden. The final moment is sudden, but the process has often been developing for years.

The stream was weakening. The bladder was pushing harder. Urine was being left behind. Nighttime urination was worsening. The prostate was enlarging. The patient was taking medication but not truly emptying. Then a trigger pushed him over the edge: cold medicine, anesthesia, alcohol, constipation, infection, travel, dehydration, or simply progression of the obstruction.

Retention is often the end of a story, not the beginning. That is why I do not like waiting for retention before taking BPH seriously. A catheter should not be the first serious prostate plan.

AFTER A CATHETER

Once a catheter is placed for retention, the next question is whether the patient can urinate again after it is removed. This is called a voiding trial. The bladder is filled or allowed to fill, the catheter is removed, and the patient tries to urinate. If he empties well, that is encouraging. If he cannot urinate or leaves too much urine behind, the problem is still active.

Medication may help some men pass a voiding trial, especially if the obstruction has a relaxable component. But if the prostate is large, the stream has been poor for years, urine was being left behind, or the bladder is weak, medication may not be enough.

At that point, the doctor must ask whether the prostate needs treatment, whether the bladder can recover, and whether additional testing is needed. The patient should not be told simply, "Try again later," without a strategy. Retention changes the urgency of the conversation.

BLADDER PRESSURE TESTING

Sometimes we need to know whether the bladder is strong enough to empty. This is where bladder pressure testing becomes important. Doctors may call this urodynamics. The patient-friendly explanation is that the test measures how the bladder stores urine, how much pressure it generates, and whether it can empty properly.

This test is not needed for every man with BPH. It is not a routine test for every weak stream. But in selected patients, it can be extremely valuable.

A man with very high urine left behind after urination may need it. A man who has gone into retention may need it. A man who fails catheter removal may need it. A man whose symptoms do not match his prostate size may need it. A man who had a procedure but still cannot empty may need it. A man with neurologic disease may need it.

The key question is simple: if we open the prostate channel, can the bladder push? If the answer is yes, treating the prostate may produce a strong result.

If the answer is no, the plan must be more cautious. The prostate may still need treatment, but the patient has to understand that bladder weakness may limit improvement. Testing prevents false promises.

PERSISTENT SYMPTOMS AFTER PROSTATE TREATMENT

Persistent symptoms after prostate treatment can happen for several reasons. The first possibility is that the prostate is still obstructing. Maybe not enough tissue was treated. Maybe a middle portion of the prostate is still blocking the bladder opening. Maybe scar tissue, narrowing, or bladder neck tightness developed. Maybe the original procedure did not match the anatomy well enough.

The second possibility is that the prostate obstruction improved, but the bladder is still irritated. This is common after years of obstruction. The bladder may continue to send urgency signals even after the outlet is more open.

The third possibility is bladder weakness. The channel may be open, but the bladder may not push well enough to empty.

The fourth possibility is that another problem was present all along. Constipation, pelvic floor tension, sleep apnea, diabetes, medications, infection, stones, or fluid habits may still be driving symptoms. This is why persistent symptoms should be evaluated, not dismissed.

The patient should not be told, "The procedure worked, so you must be fine," if he is still suffering. The doctor should ask what part of the system remains abnormal.

A better stream is good. But a better stream is not the story.

HEALING TAKES TIME

Not every symptom after treatment means failure. After a prostate procedure, the prostate and bladder may need time to heal. Depending on the treatment, there may be swelling, inflammation, burning, urgency, frequency, blood in the urine, or temporary worsening before improvement.

The bladder may also take time to calm down. If it spent years pushing against resistance, it may not immediately behave normally just because the outlet is improved. Urgency and nighttime urination can take longer to settle than the stream.

In many cases, I like to give the bladder time after a prostate procedure before labeling symptoms as persistent overactive bladder. A rough window of several months is often reasonable, depending on the procedure, the prostate anatomy, and the patient's baseline condition. But waiting should be guided.

If symptoms are severe, if the patient cannot urinate, if infection is suspected, if urine is being left behind, or if symptoms worsen unexpectedly, the patient should be evaluated earlier. Healing takes time. Neglect is not healing.

WHEN URGENCY PERSISTS

Urgency after prostate treatment can be extremely frustrating. The patient may say, "My stream is better, but I still have to run to the bathroom."

This can happen because the bladder was overactive before treatment and remains overactive afterward. Sometimes it improves gradually. Sometimes it needs treatment.

Before treating persistent urgency, I want to know whether the bladder empties. If a large amount of urine is still left behind, bladder-calming medication may not be safe or may not address the root problem. If the bladder empties well and the outlet is open, then bladder-directed treatment makes more sense.

Treatment may include lifestyle changes, reducing bladder irritants, treating constipation, pelvic floor therapy, medications that relax bladder activity, or procedures such as bladder Botox in selected patients. The right treatment depends on the mechanism. Urgency is a symptom. The cause must be identified.

BLADDER MEDICATIONS AFTER PROSTATE TREATMENT

Bladder medications can be helpful after prostate treatment when the bladder remains overactive and emptying is safe. Some medications calm bladder contractions. Others help the bladder relax during filling. These drugs may reduce urgency, frequency, nighttime urination, and urge leakage. But they must be used intelligently.

If the patient is still retaining urine, the medication could worsen emptying. If constipation is severe, certain bladder medications may worsen it. If the patient has dry mouth, cognitive concerns, glaucoma, or other medical issues, the choice of medication matters.

Modern bladder treatment should not be automatic. It should be personalized. The goal is to calm the bladder without creating a new problem.

BLADDER BOTOX

Bladder Botox can be effective for selected patients with persistent overactive bladder symptoms. The concept is straightforward. Botox is injected into the bladder muscle to reduce overactivity. It can help patients who have severe urgency, frequency, or urge leakage that has not responded well enough to medication.

But bladder Botox has to be used with caution in men who do not empty well. If a bladder is already weak or if the patient leaves too much urine behind, Botox can increase the risk of retention. Some patients may need to catheterize temporarily or, rarely, longer. This is why bladder emptying must be checked before and after treatment.

Botox can be excellent when the problem is bladder overactivity and the bladder can still empty safely. It can be risky if the bladder is already failing. Again, the treatment must match the mechanism.

NEUROMODULATION AND OTHER BLADDER TREATMENTS

Some men with persistent bladder symptoms may benefit from nerve-based treatments. These therapies attempt to calm bladder signaling by influencing the nerves that help control bladder function. Options may include tibial nerve stimulation, sacral neuromodulation, or other approaches depending on the patient and the setting.

These treatments are not first-line for every man. They are usually considered when urgency, frequency, or urge leakage persists despite more basic measures and when the bladder problem has been properly evaluated.

The principle is the same as everywhere else in this book. Do not jump to a therapy because it sounds advanced. First identify the problem.

Is the bladder overactive? Is the bladder weak? Is the prostate still blocking? Is the patient retaining urine? Are constipation or pelvic floor tension contributing? Nerve-based treatments can help the right patient, but they are not a substitute for diagnosis.

PELVIC FLOOR AFTER PROSTATE TREATMENT

Pelvic floor dysfunction can contribute to persistent symptoms after prostate treatment. Some men tighten the pelvic floor because they have been straining for years. Some develop pelvic discomfort after procedures. Some have urgency and frequency that are amplified by muscle tension. Some have leakage after prostate cancer surgery and need strengthening and coordination. Others have pain and need relaxation rather than strengthening.

This is why pelvic floor therapy should be individualized. A man with leakage after radical prostatectomy may need a different program than a man with chronic pelvic pain and tight muscles. A man with urgency and pelvic tension may need relaxation, breathing, and coordination. A man with weakness may need strengthening.

The pelvic floor should not be ignored. But it also should not be blamed for everything. If urine is still being left behind or the prostate channel is still blocked, that must be addressed.

CONSTIPATION AFTER TREATMENT

Constipation can worsen urinary symptoms after prostate treatment. Pain medication, anesthesia, reduced activity, stress, dehydration, and diet changes can all contribute. A constipated patient may feel more urgency, pelvic pressure, and difficulty urinating. He may strain, which can irritate the pelvic floor and worsen symptoms.

This is one of the simplest things to overlook and one of the easiest things to address. A good post-procedure plan should include bowel management. The patient should avoid severe constipation, stay hydrated appropriately, use stool softeners or other measures when advised, and report significant bowel issues.

The prostate and bladder do not recover in a vacuum. The bowel is part of the neighborhood.

SLEEP AND PERSISTENT NIGHTTIME URINATION

Nighttime urination may persist after prostate treatment if the cause was not only prostate obstruction. Some men produce too much urine at night because of sleep apnea, leg swelling, heart or kidney issues, diabetes, medications, or evening fluid and alcohol patterns. Others wake for sleep reasons and urinate because they are awake, not because the bladder woke them. This is important.

If the stream improves after prostate treatment but nighttime urination remains, the next step is not always another prostate procedure. The doctor should ask whether the man is making too much urine at night, whether sleep apnea is present, whether legs swell during the day, whether fluid intake is late, whether alcohol is involved, and whether diabetes or medications play a role.

Nocturia is not always a prostate symptom. It is often a sleep, kidney, bladder, and whole-body symptom.

WHEN TO RECHECK THE ANATOMY

If symptoms persist after prostate treatment, the anatomy may need to be rechecked. A small camera test can show whether the urine channel is open, whether scar tissue is present, whether the bladder neck is tight, whether residual prostate tissue remains, whether stones are present, or whether the bladder shows signs of long-standing obstruction.

A urine flow test can show whether the stream actually improved. A bladder scan can show whether urine is still being left behind. Urine testing can evaluate infection or blood. Bladder pressure testing may help if bladder weakness is suspected. The goal is not to blame the patient or the procedure.

The goal is to identify what remains. Persistent symptoms should lead to analysis, not dismissal.

THE EMOTIONAL SIDE

Men can feel defeated when symptoms persist after treatment. They may think they made the wrong decision. They may worry that nothing will help. They may become angry at the doctor, the procedure, or themselves. They may feel embarrassed that they still have urgency or leakage. They may stop reporting symptoms because they do not want to seem like a difficult patient. This is why pre-treatment counseling matters.

A man should know before treatment that some symptoms improve faster than others. The stream may improve before urgency. Emptying may improve before nighttime urination. Bladder irritation may take time. If the bladder was damaged, full recovery may not be possible. If other factors are involved, they may need to be treated separately.

Honest counseling does not scare patients. It prepares them. Prepared patients recover better emotionally because they understand what is happening.

THE GOAL IS A SYSTEM PLAN

Persistent symptoms after prostate treatment are not a reason to give up. They are a reason to think in systems.

The prostate may need reassessment. The bladder may need

calming. The bladder muscle may need testing. The pelvic floor may need therapy. Constipation may need treatment. Sleep apnea may need evaluation. Diabetes may need control. Medications may need review. Infection or stones may need to be ruled out.

This is modern urology. Not one organ. Not one pill.

Not one procedure. A system. When the prostate-bladder system is evaluated properly, many men can still improve even after an incomplete response to treatment. The key is not to stop at the first explanation.

DR. SHUSTERMAN'S MODERN PROSTATE TAKEAWAY

Overactive bladder, bladder weakness, and persistent symptoms after prostate treatment are some of the most misunderstood parts of men's urinary health. The bladder is a muscle. If it spends years pushing against a blocked prostate, it can become irritated, overactive, stretched, or weak. Treating the prostate may relieve the obstruction, but the bladder may need time or additional treatment to recover.

Urgency, frequency, and nighttime urination do not always disappear immediately after a prostate procedure. Sometimes healing takes time. Sometimes the bladder remains overactive. Sometimes the bladder is weak. Sometimes obstruction remains. Sometimes constipation, pelvic floor tension, sleep apnea, diabetes, medication, or another factor is still driving symptoms.

The answer is not to dismiss the patient. The answer is to re-evaluate the system. A better stream is important, but the real goal is better function.

Treat the prostate before the bladder becomes the disease. And if the bladder has already become part of the disease, treat the bladder too.

CHAPTER 24

THE PROSTATE AND SEXUAL FUNCTION

FIGURE 24.1

Prostate-Bladder-Sexual Function Link

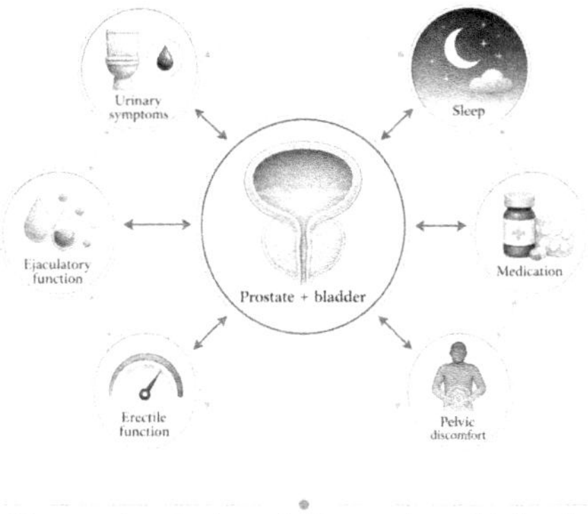

Urinary symptoms, sleep loss, medications, procedures, pelvic discomfort, and cancer treatment can all affect sexual function.

FIGURE 24.1 - PROSTATE-BLADDER-SEXUAL *Function Link. Urinary symptoms, sleep, medications, procedures, and confidence affect sex.*

Men often separate urination and sex in their minds. They think of urinary symptoms as a prostate problem and erections as a sexual problem. They think of ejaculation as something different again. They think of testosterone as another category. They think of prostate cancer as a separate fear entirely.

In real life, these issues overlap. The prostate sits in the middle of the male pelvis, surrounded by the bladder, urine channel, pelvic floor muscles, nerves, blood vessels, and structures involved in ejaculation. It is not the organ that creates erections, but it lives in the same neighborhood as the systems that make sex possible. When the prostate enlarges, becomes inflamed, is treated with medication, or is treated for cancer, sexual function can be affected.

That does not mean every sexual problem is caused by the prostate. Most erectile dysfunction is not simply a prostate problem. Erections are mainly about blood flow, nerve function, hormones, the brain, vascular health, medications, diabetes, blood pressure, smoking, weight, sleep, and emotional state. A man with erectile dysfunction should not assume his prostate is the only explanation.

But it is also wrong to pretend the prostate has nothing to do with sexual life. BPH can affect sleep, confidence, urinary control, and ejaculation. Prostate medications can change ejaculation or libido. Prostatitis can cause pain with ejaculation. Prostate cancer treatments can affect erections, ejaculation, orgasm, continence, and sexual identity. Pelvic floor tension can create pain and interfere with sexual function. Testosterone therapy must be monitored with PSA and prostate evaluation.

The prostate is not the whole sexual system. But it is part of the male function system. A modern urologist should treat the man, not just the gland.

ERECTIONS ARE NOT MADE BY THE PROSTATE

The first thing men should understand is that the prostate does not directly create erections. An erection depends on blood flowing into the penis and being trapped there long enough to create rigidity. That process depends on healthy blood vessels, nerve signaling, smooth muscle relaxation, hormones, and the brain. Cardiovascular health matters. Diabetes matters. Blood pressure matters. Cholesterol matters. Smoking matters. Sleep matters. Testosterone can matter. Stress and anxiety can matter. Medications can matter.

That is why erectile dysfunction is often a vascular warning sign. A man with new erectile dysfunction should not simply receive a pill and be sent away. He may benefit from medication, but the doctor should also think about the heart, blood vessels, blood sugar, blood pressure, hormones, weight, sleep, and overall metabolic health.

The penis can be a check-engine light for the vascular system. That idea is important because men often come to the urologist for erections and discover a broader health issue. Erectile dysfunction may appear before a heart problem is diagnosed. It may be the first sign of diabetes, vascular disease, low testosterone, or medication side effects. So, no, the prostate does not make erections.

But the same aging male body that develops prostate problems often develops sexual and vascular problems at the same time. That is why the conversation belongs together.

BPH AND ERECTILE DYSFUNCTION OFTEN TRAVEL TOGETHER

Many men with prostate enlargement also have erectile dysfunction. This does not mean one always causes the other directly. Aging itself increases the chance of both. Vascular disease, diabetes, obesity, low activity, poor sleep, inflammation, medication use, and hormone changes can contribute to both urinary symptoms and sexual dysfunction. But the overlap is real.

A man with BPH may wake up several times per night. Poor sleep affects energy, testosterone, mood, and sexual desire. He may have urgency and worry about needing the bathroom during intimacy. He may feel older, less confident, and less in control. He may avoid sex because urinary symptoms make him uncomfortable. If he takes certain prostate medications, ejaculation may change. If he has pelvic discomfort or prostatitis, ejaculation may hurt.

In that way, the prostate affects sex even when it is not directly affecting the erection nerves. Sexual function is not only blood flow. It is confidence, comfort, sleep, energy, pelvic sensation, urinary control, and body trust.

A man who does not trust his bladder may not feel sexually free. That matters.

THE CONFIDENCE PROBLEM

Patients often underestimate how much urinary symptoms affect confidence. A man may not describe it as sexual dysfunction. He may simply say he is tired, less interested, or not as spontaneous. But when you ask more questions, the urinary system is part of the story.

He wakes up at night and feels exhausted. He has urgency and worries he might need to urinate. He feels pressure in the pelvis. He dribbles after urination. He has to go back to the bathroom soon after finishing. He is embarrassed by the idea that his body is not as reliable as it used to be. That creates hesitation.

Sex requires a certain amount of confidence in the body. If a man is constantly thinking about his bladder, he is not fully present. Even if his erections are physically possible, the experience may be affected.

This is one reason I take urinary symptoms seriously even when they are not medically dangerous yet. Quality of life is not cosmetic. A man's sleep, confidence, and sexual comfort are part of health. If prostate treatment improves sleep, reduces urgency, restores a better stream, and gives a man back confidence, sexual function may improve indirectly.

The goal is not just to open the urine channel. The goal is to give the man back control.

EJACULATION AND THE PROSTATE

The prostate plays a direct role in ejaculation. Sperm are made in the testicles. Seminal vesicles add much of the fluid. The prostate contributes additional fluid and proteins, including PSA, which helps semen liquefy after ejaculation. During orgasm, these fluids pass through the prostate area and out through the urine channel.

This is why prostate disease and prostate treatment can affect ejaculation. If the prostate is inflamed, ejaculation may be painful. If the pelvic floor muscles are tight, orgasm or ejaculation may trigger discomfort. If a man takes certain prostate medications, semen volume may decrease or semen may go backward into the bladder instead of out through the penis. If the prostate is removed for cancer, normal ejaculation is eliminated because the prostate and seminal vesicles are removed.

Men need to know this before treatment. Too often, ejaculation is treated as a minor issue, especially in older men. That is wrong. Ejaculation may not be necessary for survival, but it can be important for sexual identity, satisfaction, fertility, and quality of life.

A doctor should never assume that ejaculation does not matter because a man is over sixty. Men deserve to know what may change.

RETROGRADE EJACULATION

Retrograde ejaculation means semen goes backward into the bladder during orgasm instead of coming out through the penis. This can happen with certain prostate medications and after some prostate procedures. The orgasm sensation may still occur, but little or no semen comes out. Some men describe it as a dry orgasm.

Medically, retrograde ejaculation is usually not dangerous. The semen mixes with urine and later leaves the body during urination. But the experience can be disturbing if the man was not warned. It can also affect fertility because semen is not exiting normally.

Some men do not care much about this side effect. Others care a lot. Both reactions are valid. The important point is informed choice.

If a medication or procedure has a significant chance of changing ejaculation, the patient should know before he agrees to it. It should not be discovered afterward as an unpleasant surprise. Sexual function is part of consent.

ALPHA BLOCKERS AND EJACULATION

Common prostate-relaxing medications can affect ejaculation. Tamsulosin, silodosin, and similar medications can reduce semen volume or cause retrograde ejaculation in some men. The mechanism is related to relaxation of smooth muscle around the prostate and bladder neck. If that area does not close normally during ejaculation, semen may not move forward in the usual way.

This side effect is often reversible when the medication is stopped, but the patient should not stop medication without speaking to his doctor. The key point is that the patient should know why it is happening. A man who suddenly has a dry orgasm after starting a prostate medication may fear something terrible has occurred. In reality, it may be a known medication effect.

That does not mean he has to accept it forever. If the side effect bothers him, the doctor can discuss switching medication, changing strategy, or considering a different treatment plan. The purpose of treatment is not only to make urination slightly better while quietly damaging the man's sexual satisfaction. The tradeoff should be discussed openly.

FINASTERIDE, DUTASTERIDE, AND SEXUAL SIDE EFFECTS

Medications that slowly shrink selected enlarged prostates can also affect sexual function in some men. Finasteride and dutasteride work by reducing the conversion of testosterone into DHT, a stronger hormone involved in prostate growth. These medications can be useful for selected men with larger prostates, but they can also cause decreased libido, erectile difficulties, ejaculation changes, breast tenderness, mood changes, or other side effects in some patients.

Not every man has these side effects. Some tolerate the medications well.

But the possibility should be discussed before treatment begins. This is especially important in men who are sexually active, concerned about libido, trying to preserve performance, or already dealing with erectile dysfunction.

A man should understand the tradeoff. If the prostate is large and the goal is to reduce future retention risk, the benefit may be worth it. If the prostate is only mildly enlarged and the man is placed on a medication that affects sexual function without a strong reason, the plan should be questioned.

Mechanism matters. So does the man's life.

PROSTATITIS AND PAIN WITH EJACULATION

Pain with ejaculation is one of the most upsetting prostate-related sexual symptoms. It can happen with prostatitis, pelvic floor tension, inflammation, infection, seminal vesicle irritation, or chronic pelvic pain syndromes. The pain may be sharp, aching, burning, deep, or pressure-like. It may occur during ejaculation, after ejaculation, or for hours afterward.

Men often worry that this means cancer. Usually, pain with ejaculation is not a prostate cancer symptom. It is more commonly related to inflammation, pelvic floor dysfunction, infection, or irritation. But new, severe, persistent, or recurrent symptoms should still be evaluated, especially if there is blood in the semen, urinary symptoms, fever, elevated PSA, or other concerns.

The worst approach is to ignore it or treat it forever with the same antibiotic without understanding the cause. If infection is present, treat it. If pelvic floor tension is driving the pain, therapy may help. If constipation is contributing, address it. If the prostate is obstructing and the bladder is not emptying, evaluate that too.

Pain with ejaculation is not just a sexual complaint. It is a pelvic health signal.

BLOOD IN THE SEMEN

Blood in the semen is frightening because men do not expect to see it. It may look red, brown, rusty, or dark. Many men immediately think of cancer. In many cases, blood in the semen is benign and related to inflammation, infection, irritation, recent sexual activity, or a recent prostate procedure. It can also occur after biopsy. But context matters.

In a younger man with one episode and no other symptoms, the evaluation may be limited. In an older man, or in a man with recurrent blood in the semen, elevated PSA, blood in the urine, pelvic pain, or other symptoms, a more careful evaluation may be needed.

The prostate and seminal vesicles contribute fluid to semen, so irritation in that system can show up visibly. The rule is the same as elsewhere in this book.

Do not panic. Do not ignore. Understand the signal.

PROSTATE PROCEDURES AND SEXUAL FUNCTION

Different BPH procedures have different sexual side-effect profiles. Some are more likely to affect ejaculation. Some are designed to preserve ejaculation in selected men. Some are more anatomy-preserving. Some remove tissue. Some heat tissue. Some reduce blood supply. Some pull tissue aside.

Patients often focus on whether a procedure causes erectile dysfunction. That is important, but ejaculation should also be discussed. A man may maintain erections but lose forward ejaculation. For some men, that is acceptable. For others, it is deeply bothersome.

Traditional tissue-removing procedures such as TURP and HoLEP commonly affect ejaculation. Rezūm may preserve ejaculation in many properly selected men, but no procedure should be described as having zero risk. PAE is often attractive because it treats the prostate through the blood supply and tends to preserve anatomy, which may be favorable for sexual function in many men. UroLift has been marketed heavily around ejaculation preservation in selected patients, although its durability and effectiveness depend heavily on anatomy.

The best sexual outcome comes from matching the treatment to the anatomy and discussing priorities before treatment. A man should not choose a procedure without asking what it may do to erections, ejaculation, orgasm, and sexual confidence.

RADICAL PROSTATECTOMY AND SEXUAL FUNCTION

Radical prostatectomy is a different category because it is performed for prostate cancer, not BPH. In radical prostatectomy, the entire prostate and seminal vesicles are removed. That means normal ejaculation is gone. The orgasm sensation may remain, but semen does not come out because the organs producing the fluid have been removed.

Erections can also be affected because the nerves involved in erections run close to the prostate. Even with robotic surgery and nerve-sparing technique, erectile dysfunction is a major risk. Recovery can take time, and some men need medications, injections, vacuum devices, penile rehabilitation, or other treatments afterward. Some men recover well. Others do not.

Urinary leakage can also affect sexual confidence. This is one reason I am cautious about radical prostatectomy as an automatic recommendation. For some men, surgery may be appropriate. But the patient should understand the functional cost before choosing it. Removing the prostate is not just removing a cancer-bearing organ.

It is changing the male pelvic system. That decision deserves respect.

RADIATION AND SEXUAL FUNCTION

Radiation therapy can also affect sexual function, although the pattern may be different from surgery. Erections may decline gradually over time after radiation. Some men maintain function for years. Others notice worsening erections months or years later. Age, baseline erectile function, diabetes, vascular health, smoking, hormone therapy, and radiation dose all matter.

If hormone therapy is used with radiation, sexual function may be affected more significantly during treatment. Testosterone suppression can reduce libido, erections, energy, mood, muscle, and sexual desire.

Ejaculation may also change after radiation. Semen volume may decrease. Orgasm may feel different. Some men develop urinary or bowel symptoms that affect sexual confidence.

Radiation can be an excellent cancer treatment. It should not be dismissed. But it also should not be presented as side-effect free. The right cancer treatment discussion includes both cancer control and function.

FOCAL THERAPY AND FUNCTION PRESERVATION

Focal therapy is attractive because it attempts to treat the cancerous area while preserving more of the prostate and surrounding structures. The goal is cancer control with less damage to urinary and sexual function. That idea is powerful.

For selected men with localized, visible, well-mapped cancer, focal therapy may offer a way to treat the important lesion while reducing the risk of side effects associated with whole-gland treatment. This can be especially appealing to men who want to preserve erections, ejaculation, and urinary control.

But focal therapy is not right for everyone. The cancer must be properly mapped. The patient must understand follow-up. PSA does not drop to zero because the prostate remains. MRI and repeat biopsy may be needed. If cancer exists elsewhere in the gland, focal therapy may miss it.

The function-preserving promise is real in selected patients. But the selection must be careful. The treatment is only as good as the map.

TESTOSTERONE, PSA, AND SEXUAL FUNCTION

Testosterone is central to many aspects of male sexual health: libido, energy, erections, mood, muscle, and overall vitality. For many years, men were told that testosterone was dangerous for the prostate. The relationship is more nuanced. Testosterone is not automatic cancer fuel in the simplistic way many men were taught. But testosterone therapy should never be casual.

A man on testosterone needs prostate monitoring. PSA should be checked. Urinary symptoms should be reviewed. Prostate cancer risk should be considered. If PSA rises in a concerning way, the answer is not to ignore it. The answer is to evaluate it properly.

In my practice, I do not treat testosterone as automatic prostate cancer danger. I treat PSA movement as a signal. That distinction matters.

A man with low testosterone and sexual symptoms deserves a thoughtful discussion, not fear. But he also deserves monitoring. Hormones are medicine. Monitoring is not optional.

FERTILITY CONSIDERATIONS

Sexual function and fertility are not the same thing. A man may have erections and orgasms but still have impaired fertility. Prostate medications and treatments can affect ejaculation. Testosterone therapy can suppress sperm production by reducing the brain's signal to the testicles. Prostate cancer surgery eliminates ejaculation. Some procedures may cause semen to go backward into the bladder.

This matters for younger men and for older men who still want fertility. Doctors should not assume fertility is irrelevant. A man in his forties, fifties, or beyond may still want children. If fertility matters, the treatment plan changes. Sperm banking may be considered before certain treatments. Alternatives to testosterone therapy may be discussed. Ejaculation-preserving strategies may be prioritized. A modern men's health conversation should ask about fertility before making decisions that may affect it.

THE PELVIC FLOOR AND SEXUAL FUNCTION

The pelvic floor muscles affect ejaculation, orgasm, erection quality, and pelvic comfort. When these muscles are tight or painful, sex can become uncomfortable. A man may develop pain during or after ejaculation. He may have testicular discomfort, penile pain, rectal pressure, or urinary urgency after sex. He may be told he has prostatitis, but the real driver may be pelvic floor tension.

Pelvic floor therapy can help selected men, especially when infection has been ruled out, urine cultures are negative, and symptoms are linked to sitting, stress, constipation, or ejaculation. The goal is not to make men afraid of sex. The goal is to restore normal pelvic function so sex does not trigger pain. Sexual symptoms are often the clue that the pelvis is not relaxing properly.

ED AS A HEALTH SIGNAL

Erectile dysfunction should never be treated as only a bedroom problem. It may be the first warning sign of vascular disease. The arteries of the penis are small. Problems with blood flow may show up there before they show up in the heart. A man with new erectile dysfunction should think beyond performance. He should ask whether his blood pressure, cholesterol, blood sugar, weight, sleep, smoking, testosterone, medications, and cardiovascular risk have been evaluated.

This is why urology is often the front door to men's health. A man comes in for erections and discovers diabetes. He comes in for urinary symptoms and discovers sleep apnea. He comes in for low libido and discovers low testosterone, metabolic syndrome, or depression. He comes in for prostate care and ends up getting a broader male health evaluation. That is exactly how modern urology should work.

The goal is not simply to prescribe a sex pill. The goal is to understand the man.

DAILY TADALAFIL: WHERE URINATION AND ERECTIONS MEET

Daily tadalafil is one of the medications that sits directly at the intersection of urinary and sexual function. At low daily doses, tadalafil can help some men with erectile dysfunction and urinary symptoms. It may improve erections and provide some urinary benefit. For men with both issues, it can be a useful option. But it has limits.

It does not remove prostate tissue. It does not shrink a large gland. It does not erase a ball-valve prostate growth at the bladder opening. It does not prove the bladder is emptying safely.

Daily tadalafil can be helpful when the symptoms fit. It is less convincing when the man has significant obstruction, a very slow stream, or a large amount of urine left behind. Again, mechanism matters. A medication that helps erections and mild urinary symptoms should not be used to ignore serious prostate obstruction.

TALKING ABOUT SEX DIRECTLY

Doctors need to ask about sexual function directly. Many men will not bring it up. They may be embarrassed. They may assume the doctor is too busy. They may think it is not relevant. They may think sexual concerns are superficial compared with cancer or urination. They are wrong.

Sexual function is part of health. It affects relationships, confidence, mood, identity, and quality of life. A man's urinary plan, prostate medication, BPH procedure, testosterone plan, or cancer treatment may all affect sexual function. If the doctor does not ask, the patient may suffer silently.

A good urologist should ask about erections, ejaculation, libido, orgasm, pain with ejaculation, fertility goals, medication side effects, and the patient's priorities. That conversation should be normal. Men should not have to apologize for wanting to preserve sexual function.

WHAT A MAN SHOULD ASK BEFORE PROSTATE TREATMENT

Before starting medication, a man should ask whether it may affect erections, libido, ejaculation, or semen volume. Before a BPH procedure, he should ask about ejaculation preservation, erectile risk, orgasm changes, recovery time, and future treatment options. Before prostate cancer treatment, he should ask about urinary control, erections, ejaculation, orgasm, hormone therapy, penile rehabilitation, and quality-of-life outcomes.

He does not need to know every technical detail. He needs to know what may change in his life. The best time to discuss sexual side effects is before treatment, not after the patient is living with them. Informed consent should include function.

DR. SHUSTERMAN'S MODERN PROSTATE TAKEAWAY

The prostate is not the organ that creates erections, but prostate health and sexual health are deeply connected. BPH can affect sleep, confidence, urinary control, and ejaculation. Prostate medications can change ejaculation, libido, or erections. Prostatitis and pelvic floor tension can cause pain with ejaculation. Prostate cancer treatments can affect erections, ejaculation, orgasm, urinary control, and sexual identity. Testosterone therapy can improve sexual symptoms in selected men, but it requires prostate monitoring.

A man should not accept prostate treatment without understanding the sexual consequences. He should ask about erections, ejaculation, orgasm, libido, fertility, and recovery before starting medication or choosing a procedure.

Preserving function is not cosmetic. It is part of treating the man.

CHAPTER 25

TESTOSTERONE AND THE PROSTATE

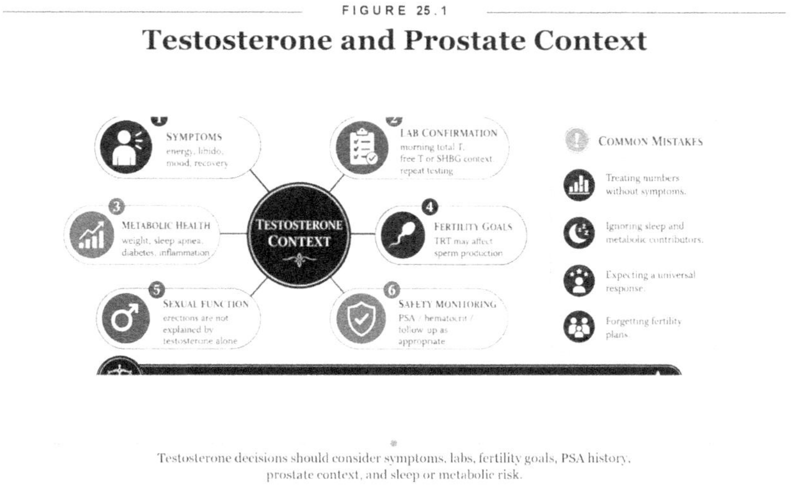

FIGURE 25.1 - TESTOSTERONE *and Prostate Context. Testosterone decisions should consider PSA, symptoms, fertility, and risk.*

Few topics in men's health create more confusion than testosterone and the prostate. A man feels tired. His libido is lower. His erections are weaker. He has less muscle, more belly fat, less motivation, and less drive. He checks his testosterone and finds out it is low. Then he asks the question that has frightened men for decades:

"Doctor, is testosterone bad for my prostate?" The old answer was usually simple. Yes. Be careful. Testosterone feeds the prostate. Testosterone causes prostate cancer. Testosterone makes BPH worse. Avoid it if you are worried about your prostate. That answer was too simple.

The relationship between testosterone and the prostate is more complicated than that. Testosterone is not automatic cancer fuel in the simplistic way many men were taught. At the same time, testosterone therapy is not a casual wellness supplement. It is real medicine. It affects the whole man. It should be prescribed with a diagnosis, a plan, and monitoring. This is the balance patients need to understand.

I do not treat testosterone as something men should fear automatically. I also do not treat it like candy.

Testosterone can be life-changing for the right man. It can improve libido, energy, mood, muscle, motivation, sexual function, and overall quality of life. But the prostate must be respected. PSA must be monitored. Urinary symptoms must be reviewed. Prostate cancer risk must be considered. The treatment must be supervised.

Hormones are medicine. Monitoring is not optional.

WHY TESTOSTERONE BECAME SO FEARED

The fear around testosterone and prostate cancer comes from a real historical observation. Advanced prostate cancer often responds to lowering testosterone. When testosterone signaling is suppressed, many prostate cancers shrink or slow down. This is the basis of hormone therapy, also called androgen deprivation therapy, for advanced or high-risk prostate cancer.

That treatment works. It is one of the most important tools in prostate cancer care.

But a conclusion was drawn from that observation that became too broad. If lowering testosterone helps treat advanced prostate cancer, then giving testosterone must cause prostate cancer or make all prostate cancer worse. That leap is not accurate.

Advanced prostate cancer biology is not the same as carefully treating a man with documented low testosterone under medical supervision. A metastatic cancer responding to hormone deprivation does not prove that restoring a low testosterone level to a normal range in a properly selected man causes cancer.

The prostate is hormone-sensitive. That is true. But hormone-sensitive does not mean testosterone therapy automatically creates prostate cancer. This distinction changed the way many modern urologists think about testosterone.

THE SATURATION IDEA

One way physicians have tried to explain testosterone and the prostate is through what is often called the saturation model. The patient-friendly version is this: prostate tissue appears to need a certain amount of androgen signaling to function and grow, but once that signaling reaches a certain level, adding more testosterone may not keep stimulating the prostate in a straight-line way.

In other words, going from severely low testosterone to normal may matter biologically. But once the receptors are already sufficiently stimulated, more testosterone does not necessarily mean more prostate growth or more prostate cancer growth in a simple linear fashion. This model helps explain why the old fear — more testosterone automatically equals more prostate cancer — is too simplistic.

But it is still a model. It is not a free pass. The relationship between hormones and prostate biology is complex. Different men have different risks. Some have undiagnosed prostate cancer. Some have rising PSA. Some have severe urinary symptoms. Some have a prior prostate cancer history.

So I use the saturation concept as a framework, not as an excuse to stop monitoring. The practical message is this: testosterone is not automatically forbidden in every man with prostate concerns, but it must be managed intelligently.

LOW TESTOSTERONE IS ALSO A MEDICAL PROBLEM

Low testosterone is not just a number. A man with true testosterone deficiency may have low libido, erectile dysfunction, fatigue, depressed mood, poor concentration, loss of muscle, increased fat, lower motivation, reduced exercise recovery, anemia, low bone density, and a general sense that he is not himself.

Not every tired man has low testosterone. Not every man with low testosterone needs treatment. Symptoms matter, and the lab result should be interpreted correctly. Testosterone should generally be checked in the morning, and abnormal results are often confirmed. Free testosterone, sex hormone binding globulin, luteinizing hormone, prolactin, thyroid function, metabolic health, medications, sleep, obesity, alcohol, and chronic illness may all be relevant.

But when a man truly has testosterone deficiency, ignoring it is not automatically safer. A man with low testosterone may lose muscle, gain fat, lose sexual function, and feel older than he is. He may exercise less, sleep worse, become more insulin resistant, and lose confidence. Those things matter.

Men's health should not be reduced to prostate fear. The prostate matters. So does the rest of the man.

THE BASELINE PROSTATE CHECK

Before starting testosterone therapy, a man needs a baseline evaluation. At minimum, the doctor should understand the patient's PSA, urinary symptoms, prostate history, family history, and cancer risk. In many men, especially older men or men with urinary complaints, it also makes sense to understand prostate size and whether the bladder is emptying safely.

The patient should not begin testosterone from a casual online clinic, gym source, or wellness program without prostate monitoring. That is not modern medicine.

A baseline PSA is essential in appropriate men. If the PSA is elevated, rising, or inappropriate for age, the answer is not to ignore it and start testosterone anyway. The PSA should be evaluated. That may mean repeating the test, checking for infection or retention, measuring the prostate, using an advanced blood test, obtaining MRI, or performing biopsy if the risk justifies it.

A man should know where he stands before hormones are started. Testosterone may be reasonable. Blind testosterone is not.

PSA MOVEMENT IS THE SIGNAL

I do not treat testosterone as automatic cancer fuel. I treat PSA movement as a signal. That is the key difference. If a man starts testosterone and his PSA remains stable, his urinary symptoms are stable, and he is monitored properly, that is a different situation from a man whose PSA rises in a concerning way.

If PSA rises, the answer is not panic. It is also not denial. The answer is evaluation.

Was the PSA repeated? Is there infection? Is there inflammation? Is the prostate enlarged? Is the bladder retaining urine? Has the testosterone level become too high? Is the patient taking other hormones or supplements? Is MRI needed? Is biopsy needed? PSA can rise for reasons other than cancer, but a concerning rise should not be ignored because the man feels better on testosterone.

The hormone plan must respect the cancer-risk signal. That is the modern balance.

MONITORING AFTER STARTING TESTOSTERONE

Monitoring is part of testosterone therapy. A man should expect follow-up bloodwork. Testosterone level should be checked to ensure the dose is appropriate. Blood count should be monitored because testosterone can raise red blood cell levels. PSA should be monitored in appropriate men. Liver function, lipids, metabolic markers, estradiol, and other labs may be considered depending on the patient and treatment plan.

The American Urological Association's testosterone deficiency guideline states that PSA should be measured in men over forty before starting testosterone therapy to exclude a prostate cancer diagnosis, and that men with prior prostate cancer should be informed that evidence is inadequate to quantify the risk-benefit ratio of testosterone therapy. The guideline also notes that PSA monitoring in men on testosterone should follow shared decision-making and prostate cancer screening guidance. ()

The Endocrine Society guideline similarly emphasizes prostate monitoring in men who choose prostate cancer screening, including baseline assessment and follow-up after starting therapy, with urologic consultation for concerning PSA changes. () The exact monitoring schedule should be individualized. A younger low-risk man may not need the same intensity as an older man with PSA concerns. A man with prior prostate cancer requires a different discussion than a man with no cancer history. But the principle is universal. If you are taking testosterone, someone should be watching the prostate.

TESTOSTERONE AND BPH SYMPTOMS

Another common fear is that testosterone will make urinary symptoms worse. The answer is not simple, but the old fear is often overstated.

Some men worry that testosterone will automatically enlarge the prostate and cause retention. In carefully selected and monitored men, testosterone therapy does not appear to routinely worsen mild to moderate urinary symptoms. Recent regulatory and evidence reviews have also moved away from the older blanket warning that testosterone therapy generally increases prostate cancer risk or necessarily worsens mild-to-moderate prostate enlargement symptoms, while still emphasizing assessment and monitoring. ()

But that does not mean urinary symptoms can be ignored. If a man already has severe BPH symptoms, a very slow stream, a large amount of urine left behind after urination, retention, or a prostate that is physically blocking the bladder opening, testosterone should be handled carefully. The urinary situation should be evaluated. The bladder should be protected.

Testosterone should not be blamed for every urinary symptom, but it also should not be started in a vacuum. The prostate-bladder system still matters.

TESTOSTERONE AFTER PROSTATE CANCER TREATMENT

This is one of the most controversial areas. Years ago, many doctors considered testosterone therapy absolutely forbidden after prostate cancer. That view has softened in modern practice, especially for carefully selected men who have been definitively treated and remain disease-free.

A man who had prostate cancer treated with surgery, radiation, or focal therapy and has stable follow-up may be considered for testosterone therapy in selected situations after a careful discussion of risks, uncertainty, and monitoring. The evidence is not perfect, but multiple retrospective studies and reviews suggest that testosterone therapy in selected men after definitive prostate cancer treatment has not consistently shown a major increase in recurrence risk. Still, long-term randomized data remain limited, and patients need honest counseling. This is where individualized medicine matters.

What was the original cancer risk? Was it low risk or high risk? How was it treated? How long has the PSA been stable? Is the PSA undetectable after surgery or appropriately stable after radiation? Is the patient symptomatic from low testosterone? How important are libido, energy, muscle, mood, and sexual function? Is he willing to follow closely?

There is no one-size-fits-all answer. But the old automatic "never" is no longer how many modern urologists think.

TESTOSTERONE DURING ACTIVE SURVEILLANCE

Testosterone therapy during active surveillance for prostate cancer is even more nuanced. Active surveillance means the man has prostate cancer that is being monitored rather than treated immediately, usually because it is low risk or carefully selected favorable disease. Giving testosterone in that setting requires a serious conversation.

Some modern experts believe testosterone may be reasonable in selected symptomatic men on active surveillance, especially if the cancer is low-risk, well-characterized, and closely followed. Available literature is limited, and the decision remains controversial. Some reviews conclude that early evidence is reassuring, but prospective randomized trials are lacking and caution is appropriate. ()

My view is that patient autonomy matters. If a man has significant symptoms of low testosterone, understands the uncertainty, has low-risk cancer, is monitored carefully, and accepts the risks, the discussion can be reasonable. But it should never be casual.

Active surveillance plus testosterone requires discipline. PSA must be followed. MRI may be needed. Repeat biopsy may be needed. Any change in risk must be taken seriously. This is not a setting for sloppy hormone prescribing.

METASTATIC OR ADVANCED PROSTATE CANCER

Testosterone therapy is a different issue in advanced or metastatic prostate cancer. In men with metastatic prostate cancer, testosterone therapy is generally contraindicated. These cancers are often treated by lowering testosterone signaling because androgen deprivation can control disease. Giving testosterone in that setting can be dangerous. This is where the distinction becomes important.

Testosterone therapy in a carefully selected man with low testosterone and no prostate cancer is not the same as testosterone therapy in a man with metastatic prostate cancer. Testosterone therapy after successful treatment of low-risk localized disease is not the same as testosterone therapy in active advanced disease.

The risk is not the same in every prostate situation. That is why broad fear and broad enthusiasm are both wrong. Risk category matters.

TESTOSTERONE, FERTILITY, AND THE TESTICLES

Many men do not realize that testosterone therapy can reduce fertility. When testosterone is taken from outside the body, the brain may reduce the signals that tell the testicles to produce testosterone and sperm. The testicles may shrink. Sperm production may fall significantly. Some men become temporarily or sometimes persistently infertile while on therapy. This matters for any man who wants children.

A man should not start testosterone without being asked about fertility goals. If fertility matters, alternatives may be considered. Medications such as clomiphene or other approaches may stimulate the body's own testosterone production in selected men. Human chorionic gonadotropin may be used in some settings to support testicular function. Certain testosterone delivery approaches may have different effects on sperm production, but no strategy should be assumed safe for fertility without evaluation.

If a man wants children soon, sperm testing and fertility planning should happen before treatment. Sexual function and fertility are not the same thing. A man can feel better sexually and still lose sperm production if the plan is not designed carefully.

DELIVERY METHODS

Testosterone can be delivered in several ways. Injections are common. They can be effective and flexible, but levels may rise and fall depending on the dosing schedule. Some men feel peaks and troughs. Some do well with weekly or more frequent dosing.

Topical gels can provide more steady absorption for some men, but they require daily use and carry a risk of transferring testosterone to a partner or child through skin contact if precautions are not followed. Patches are less commonly used but remain an option for some patients.

Pellets are placed under the skin and release testosterone slowly over months. Many men like the convenience and steady levels. In my practice, pellets can be a good option for selected men because they reduce the burden of frequent dosing and can provide stable symptom control.

Auto-injector products can also be useful, though cost and insurance coverage may be limiting. There is no perfect delivery method for every man. The choice depends on symptoms, testosterone levels, lifestyle, cost, insurance, preference, side effects, fertility goals, blood count response, estradiol response, and follow-up reliability. The right treatment is the one the patient can use safely and consistently.

ESTRADIOL, DHT, AND THE HORMONE ECOSYSTEM

Testosterone does not act alone. Some testosterone converts to estradiol, a form of estrogen. Men need some estradiol for bone health, libido, mood, and vascular function, but too much or too little can create symptoms. Some testosterone converts to DHT, a stronger androgen involved in prostate biology, hair biology, and sexual function. Sex hormone binding globulin affects how much testosterone is available to tissues.

This is why good hormone management is more than simply prescribing testosterone and checking one number. A man may have normal total testosterone but low free testosterone because of high binding protein. Another may have high estradiol symptoms. Another may have rising blood count. Another may have worsening acne, hair changes, mood changes, or fluid retention. Another may feel no better because sleep apnea, depression, obesity, or medications were the real issue.

The goal is not to chase a number. The goal is to treat the man.

THE ONLINE TESTOSTERONE PROBLEM

Testosterone has become a major business. Online clinics, wellness centers, anti-aging programs, gyms, and cash-pay hormone shops often market testosterone aggressively. Some provide good care. Others are too casual. The danger is not testosterone itself.

The danger is testosterone without diagnosis, monitoring, or prostate awareness. A man should be cautious if he is offered testosterone without proper labs, without repeat confirmation when needed, without PSA evaluation in appropriate men, without blood count monitoring, without fertility discussion, without sleep apnea consideration, and without a plan for follow-up.

Feeling better is not enough if the therapy is being managed recklessly. A modern testosterone program should include prostate safety, cardiovascular and metabolic context, fertility discussion, blood count monitoring, symptom tracking, and dose adjustment. Hormones should be treated with the same seriousness as any other prescription medicine.

TESTOSTERONE AND UROLONGEVITY

In a modern men's health model, testosterone belongs in a broader conversation. It is not just about libido. It is not just about gym performance. It is not just about erections. Testosterone intersects with muscle, bone, mood, metabolism, sexual function, energy, sleep, body composition, and confidence. But testosterone also intersects with the prostate.

That is why hormone optimization should be connected to prostate care. A man should not optimize testosterone while ignoring PSA, urinary symptoms, prostate size, bladder emptying, or cancer risk. He should not treat the body like separate departments. The prostate, bladder, hormones, sexual function, metabolic health, and longevity are connected.

That is the UroLongevity idea. The goal is not simply to raise testosterone. The goal is to help a man function longer and better, safely.

WHAT A MAN SHOULD ASK BEFORE STARTING TESTOSTERONE

A man considering testosterone should ask whether he truly has testosterone deficiency and whether the diagnosis has been confirmed properly. He should ask what symptoms the treatment is meant to improve. He should ask what his baseline PSA is and whether it is appropriate for his age. He should ask whether urinary symptoms or prostate enlargement need evaluation first. He should ask how often PSA and blood count will be monitored. He should ask whether fertility matters and how treatment may affect sperm production. He should ask what delivery method fits his life and risk profile. He should ask what would happen if PSA rises.

Those questions are not obstacles to treatment. They are what make treatment safe.

A man should not be afraid of testosterone when it is appropriate. He should be afraid of careless testosterone.

DR. SHUSTERMAN'S MODERN PROSTATE TAKEAWAY

Testosterone is not the simple prostate villain many men were taught to fear. It is also not a casual wellness supplement.

Testosterone therapy can be helpful for properly selected men with true testosterone deficiency. It may improve libido, energy, mood, muscle, sexual function, and quality of life. But it must be prescribed with prostate awareness and ongoing monitoring.

I do not treat testosterone as automatic cancer fuel. I treat PSA movement as a signal.

Before starting therapy, a man should understand his PSA, urinary symptoms, prostate history, fertility goals, and risk factors. During therapy, PSA and blood count should be monitored. If PSA rises in a concerning way, the answer is not panic and not denial. The answer is evaluation.

Men with prior prostate cancer, men on active surveillance, and men with significant urinary symptoms require individualized discussion. Men with metastatic prostate cancer are in a different category and generally should not receive testosterone therapy.

Hormones are medicine. Monitoring is not optional.

The modern goal is not to fear testosterone. The goal is to use it intelligently, safely, and in the context of the whole man — prostate, bladder, sex, metabolism, and longevity.

CHAPTER 26

DAILY TADALAFIL, ED, AND BPH

SOME MEDICATIONS SIT at the intersection of two problems. Daily tadalafil is one of them.

Most men know tadalafil by its brand name, Cialis. They think of it as an erectile dysfunction medication, and that is true. Tadalafil can help men get and maintain erections by improving blood flow and smooth muscle relaxation in the penis.

But tadalafil also has a role in urinary symptoms related to prostate enlargement. At a low daily dose, it can help some men with both erectile dysfunction and BPH symptoms. That makes it one of the more interesting medications in men's health because it crosses the boundary between sexual function and urination. That boundary is artificial anyway.

Men do not experience their body in separate departments. A man who wakes up three times a night to urinate does not feel sexually optimized. A man with erectile dysfunction may also have urinary symptoms, metabolic issues, vascular disease, low testosterone, poor sleep, or prostate enlargement. A man who is tired, anxious about urgency, and worried about his bladder is not living in a purely urologic problem or a purely sexual problem. He is living in both.

Daily tadalafil fits into that overlap. But like every medication in this book, it has to be understood correctly.

Tadalafil can help. It can be useful in selected men. But it is not magic. It is not a substitute for measuring the prostate. It does not remove tissue. It does not shrink a large prostate. It does not make a ball-valve blockage at the bladder opening disappear. It does not prove the bladder is emptying safely.

It is a useful medication when the mechanism matches the problem. It is not a replacement for diagnosis.

WHY ED AND URINARY SYMPTOMS OFTEN OVERLAP

Erectile dysfunction and urinary symptoms often travel together as men age. That does not mean one always causes the other directly. The relationship is more complicated. Aging affects blood vessels, nerves, hormones, smooth muscle, sleep, metabolism, inflammation, body weight, and the prostate-bladder system. Those same factors can influence both erections and urination.

A man with poor vascular health may develop erectile dysfunction because blood flow to the penis is impaired. That same man may also have metabolic syndrome, weight gain, inflammation, and worsening urinary symptoms. A man with prostate enlargement may wake up repeatedly at night, damaging sleep and reducing energy and libido. A man with low testosterone may have less sexual desire and may also have poorer body composition, worse metabolic health, and reduced motivation to exercise.

These issues overlap because the body is one system. That is why I do not like treating erectile dysfunction as only a bedroom problem. ED can be a check-engine light for a man's overall health. It may be the first visible sign of vascular disease, diabetes, high blood pressure, low testosterone, medication side effects, poor sleep, depression, stress, or metabolic dysfunction.

The penis often tells the truth before the rest of the body admits it. When a man comes in for ED, he deserves more than a prescription. He deserves a real men's health evaluation.

HOW TADALAFIL WORKS

Tadalafil is part of a class of medications called PDE5 inhibitors. Patients do not need to remember the acronym, but the mechanism is useful to understand.

Sexual arousal triggers chemical signals that relax smooth muscle and allow blood to flow into the penis. Tadalafil helps preserve one of those signaling pathways, allowing better blood flow and improved erectile response. It does not create desire by itself. It does not replace testosterone if testosterone is truly low. It does not fix severe vascular disease. It helps the erection mechanism work better when the underlying system can still respond.

That same smooth muscle and blood-flow biology may also explain why tadalafil can improve urinary symptoms in selected men. The lower urinary tract contains smooth muscle in and around the prostate, bladder neck, bladder, and blood vessels. Tadalafil may improve urinary symptoms through effects on smooth muscle tone, blood flow, nerve signaling, and inflammation-related pathways.

The patient-friendly explanation is simple: tadalafil can help relax and improve function in tissues involved in erections and urination. That is why it can help both ED and urinary symptoms. But the same explanation also shows its limits.

If the prostate is physically too large, or if tissue is bulging into the bladder opening and blocking the exit, tadalafil cannot remove that tissue. It may improve symptoms, but it does not change the anatomy enough when anatomy is the dominant problem.

DAILY DOSE VERSUS AS-NEEDED USE

Many men know ED medication as something taken before sex. Tadalafil can be used that way, but it can also be taken daily at a lower dose. The daily approach is often used when a man has both erectile dysfunction and urinary symptoms, or when he wants more spontaneity rather than timing a pill before sexual activity.

The daily dose creates a steady level of medication in the body. For some men, this improves sexual confidence because they do not have to plan intimacy around a pill. It may also provide ongoing urinary symptom benefit. This can be helpful for the right patient.

A man with mild or moderate urinary symptoms and erectile dysfunction may do well with daily tadalafil. He may notice better erections, improved confidence, and some improvement in urinary urgency or flow. For men who dislike the idea of taking separate medications for sex and urination, it can feel like one medication addresses two issues. But again, the key phrase is selected patients. A daily pill is not a universal prostate solution.

TADALAFIL FOR BPH SYMPTOMS

Tadalafil 5 mg daily is recognized in urology guidelines as a treatment option for urinary symptoms attributed to BPH, including in men with or without erectile dysfunction. The AUA BPH guideline states that 5 mg daily tadalafil should be discussed as a treatment option for patients with urinary symptoms from BPH, and updated guideline material also supports discussing combination therapy with selected alpha blockers in appropriate patients. (,) That is the guideline-level statement.

The practical statement is this: tadalafil can improve symptoms and quality of life in some men, especially when urinary symptoms and ED overlap. But the improvement is usually symptom improvement. It should not be confused with fixing every mechanical cause of BPH. If a man has severe obstruction, significant urine left behind after urination, a very slow stream, recurrent retention, bladder stones, or a large amount of prostate tissue blocking the bladder opening, tadalafil should not be treated as enough without further evaluation. It may be part of the plan. It should not be the whole plan when the bladder is at risk.

TADALAFIL IS ED-FIRST, BPH-SECOND

In my clinical thinking, tadalafil is often ED-first and BPH-second. That does not mean its urinary benefit is fake. It can be real. But when I see a man with both erectile dysfunction and mild or moderate urinary symptoms, tadalafil is attractive because it can address both areas at once.

If the man's main problem is severe prostate obstruction, tadalafil is usually not the strongest BPH tool. An alpha blocker may relax the outlet more directly. A procedure may be needed if anatomy is driving the problem. PAE, Rezūm, or tissue-removing surgery may be more appropriate depending on size, shape, bladder function, and goals. This distinction helps prevent overpromising.

A man with ED and mild urinary symptoms may do well with tadalafil. A man with a large obstructing prostate and a bladder that is not emptying should not be told tadalafil is the solution because it is easy to prescribe.

The medication has a role. It also has a ceiling.

WHEN TADALAFIL MAKES THE MOST SENSE

Daily tadalafil often makes the most sense when the urinary symptoms are mild to moderate, the bladder is emptying safely, and erectile dysfunction is also present. This is the man who says, "My erections are not as reliable, and I am also getting up at night or noticing some urinary changes." If his prostate evaluation does not show dangerous blockage, if urine is not being left behind in a concerning amount, and if his stream is not severely slow, tadalafil may be a reasonable option.

It can improve sexual confidence and may help urinary comfort. That matters because confidence is part of function. Men often underestimate the psychological relief of knowing they have support every day rather than only before sex. A daily medication can reduce performance pressure because the man is not waiting to see whether a timed dose will work. It can make intimacy feel more natural.

That psychological benefit is not trivial. Sex is not purely mechanical. Urination is not purely mechanical either. Both involve confidence in the body.

WHEN TADALAFIL IS NOT ENOUGH

Tadalafil is not enough when the prostate problem is mainly mechanical and significant. If a man has a very slow urinary stream, a large amount of urine left behind after urination, recurrent urinary retention, bladder stones, recurrent infections, or prostate tissue growing into the bladder opening like a ball valve, then tadalafil alone is not a serious plan.

It may make the man feel somewhat better. But better is not fixed.

That phrase matters here. A man may have slightly less urgency or a little better flow while the bladder is still struggling. He may feel more sexually confident while the prostate continues to obstruct. He may confuse symptom improvement with bladder protection.

The bladder does not care that a medication helped erections. The bladder cares whether it can empty.

That is why a man taking tadalafil for urinary symptoms should still be evaluated if symptoms persist or if there are danger signs. The doctor should know prostate size, whether tissue is blocking the bladder opening, how much urine is left behind, and how fast the urine comes out. A sex pill should not become a way to ignore a prostate blockage.

COMBINING TADALAFIL WITH OTHER ED MEDICATION

Some men ask whether they can take daily tadalafil and still use another ED medication before sex. In selected patients, under physician supervision, combination strategies may be used. For example, a man may take daily tadalafil for baseline support and occasionally use sildenafil before sex if additional help is needed. But this should not be done casually.

Both medications affect blood vessel relaxation and blood pressure. The patient's heart health, blood pressure, medication list, nitrate use, alpha blocker use, and overall risk must be reviewed. Dosing matters. Timing matters. Side effects matter. The man should not create his own combination from leftover pills, online prescriptions, or advice from friends.

ED medication is common, but common does not mean risk-free. A man who needs escalating ED medication should also be evaluated for the reason. Is the issue vascular? Hormonal? Medication-related? Psychological? Neurologic? Is there diabetes, high blood pressure, sleep apnea, low testosterone, depression, or cardiovascular disease?

More pills are not always the answer. Sometimes ED is the clue.

TADALAFIL AND ALPHA BLOCKERS

Alpha blockers are common prostate medications that relax the prostate opening and bladder neck. Tadalafil can also affect smooth muscle and blood pressure. Combining them can be useful in selected patients, but it requires attention.

Historically, there was concern about blood pressure drops when PDE5 inhibitors like tadalafil were combined with alpha blockers. More recent guideline updates have become more open to discussing low-dose tadalafil with alpha blockers in selected men, but patient selection and monitoring remain important. ()

The practical message for patients is this: do not combine

prostate and erection medications without medical guidance. A man taking tamsulosin, alfuzosin, doxazosin, terazosin, silodosin, blood pressure pills, nitrates, or multiple heart medications should tell his doctor before starting tadalafil. The goal is not to scare men away from combination therapy. The goal is to use it safely.

THE NITRATE WARNING

The most important safety rule with tadalafil is nitrates. Men taking nitrates for chest pain or certain heart conditions should not use tadalafil because the combination can cause a dangerous drop in blood pressure. This is not a minor warning. It is one of the most important contraindications in ED medication prescribing.

Patients may not always recognize that a medication is a nitrate. They may know it as nitroglycerin or by another name. They may have pills, sprays, patches, or emergency medication. They must tell the prescribing doctor. Tadalafil should also be used carefully in men with unstable heart disease, very low blood pressure, certain complex cardiovascular conditions, or situations where sexual activity itself may not be safe.

A man with ED deserves treatment, but he also deserves cardiovascular safety. The erection should not be treated separately from the heart.

SIDE EFFECTS

Tadalafil is generally well tolerated, but it can cause side effects. Some men develop headache, flushing, nasal congestion, heartburn, back discomfort, muscle aches, or lightheadedness. Rarely, men can experience vision or hearing changes, prolonged erection, or more serious reactions that require urgent medical attention.

Most side effects are manageable, but patients should know what to expect. Backache and muscle aches are particularly associated with tadalafil in some men. They are usually temporary but can be bothersome. Heartburn can also occur. Men who take blood pressure medications should be aware of dizziness or lightheadedness.

Again, the goal is not fear. It is informed use.

ED AS A CARDIOVASCULAR WARNING

When a man comes in for erectile dysfunction, I think about blood vessels. The penile arteries are small. They may show vascular dysfunction before larger arteries create symptoms. This is why ED can appear before a heart attack, stroke, or diagnosis of coronary artery disease in some men.

A man with new erectile dysfunction, especially if he has risk factors, should be evaluated beyond the penis. Blood pressure, cholesterol, diabetes, weight, smoking, sleep apnea, medications, exercise, and family history matter. The AUA erectile dysfunction guideline describes ED as a condition requiring clinical evaluation and shared decision-making, and many clinical discussions of ED emphasize its association with cardiovascular risk factors. ()

A prescription can help the symptom. But the symptom may be pointing to a bigger health issue.

This is one reason I consider ED care part of men's longevity care. The erection problem may be the reason a man finally walks into the office. The real opportunity is to evaluate the man's vascular, metabolic, hormonal, prostate, and bladder health together.

TADALAFIL AFTER PROSTATE PROCEDURES

Some men benefit from tadalafil after prostate procedures. This is not because PAE or Rezūm typically cause erectile dysfunction in my experience. In fact, one of the goals of those treatments is to improve urination while preserving sexual function as much as possible.

But after any prostate treatment, men may experience anxiety, temporary changes in urination, catheter concerns, inflammation, or loss of confidence. Tadalafil may support erections and confidence during recovery. In some men, it may also help urinary comfort.

The purpose is not to treat damage. The purpose is to support function. A man who urinates better, sleeps better, and feels sexually supported may recover with more confidence. This is part of treating the whole man rather than just the channel.

TADALAFIL AFTER PROSTATE CANCER TREATMENT

Tadalafil also has a role after prostate cancer treatment, especially in penile rehabilitation after radical prostatectomy or radiation-related erectile changes. After radical prostatectomy, the nerves involved in erections may be stretched, bruised, or partially injured even when a nerve-sparing technique is used. Erections may take time to recover. Some men use PDE5 inhibitors like tadalafil or sildenafil as part of a rehabilitation strategy. Others may need vacuum devices, injections, or additional treatments.

After radiation, erectile function may decline gradually over time, and tadalafil may help selected men depending on vascular and nerve function. The key is expectation.

Tadalafil works best when the erectile system can still respond. If nerve injury is severe, vascular disease is advanced, testosterone is low, or the patient has major diabetes or pelvic damage, pills may not be enough.

Men should not be shamed if pills fail. There are other treatments.

TESTOSTERONE AND TADALAFIL

Tadalafil helps the erection mechanism. Testosterone influences libido, energy, mood, sexual interest, and sometimes erectile function. A man with low testosterone may not respond as well to ED medication because the desire and hormonal environment are not optimized.

That does not mean every man with ED needs testosterone. It means testosterone should be checked when the clinical picture fits: low libido, fatigue, reduced morning erections, low energy, loss of muscle, weight gain, depressed mood, or poor response to ED medication.

If testosterone is low, treatment may help selected men, but it must be done with prostate monitoring and proper evaluation. Tadalafil and testosterone are not the same treatment. One supports the erection pathway. The other addresses hormone deficiency.

Some men need one. Some need the other. Some need both. Some need neither and instead need vascular, metabolic, psychological, or medication-related evaluation. Again, mechanism matters.

THE MAN WHO WANTS ONE PILL TO FIX EVERYTHING

Some men want tadalafil to solve the whole problem. They want better erections, better urination, better confidence, better sleep, and no further evaluation.

I understand the desire. But one pill cannot replace a real diagnosis.

If a man's urinary symptoms are mild and his bladder is safe, tadalafil may be a reasonable place to start. If he has serious prostate anatomy, a very slow stream, urine left behind, recurrent infections, or retention risk, tadalafil should not become a comfort blanket.

The same is true sexually. If a man has new ED, tadalafil may help, but the doctor should still ask why the ED developed. Is this vascular disease? Diabetes? Low testosterone? Medication effect? Sleep apnea? Depression? Pelvic surgery? Prostate cancer treatment? Tadalafil can be part of excellent care. It should not be used to avoid excellent care.

WHAT A MAN SHOULD ASK BEFORE TAKING DAILY TADALAFIL

A man considering daily tadalafil should understand why it is being prescribed. Is it mainly for erections, urinary symptoms, or both? Is the bladder emptying safely? Has the prostate been evaluated? Is urine being left behind? Is the stream severely slow? Is there prostate tissue blocking the bladder opening? Is he taking nitrates? Is his heart healthy enough for sexual activity? Is he taking alpha blockers or blood pressure medications? What side effects should he expect? What happens if the medication helps erections but urinary symptoms persist?

These questions are practical. They do not make the patient difficult. They make the treatment safer.

DR. SHUSTERMAN'S MODERN PROSTATE TAKEAWAY

Daily tadalafil is one of the most useful crossover medications in men's health because it can help erectile dysfunction and urinary symptoms in selected men. It is especially attractive when ED and mild or moderate prostate-related urinary symptoms overlap. It can support erections, confidence, spontaneity, and sometimes urinary comfort.

But tadalafil is not a substitute for prostate evaluation. It does not shrink a large prostate. It does not remove tissue. It does not make a ball-valve blockage at the bladder opening disappear. It does not prove the bladder is emptying safely.

If urinary symptoms are significant, the prostate and bladder still need to be measured. If ED is new or worsening, the man's vascular, metabolic, hormonal, sleep, and cardiovascular health should be reviewed. Tadalafil can help the right man. But the right man still needs the right diagnosis.

CHAPTER 27

THE PROSTATE-LONGEVITY CONNECTION

FIGURE 27.1

Prostate Healthspan System

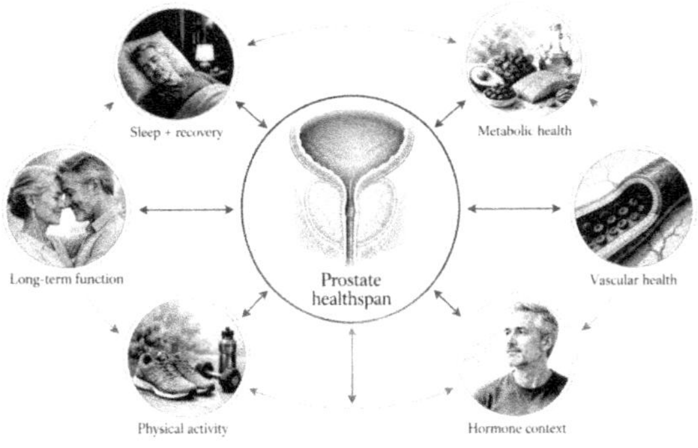

Prostate care connects to sleep, sexual function, metabolic health, hormones, vascular risk, and long-term function.

FIGURE 27.1 - PROSTATE HEALTHSPAN SYSTEM. *Prostate care connects to sleep, sex, metabolism, hormones, and function.*

A man can have every modern health gadget and still miss the organ that is quietly controlling his life. He tracks his sleep on a ring. He wears a glucose monitor. He checks his heart rate variability. He takes supplements. He has a trainer. He gets bloodwork. He talks about longevity, peptides, testosterone, weight loss, VO_2 max, inflammation, and biological age. Then I ask him a simple question.

"How many times do you wake up at night to urinate?" He pauses. "Three or four." That is when the conversation changes. Because a man who wakes up three or four times every night is not optimized. He may have excellent intentions. He may be working hard on his health. But if his bladder is waking him repeatedly, his sleep is being fractured. If his sleep is fractured, his recovery is impaired. His energy, mood, testosterone, metabolism, cardiovascular health, mental sharpness, and sexual function can all suffer.

No man is optimized if his bladder controls his sleep. This is why prostate care belongs in the longevity conversation.

For too long, prostate care has been treated as something separate from men's health. The prostate was discussed only when the stream became weak, PSA rose, cancer was suspected, or a man could not urinate. Longevity medicine, meanwhile, often focused on hormones, weight, nutrition, exercise, sleep, and biomarkers while ignoring the prostate-bladder system. That separation makes no sense.

The prostate affects sleep. The bladder affects recovery. Urinary symptoms affect exercise, sex, travel, confidence, and quality of life. PSA affects cancer-risk strategy. Testosterone therapy requires prostate monitoring. Erectile dysfunction may signal vascular disease. Weight, insulin resistance, inflammation, and metabolic syndrome may worsen urinary symptoms. Pelvic health affects sexual and urinary function.

The prostate is not isolated from longevity. It is one of the gateways into it.

LIFESPAN IS NOT ENOUGH

Living longer is not the same as living well. Most men do not simply want more years. They want useful years. They want strength, sexual function, energy, sleep, urinary control, mental clarity, independence, and the ability to move through life without being controlled by medications, procedures, fear, or the bathroom. That is healthspan.

A man can live a long time and still spend years waking up all night, avoiding travel, losing sexual confidence, and worrying about prostate cancer. That is not the goal.

The goal is not merely to extend life. The goal is to extend function.

This is why prostate health matters so much. The prostate may not be the organ men think about first when they hear the word longevity, but it affects some of the most practical parts of aging. Can the man sleep? Can he urinate normally? Can he have sex? Can he monitor cancer risk intelligently? Can he use testosterone safely if he needs it? Can he avoid the catheter, the emergency room, and the slow loss of bladder function? These are not minor issues. They are the difference between being alive and living well.

THE PROSTATE-BLADDER-SLEEP CONNECTION

Sleep is one of the most important pillars of longevity. That statement has become popular, but in urology we see the practical side of it every day. Men with nighttime urination often do not sleep normally. They may wake up once, twice, three times, or more. They may fall back asleep quickly or they may not. They may spend years in fragmented sleep and call it normal because so many men around them have the same problem. But common is not the same as healthy.

Nighttime urination can come from several sources. The prostate may be blocking the bladder outlet. The bladder may be irritated or overactive. The body may produce too much urine at night. Sleep apnea, diabetes, leg swelling, heart issues, kidney issues, medications, evening alcohol, and late fluids can all contribute.

This is exactly why nocturia should not be treated casually. It is not always just the prostate, but it is often a sign that the prostate-bladder-sleep system needs evaluation.

If the prostate is blocking and the bladder is not emptying, treating sleep alone will not solve the problem. If sleep apnea is driving nighttime urine production, treating only the prostate may not be enough. If both are present, both need to be addressed. That is the point. Longevity medicine cannot ignore the bladder, and urology cannot ignore sleep.

THE PROSTATE AND METABOLIC HEALTH

The prostate does not age in isolation. A man's weight, insulin resistance, blood pressure, cholesterol, inflammation, activity level, and hormonal environment all influence the way he ages. These same factors can overlap with urinary symptoms and benign prostate enlargement.

Research has increasingly connected obesity, metabolic syndrome, diabetes, dyslipidemia, hypertension, and inflammation with lower urinary tract symptoms and benign prostate enlargement. The relationship is complex, but the clinical message is straightforward: the same metabolic problems that damage the heart, blood vessels, erections, sleep, and energy may also worsen the prostate-bladder system.

This does not mean every man can diet his way out of prostate obstruction. A man with a large prostate growing into the bladder opening still needs proper urologic evaluation. A man leaving a large amount of urine behind after urination should not be told to simply lose weight and come back in a year. But metabolic health matters.

Weight loss may reduce inflammation, improve insulin sensitivity, improve sleep apnea, improve testosterone, improve erectile function, improve energy, and reduce pressure on the bladder and pelvis. Exercise may improve vascular health and sexual function. Better blood sugar control may reduce excessive urination. Alcohol reduction may improve nighttime urination and bladder irritation. Treating constipation may reduce pelvic pressure.

These interventions do not replace prostate care. They make prostate care more complete.

THE GLP-1 ERA AND MEN'S HEALTH

The rise of GLP-1 medications changed the weight-loss conversation. For years, men were told to eat less and exercise more, which is not wrong but is often incomplete. Obesity is a biological condition, not simply a willpower failure. GLP-1 medications and related therapies have given many patients a powerful medical tool to lose weight, improve metabolic markers, and change the trajectory of chronic disease.

In a prostate-longevity model, weight loss is not cosmetic. It can be part of urinary and sexual health. A man who loses significant weight may sleep better, move better, improve blood pressure, improve blood sugar, reduce inflammation, improve erections, raise confidence, and reduce the severity of sleep apnea. Those changes can indirectly improve nighttime urination, energy, and sexual function. But GLP-1 medications are not prostate treatments.

They do not remove a ball-valve prostate obstruction. They do not measure PSA. They do not empty the bladder. They do not replace a urine flow test or prostate imaging.

This is the modern balance. Weight loss medicine may be a major part of men's longevity, but it should be integrated with prostate and bladder evaluation, not used as a distraction from it.

A man can be losing weight beautifully and still have an obstructing prostate. Both truths can exist at the same time.

ERECTILE DYSFUNCTION AS A LONGEVITY SIGNAL

Erectile dysfunction is often the symptom that brings a man into the office, but it may not be the biggest issue. The penis is a vascular organ. Erections depend on healthy blood flow, nerve signaling, hormones, smooth muscle relaxation, and psychological readiness. When erections decline, the problem may be local, but it may also reflect broader vascular or metabolic disease.

ED can be a warning light. A man with new erectile dysfunction should not only receive a prescription. He should be evaluated for blood pressure, diabetes, cholesterol, weight, sleep apnea, testosterone deficiency, smoking, medications, cardiovascular risk, depression, stress, and overall health. This is where urology becomes preventive medicine.

The patient comes in because sex is not working. The doctor has an opportunity to detect diabetes, vascular disease, low testosterone, poor sleep, metabolic syndrome, medication effects, and prostate problems. A thoughtful urology visit can become the doorway into a longer functional life.

That is why I do not separate sexual function from longevity. A man's erections may reveal what his blood vessels are trying to tell him.

TESTOSTERONE AND PROSTATE MONITORING

Testosterone is one of the central topics in men's longevity medicine. When used appropriately, testosterone therapy can help selected men with true testosterone deficiency. It may improve libido, energy, mood, muscle, sexual function, and quality of life. But testosterone therapy must be done with prostate awareness.

A man should not start testosterone without knowing his PSA when appropriate. Urinary symptoms should be reviewed. Prostate cancer history should be discussed. The bladder should be evaluated if symptoms suggest obstruction. Blood count should be monitored. Fertility goals should be addressed. This is where some wellness models fail.

They treat testosterone as a performance product, not as medicine. They may focus on energy, libido, and muscle while giving too little attention to PSA, prostate size, urinary symptoms, blood count, sleep apnea, and long-term monitoring. That is not modern urology.

A UroLongevity approach connects the pieces. Testosterone is not automatically dangerous for the prostate, but it is also not casual.

PSA movement is a signal. Urinary symptoms matter. Cancer-risk assessment matters. The prostate has to be watched. Hormone optimization without prostate monitoring is incomplete.

PSA AND CANCER RISK AS LONGEVITY CARE

Many men think of PSA only as a cancer scare. I think of PSA as part of intelligent longevity screening.

If a man wants to live longer and function longer, he needs a rational cancer-risk strategy. That does not mean panicking over every PSA result. It does not mean rushing into biopsy for every mild elevation. It means interpreting PSA intelligently.

What is the man's age? What is the PSA trend? How large is the prostate? Has there been inflammation, infection, or retention? Is there family history? Should an advanced blood test help clarify risk? Should MRI be obtained? Does biopsy make sense?

Modern longevity is not about avoiding bad news. It is about finding important problems early enough to make intelligent decisions.

Prostate cancer is often treatable when found appropriately. Low-risk prostate cancer may not need immediate treatment. Higher-risk cancer may need timely action. The key is distinguishing one from the other. That is exactly what a modern prostate program should do.

Reduce panic. Reduce neglect. Increase precision.

THE BASELINE PROSTATE VISIT

A serious male longevity program should include a baseline prostate discussion. That does not mean every man needs every test at every age. It means men should know when prostate screening should begin, what symptoms matter, what family history means, how PSA should be interpreted, and when urinary symptoms deserve measurement.

A man over fifty with urinary symptoms should not be managed casually. A man over forty with strong family history or higher risk may need earlier PSA discussion. A man starting testosterone should know his PSA and urinary baseline. A man waking up several times a night should not be told it is just age. A man with ED should have metabolic and vascular risk considered. A man with pelvic symptoms should be asked about constipation and pelvic floor issues.

The baseline visit is not only about cancer. It is about creating a map.

Where is the prostate now? How is the bladder functioning? What is the PSA pattern? What is the sexual baseline? What is the hormone picture? What metabolic risks are present? What should be watched over time? A man cannot optimize what he has never measured.

UROLONGEVITY: THE INTEGRATED MODEL

The concept of UroLongevity is simple: urology should be one of the central specialties in male healthspan. The prostate, bladder, sexual function, hormones, fertility, pelvic health, PSA, cancer risk, sleep, metabolism, and vascular health are all connected. Men do not experience these systems separately. A man does not wake up and say, "Today I am only a bladder patient." He wakes up tired because he urinated all night, avoids sex because his erections are unreliable, worries because PSA is rising, gains weight because sleep and hormones are off, and feels older than he should.

Traditional medicine often separates those problems into different boxes. Modern men's health should connect them.

A urologist is uniquely positioned to do that because men often come to us for deeply personal symptoms: erections, urination, testosterone, PSA, prostate cancer, pelvic pain, fertility, and sexual function. These concerns open the door to a broader conversation about the man's health trajectory.

That does not mean urologists replace cardiologists, endocrinologists, sleep doctors, nutrition experts, or primary care physicians. It means urology can serve as a powerful front door into men's health optimization. The prostate visit can become the longevity visit.

THE 360-DEGREE MALE HEALTH VIEW

A complete male health evaluation should not stop at PSA and testosterone. Depending on the patient, it may include metabolic markers, blood sugar, insulin resistance, cholesterol, blood pressure, kidney function, liver function, inflammation markers, hormone panels, blood count, vitamin levels, body composition, sleep assessment, cardiovascular risk, sexual function, urinary function, and cancer-risk screening.

Not every test is needed for every man. But the philosophy matters.

A man is not just a PSA. He is not just a testosterone number. He is not just a prostate size. He is not just an erection score. He is a system.

If his sleep is destroyed, his testosterone may suffer. If his metabolic health is poor, his erections may suffer. If his prostate blocks the bladder, his sleep may suffer. If he takes testosterone without monitoring, PSA interpretation may become more important. If he has ED, his vascular health may need attention. If he has urinary symptoms, bladder safety matters.

The body does not care about medical silos. The body is integrated.

PEPTIDES AND THE MECHANISM RULE

Peptides have become popular in longevity medicine. Patients ask about them frequently. Some are interested in growth hormone secretagogues, recovery peptides, sexual performance peptides, weight-related peptides, and other compounds marketed through wellness clinics. My approach to peptides is the same as my approach to supplements, medications, devices, and procedures.

Mechanism first. Endpoint second. Marketing last.

A peptide should not be used because it sounds advanced. The patient should know what it is supposed to do, what receptor or pathway it affects, what endpoint is expected to improve, what evidence exists, what risks are known, whether the product is legally and safely sourced, and whether the benefit justifies the uncertainty.

When it comes to prostate health specifically, there is no routine peptide that replaces PSA screening, prostate measurement, bladder evaluation, or evidence-based treatment. If a peptide is being used for weight, recovery, sleep, sexual function, or other goals, it should still be part of a medically supervised plan.

Longevity should not become a playground for untested claims. Magic is not a mechanism of action.

INFLAMMATION: IMPORTANT, BUT NOT A BUZZWORD

Inflammation is real. It may play a role in metabolic disease, cardiovascular risk, pelvic pain, BPH symptoms, prostatitis, sexual dysfunction, and general aging. But inflammation has also become a buzzword. Patients are told that everything is inflammation, and every supplement or peptide claims to reduce it. That is not enough.

If inflammation is part of the problem, we should ask what kind of inflammation, where it is acting, and what measurable endpoint improves when we treat it. Does the patient have prostatitis? Pelvic pain? Obesity-related inflammation? Poor sleep? Gum disease? Autoimmune disease? High inflammatory markers? Bladder irritation? Recurrent infection?

A vague statement that something is "anti-inflammatory" does not create a treatment plan. Modern care should respect inflammation without turning it into marketing fog.

THE MAN WHO LOOKS HEALTHY BUT IS NOT FUNCTIONING

One of the most important patients in longevity medicine is the man who appears successful and healthy from the outside but is quietly losing function. He works hard. He has resources. He may exercise. He may look younger than his age. But he wakes up three times per night. His erections are unreliable. His testosterone is low. His PSA has not been checked properly. He has urgency. He has gained weight around the abdomen. He takes supplements but does not know his prostate size. He has never measured how much urine is left behind after urination.

This man may think he is optimized because he is doing more than most men. But optimization is not a vibe. It is measurement. If the prostate, bladder, hormones, sexual function, and metabolic system have not been evaluated, the picture is incomplete.

The goal is not to make him anxious. The goal is to give him control.

LIFESTYLE IS STILL MEDICINE

Modern urology should use technology, imaging, medications, procedures, and advanced diagnostics when appropriate. But lifestyle remains foundational.

Exercise matters. Resistance training matters. Weight management matters. Sleep matters. Alcohol reduction matters. Smoking cessation matters. Constipation treatment matters. Hydration patterns matter. Diabetes control matters. Blood pressure management matters. Nutrition matters. The mistake is thinking lifestyle is either everything or nothing.

Lifestyle cannot remove a severe prostate blockage. It cannot biopsy a suspicious MRI lesion. It cannot make a very large prostate disappear. It cannot replace a catheter when a man is in retention.

But lifestyle can improve the environment around the prostate. It can improve vascular health, sexual function, sleep, metabolism, inflammation, and resilience. It can reduce some urinary irritants. It can improve constipation. It can support hormone health.

The best care combines both sides. Modern intervention when needed. Serious lifestyle when possible.

THE FUTURE IS FUNCTIONAL

The future of men's health is not simply living to ninety. It is being able to function at seventy, eighty, and ninety. That requires earlier measurement, better prevention, smarter prostate care, safer hormone optimization, better cancer-risk stratification, more precise procedures, better weight-loss tools, improved sexual medicine, and a broader view of the male body.

A man should not wait until he has a catheter to care about his prostate. He should not wait until severe ED to care about vascular health. He should not wait until PSA panic to understand cancer risk.

He should not wait until sleep is destroyed to evaluate nighttime urination. He should not wait until testosterone is prescribed casually to ask whether his prostate is being monitored. The future is smarter, earlier, and less destructive. That is as true for longevity as it is for prostate care.

WHAT A MAN SHOULD ASK

A man interested in longevity should ask questions that connect systems. How is my sleep? How many times do I wake up to urinate? Is my bladder emptying? What is my prostate size? Is my PSA appropriate for my age and risk? Are my erections telling us something about vascular health? Is testosterone low, and if so, why? Am I metabolically healthy? Is weight affecting my urinary, sexual, or hormonal health? Is constipation worsening pelvic symptoms? Am I treating symptoms while missing the mechanism? These questions are practical.

They turn longevity from a marketing word into a medical strategy. A modern man should not chase optimization while ignoring the prostate-bladder system.

DR. SHUSTERMAN'S MODERN PROSTATE TAKEAWAY

Prostate care is longevity care. The prostate affects sleep, bladder function, sexual confidence, PSA risk, cancer screening, hormone decisions, and quality of life. The bladder affects recovery, energy, and independence. Erectile dysfunction can reveal vascular and metabolic risk. Testosterone therapy can improve function in selected men but requires prostate monitoring. Weight loss, metabolic health, sleep, and inflammation all interact with the urinary and sexual systems.

A man cannot be optimized if he wakes up all night to urinate. He cannot be optimized if his bladder is retaining urine. He cannot be optimized if his erections are failing because of undiagnosed vascular disease.

He cannot be optimized if he starts testosterone without PSA and prostate monitoring. The future of men's health is integrated: prostate, bladder, hormones, sex, metabolism, sleep, cancer risk, and functional longevity.

Do not just live longer. Function longer.

CHAPTER 28

THE 40+ PROSTATE CHECKLIST

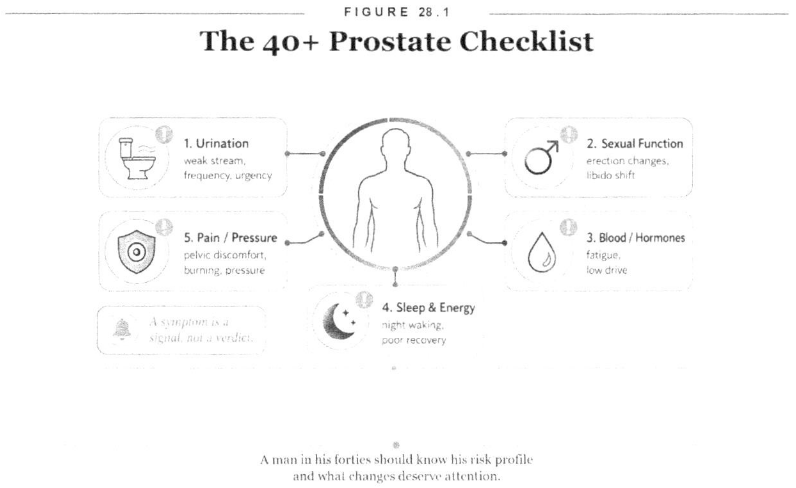

FIGURE *28.1 - The 40+ Prostate Checklist. Men in their forties should know risk profile and meaningful changes.*

A man in his forties usually does not think of himself as a prostate patient. He may be building a career, raising children, training, traveling, dating, running a business, or trying to stay competitive in a world that does not slow down. He may be thinking about weight, muscle, testosterone, sleep, stress, cholesterol, heart disease, or longevity. He may have a smartwatch, a sleep tracker, a supplement stack, or a trainer.

But the prostate is usually not on his radar. That is a mistake.

The goal in a man's forties is not to make him anxious about the prostate. It is not to turn every healthy man into a patient. It is not to order every possible test. It is to create a baseline, identify risk early, and teach men which symptoms should not be ignored.

The forties are the decade when men should stop thinking of prostate care as something that begins only after they are old. A man does not need to wait until fifty-five, sixty, or seventy to understand his urinary baseline, cancer-risk profile, family history, sexual function, hormone status, and bladder habits. By the time the prostate becomes a crisis, the opportunity for easy prevention may have already passed. The purpose of the 40+ Prostate Checklist is simple: know enough early so you are not surprised later.

FORTY IS NOT OLD, BUT IT IS A TURNING POINT

Forty is not old. But it is often when the male body starts giving quieter signals.

A man may notice that he does not recover from exercise the same way. Sleep may be less reliable. Belly fat may be harder to control. Erections may become less automatic. Energy may dip. Alcohol may affect him more. Stress may feel more physical. Blood pressure, cholesterol, blood sugar, and weight may begin to change.

The prostate may still be quiet, but the male aging system is already shifting. That is why forty is a good time to begin thinking strategically.

Not fearfully. Strategically.

If a man has no urinary symptoms, no family history, normal sexual function, and no risk factors, he may not need extensive prostate testing immediately. But he should know his risk category. He should understand when PSA screening should begin. He should know what urinary changes matter. He should not be afraid to discuss erections, testosterone, fertility, or family history.

If he does have symptoms, that changes everything. A forty-five-year-old man who wakes up three times a night, has a weak stream, or feels he does not empty should not be dismissed because he is "too young" for prostate problems. Younger men can have urinary symptoms. They can have inflammation. They can have pelvic floor dysfunction. They can have bladder problems. They can have early prostate enlargement. They can have strictures. They can have sleep apnea, diabetes, or medication-related urinary changes.

Age helps frame risk. It does not replace evaluation.

THE BASELINE CONVERSATION

The first prostate step in a man's forties should be a conversation. That sounds simple, but it is often missing. Men are not asked the right questions. They are asked whether they are "okay," and because most men do not want to complain, they say yes. But "okay" is not a prostate history.

A real baseline conversation asks how the man urinates compared with his younger normal. Does he wake at night? Does the stream start right away? Does it have good force? Does he stop and start? Does he feel empty? Does he ever rush to the bathroom? Does he dribble after urination? Does he have burning, pelvic pressure, blood in the urine, infections, or pain with ejaculation?

It also asks about family history. Did his father have prostate cancer? A brother? An uncle? At what age? Was it low-risk disease or aggressive? Did anyone have metastatic prostate cancer? Are there breast, ovarian, pancreatic, or other cancers in the family that could suggest an inherited risk pattern?

It asks about sexual function. Are erections reliable? Is libido normal? Is ejaculation painful? Is testosterone being considered? Is fertility still relevant?

It asks about healthspan. How is sleep? Weight? Blood pressure? Blood sugar? Exercise? Alcohol? Constipation? Stress? Cardiovascular risk? That conversation creates the map. Before ordering tests, the doctor should understand the man.

PSA IN THE FORTIES

PSA screening is one of the most debated areas in men's health, and different organizations recommend slightly different starting ages depending on risk. That can confuse patients. Rather than getting lost in guideline politics, men should understand the principle: PSA is a prostate cancer risk signal, and the right time to start depends on the man's risk.

A man at increased risk may need to begin the conversation in his early forties. This includes men with strong family history, known genetic risk, or higher-risk ancestry. A man with multiple close relatives diagnosed at younger ages deserves earlier attention. A man whose father or brother had prostate cancer before sixty-five should not be treated exactly like a man with no family history. A man with known inherited mutations, such as BRCA2, needs a more serious screening discussion.

For average-risk men, the conversation often begins later, but I still like the idea of men knowing where they stand rather than drifting into their fifties with no baseline. A baseline PSA in the forties can be useful because it gives context. If the PSA is low and stable, that is reassuring. If it is unexpectedly elevated for age, the man can be evaluated before the situation becomes more complicated.

The key is interpretation. A PSA number by itself is not a diagnosis. It must be interpreted based on age, trend, prostate size, inflammation, infection, urinary retention, family history, and overall risk. The goal is not to scare men into unnecessary biopsy. The goal is to create an intelligent risk strategy. A man should not ask only, "Is my PSA normal?" He should ask, "Is my PSA appropriate for my age and risk?"

FAMILY HISTORY IS NOT A FOOTNOTE

Family history can change the entire prostate plan. Many men know vaguely that someone in the family had cancer, but they do not know the details. That is not enough. For prostate cancer risk, the details matter.

A father with low-risk prostate cancer diagnosed at seventy-eight is different from a brother diagnosed with aggressive disease at fifty-two. Multiple affected relatives are different from one distant relative. Prostate cancer combined with breast, ovarian, pancreatic, or certain other cancers may suggest a hereditary cancer pattern that deserves genetic discussion.

A man in his forties should learn his family history while older relatives are still alive and able to explain it. Who had prostate cancer? How old were they? Was it treated? Did it spread? Did anyone die from it? Were genetic tests done? Were there other cancers in the family? This is not casual information.

It may determine when PSA screening starts, how often it is repeated, whether MRI or advanced testing is used earlier, and how aggressively changes are evaluated. A man cannot control his genes. But he can control whether he knows his risk.

URINARY SYMPTOMS IN THE FORTIES

Urinary symptoms in a man's forties should not be automatically dismissed. It is true that classic age-related prostate enlargement becomes more common later. But urinary symptoms can occur earlier for many reasons. The prostate may be inflamed. The pelvic floor may be tight. The bladder may be overactive. The urine channel may have a narrowing. Diabetes may be causing frequent urination. Sleep apnea may be causing nighttime urination. Medications, alcohol, caffeine, constipation, anxiety, and neurologic conditions can all contribute.

This is why a forty-five-year-old with urinary symptoms still deserves evaluation. The question is not, "Is he too young for BPH?" The question is, "Why is he urinating differently?"

If a man wakes up at night, the cause should be understood. If the stream is weak, the stream should be measured when appropriate. If he feels incomplete emptying, the bladder should be checked for urine left behind. If he has burning or urgency, urine testing matters. If there is blood, that needs evaluation. If pelvic pain is present, prostatitis, pelvic floor, bowel, and bladder causes should be considered.

Younger men are often reassured too quickly. That reassurance can be wrong.

THE AGE-25 COMPARISON

One of the simplest screening questions is not a lab test. It is a memory. How does your urination compare to when you were twenty-five?

A man in his forties can usually answer that clearly. He remembers what normal felt like. He remembers whether the stream used to start instantly, whether it had force, whether he slept through the night, whether he ever thought about bathrooms.

If the answer is, "It is different now," that does not automatically mean something dangerous is happening. But it does mean the system has changed. That change should be understood.

Men should not compare themselves only to other men their age. If all their friends wake up at night, that does not make it healthy. If all their friends joke about weak stream, that does not make it normal. The best comparison is the man's own baseline.

The body often gives warnings before it creates emergencies. The problem is that men normalize the warnings.

THE BLADDER BASELINE

Most men think prostate evaluation means PSA. But the bladder deserves a baseline too, especially if symptoms are present.

A man should know whether his bladder empties. If he urinates and a significant amount of urine remains behind, that is important. He may feel empty, but the bladder scan may tell a different story.

A man with symptoms should also know whether the urine comes out with reasonable speed. A slow stream may reflect obstruction, weak bladder function, or both.

These measurements are not complicated, but they can change the conversation. They separate the man who is mildly bothered but safe from the man whose bladder is already struggling.

In a healthy forty-year-old with no urinary complaints, these tests may not be necessary. But in a symptomatic man, they can be extremely useful. The goal is not to over-medicalize every man in his forties. The goal is to stop ignoring men who already have signals.

TESTOSTERONE BEFORE TESTOSTERONE

The forties are also when many men begin thinking about testosterone. They feel tired. Libido is lower. Gym results are worse. They gain weight more easily. Erections may be less reliable. They see ads for testosterone therapy or online men's clinics and wonder if hormones are the answer.

Sometimes testosterone deficiency is real. But testosterone should not be started blindly.

Before a man begins testosterone therapy, the prostate should be considered. PSA should be checked in appropriate men. Urinary symptoms should be reviewed. Family history should be discussed. Fertility goals should be addressed. Blood count, metabolic health, sleep apnea, and cardiovascular risk should be considered.

A man in his forties may still want children. Testosterone therapy can suppress sperm production. That discussion must happen before treatment, not afterward.

This is another reason the forty-plus prostate checklist matters. It is not only about cancer. It is about creating a safe foundation for men's health decisions. Hormone optimization without prostate awareness is incomplete.

FERTILITY AND THE PROSTATE CONVERSATION

Many men in their forties are not done with fertility. Some are starting second families. Some delayed having children. Some are unsure. Some assume fertility is still intact because sexual function is present. That assumption can be wrong.

Fertility, erections, ejaculation, and testosterone are related but different. A man can have erections and still have a low sperm count. A man can take testosterone and feel better sexually while sperm production falls. Prostate medications and procedures can affect ejaculation. Prostate cancer treatment can permanently affect fertility.

This is why fertility should be part of the conversation before testosterone therapy, before certain prostate procedures, and before cancer treatment. The question is simple: do you still want the option of having children? If the answer is yes or maybe, the plan changes.

Sperm banking, semen analysis, alternative hormone strategies, and ejaculation-preserving approaches may need to be discussed. Modern urology should not assume fertility is irrelevant because a man is over forty.

ED AS AN EARLY WARNING

Erectile dysfunction in the forties should not be dismissed as stress alone. Stress can contribute, but new ED may also be an early sign of vascular disease, diabetes, high blood pressure, cholesterol problems, low testosterone, medication effects, sleep apnea, depression, or metabolic dysfunction.

A man with ED deserves more than a prescription. He deserves a health evaluation.

The erection problem may be the first visible sign of a deeper issue. The arteries of the penis are small, and vascular problems can show up there before they become obvious elsewhere. A man who comes in for ED may be giving the doctor an opportunity to prevent bigger problems later.

This is why urology can be the front door to men's preventive health. The forty-plus checklist should include sexual function because sexual function is often where men first notice that something is changing.

CONSTIPATION AND PELVIC HEALTH

Constipation belongs on the checklist. That may surprise men, but it should not. The rectum sits directly behind the prostate and bladder area. Chronic constipation and straining can worsen urinary urgency, pelvic pressure, incomplete emptying sensations, and pelvic floor tension.

A man in his forties with urinary frequency or pelvic discomfort may not have BPH at all. He may have constipation, pelvic floor dysfunction, prostatitis, bladder irritation, or a combination. Bowel habits should be asked about directly.

How often do you move your bowels? Do you strain? Is stool hard? Do urinary symptoms worsen when you are constipated? Do you feel rectal pressure?

These questions are not embarrassing in a urology office. They are clinically relevant. The pelvis is a neighborhood, and the bowel is one of the neighbors.

LIFESTYLE THAT ACTUALLY MATTERS

By forty, lifestyle starts showing up in the urinary and sexual system. Alcohol can worsen nighttime urination and erections. Caffeine can worsen urgency. Obesity can worsen sleep apnea, testosterone levels, erections, and urinary symptoms. Diabetes can increase urinary frequency and damage nerves. Smoking harms blood vessels and erections. Poor sleep affects hormones, metabolism, and bladder control. Sedentary living worsens vascular health.

A man should not be told that lifestyle fixes every prostate problem. It does not. Lifestyle will not remove a prostate obstruction. It will not treat prostate cancer. It will not replace PSA evaluation. But lifestyle can reduce the burden on the system.

Better weight, better sleep, better bowel function, better metabolic health, and less alcohol can improve the terrain in which the prostate, bladder, and sexual system operate. This is the correct way to discuss lifestyle. Not as moral judgment. As physiology.

THE 40+ BASELINE VISIT

A strong forty-plus baseline visit should be practical. The doctor should review urinary symptoms, sexual function, family history, PSA risk, fertility goals, testosterone concerns, sleep, metabolic health, bowel habits, medications, and red flags. The man should leave understanding whether he is average risk or increased risk, whether PSA screening should start now or later, whether urinary symptoms need objective testing, and whether any lifestyle or medical issues should be addressed.

If he is asymptomatic and low risk, he may need education more than testing. If he is high risk, PSA screening may begin earlier. If he is symptomatic, the bladder and prostate should be evaluated.

If he is considering testosterone, the prostate and fertility discussion should happen first. If he has ED, cardiovascular and metabolic risk should be considered.

This is not overtesting. This is rational baseline care.

RED FLAGS IN THE FORTIES

Some symptoms should never be brushed off because of age. Blood in the urine deserves evaluation. Inability to urinate is urgent. Recurrent urinary infections in a man require explanation. A rapidly rising PSA needs follow-up. Severe nighttime urination affecting sleep should be understood. New pelvic pain with fever or significant urinary symptoms may represent infection. Bone pain or unexplained weight loss in a man with concerning prostate cancer risk requires attention. A very weak stream or large amount of urine left behind after urination should not be dismissed.

These are not symptoms to "watch for a while" without a plan. The point of a checklist is not to make men fearful. It is to tell them what deserves action.

THE MAN WHO TRACKS EVERYTHING EXCEPT HIS PROSTATE

This is the patient I see more often now. He tracks his sleep, heart rate, testosterone, workouts, body fat, supplements, glucose, and nutrition. He may know his vitamin D level, his resting heart rate, and his VO_2 max. He may have tried peptides, testosterone, GLP-1 weight loss medication, or advanced blood panels.

Then I ask his prostate size. He does not know. I ask his PSA trend.

He is not sure. I ask how much urine is left behind after he urinates. No one has checked. I ask how many times he wakes up at night to urinate.

He says, "Usually two or three." That man is not fully optimized. He is highly engaged, but the prostate-bladder system has been left out of the plan. That is exactly what modern men's health needs to correct. A man cannot call himself optimized if his bladder is waking him every night and nobody has measured why.

WHAT A MAN SHOULD KNOW BY FORTY-PLUS

By the time a man is in his forties, he should know his prostate risk category. He should know his family history. He should know when PSA screening should begin for him. He should know whether urinary symptoms are present. He should know whether erectile dysfunction is a vascular warning sign. He should know that testosterone therapy requires monitoring. He should know that fertility may be affected by hormone treatment and prostate procedures. He should know that nighttime urination is not automatically normal.

He does not need to become obsessed with the prostate. He needs to stop ignoring it. That is the difference.

DR. SHUSTERMAN'S MODERN PROSTATE TAKEAWAY

The forties are not too early to think about the prostate. They are the right decade to establish awareness, risk, and baseline function. A man over forty should know his family history, understand when PSA screening should begin, pay attention to urinary changes, take erectile dysfunction seriously, discuss testosterone safely, protect fertility if it still matters, and recognize that sleep, weight, metabolic health, constipation, and bladder function all connect to prostate health.

Not every man in his forties needs extensive testing. But every man in his forties should know what to watch for and when to act.

The goal is not fear. The goal is control. A modern man should not wait until his prostate becomes an emergency before he learns how it works.

CHAPTER 29

THE 50+ PROSTATE PROTOCOL

FIGURE 29.1

The 50+ Prostate Protocol

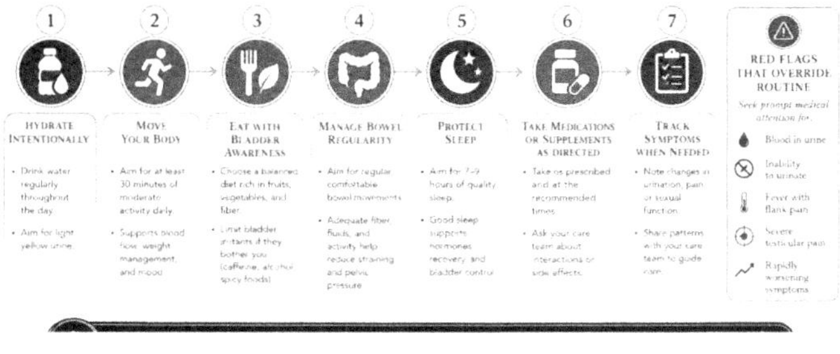

Men over fifty often need a more deliberate prostate, bladder, PSA, sexual-function, and healthspan review.

FIGURE *29.1 - The 50+ Prostate Protocol. Men over fifty often need a more deliberate prostate and bladder review.*

Fifty is the age when prostate care should become more structured. That does not mean every man turns fifty and suddenly has a prostate disease. It does not mean every man needs a procedure. It does not mean every man needs an MRI, biopsy, cystoscopy, or every test available. It means the conversation should become more serious and more organized.

By fifty, many men have already begun to notice changes. The stream may be weaker. Nighttime urination may have started. Erections may be less reliable. Sleep may be less restorative. Weight may be harder to control. PSA screening may enter the picture. Family history may become more relevant. Testosterone therapy may be considered. Longevity medicine may become more interesting.

This is the decade when men should stop drifting. A man over fifty should not be told only, "You're getting older." He should not receive automatic medication refills without measurement. He should not be reassured with vague language. He should not wait until urinary retention, bladder stones, recurrent infections, or a catheter forces the conversation.

The purpose of the 50+ Prostate Protocol is to create a clear, practical, modern approach. The goal is not fear. The goal is control. A man over fifty should understand his prostate, his bladder, his PSA risk, his urinary function, his sexual function, and his next step.

WHY FIFTY MATTERS

Fifty is not old, but it is a meaningful threshold. Benign prostate enlargement becomes more common. PSA screening becomes more relevant for many men. Erectile dysfunction becomes more common. Sleep problems become more common. Metabolic issues such as weight gain, insulin resistance, blood pressure, and cholesterol changes often become more visible. Testosterone questions become more frequent. These issues overlap.

A man may come in for urinary symptoms and discover that his sleep is being destroyed. Another may come in for erectile dysfunction and discover vascular risk. Another may come in for testosterone and discover that his PSA has never been properly followed. Another may come in for PSA and reveal that he wakes up four times a night but never mentioned it because he thought it was normal.

The prostate is often the doorway into a broader men's health evaluation. That is why fifty should not be handled casually.

At fifty, a man should know where he stands. If everything is normal, excellent. Now he has a baseline. If something is changing, it can be addressed before the bladder becomes damaged or cancer risk becomes more complicated.

Early understanding is not aggressive medicine. It is intelligent medicine.

THE FIRST VISIT SHOULD BE A PROTOCOL, NOT A CONVERSATION ONLY

Many men have had the experience of a casual prostate visit. The doctor asks a few questions. Maybe does an exam. Maybe orders or reviews a PSA. Maybe prescribes medication. The patient leaves with the phrase "enlarged prostate" but no real understanding. That is not enough.

A fifty-plus prostate visit should follow a structure. The doctor should ask about urinary symptoms in a systematic way. He should ask about nighttime urination, weak stream, urgency, incomplete emptying, stopping and starting, straining, dribbling, infections, blood in the urine, stones, and retention. He should ask about sexual function, ejaculation, libido, testosterone interest, fertility if relevant, and quality of life.

He should also ask about sleep, diabetes, medications, constipation, alcohol, caffeine, family history, and cancer risk. A man's prostate does not exist in isolation. The bladder, bowel, sleep, hormones, sexual function, and metabolic system all matter. The visit should feel like a map being created. Not like a box being checked.

THE SYMPTOM SCORE

Every man over fifty should be asked about urinary symptoms in enough detail that the doctor can tell whether the issue is mild, moderate, or severe. One way to do this is with a standardized symptom score. The specific name matters less to patients than the purpose. The questionnaire asks about the symptoms that men commonly experience: incomplete emptying, frequent urination, stopping and starting, urgency, weak stream, straining, and waking at night. This helps because men often minimize.

A patient may say, "I'm fine," then the questionnaire reveals that he wakes up three times per night, has urgency, and has a weak stream. Another man may complain loudly, but the score shows mild symptoms and points the doctor toward anxiety, bladder sensitivity, or another issue.

The score is not the diagnosis. It is the patient's report in a structured form.

It helps track whether medication or treatment is working. It also helps prevent vague follow-up. If the score remains high after medication, that should trigger a conversation. If the score improves but the bladder is still not emptying, that also matters. Symptoms are important. But symptoms are only one piece of the protocol.

URINE TESTING SHOULD NOT BE SKIPPED

A simple urine test is part of a practical fifty-plus evaluation, especially when symptoms are present. Urine can show blood, infection, glucose, protein, and other clues. Blood in the urine may require further workup. Infection changes the plan. Glucose in the urine may point toward diabetes. Protein may suggest kidney-related concerns.

This matters because urinary symptoms are not always prostate symptoms. A man with urgency and frequency may have infection. A man waking at night may have diabetes. A man with blood in the urine needs evaluation beyond BPH. A man with recurrent infections may have poor emptying, stones, or another source.

Skipping urine testing can miss basic information. Modern prostate care does not need to be complicated to be better. Sometimes it begins with doing the simple things properly.

PSA SHOULD BE INTERPRETED, NOT WORSHIPPED

For many men over fifty, PSA becomes part of the protocol. PSA is important, but it must be interpreted correctly. It is not a cancer diagnosis. It is a prostate-made protein used as a cancer-risk signal. It can rise from prostate cancer, but also from benign enlargement, inflammation, infection, urinary retention, and recent procedures or irritation.

The key is context. A fifty-five-year-old man with a PSA that has risen quickly deserves attention. A man with a very large prostate and a stable mildly elevated PSA may be different. A man with a strong family history deserves a lower threshold for concern. A man with urinary infection may need treatment and repeat testing before the PSA is interpreted. A man on medications that lower PSA needs special interpretation.

AUA/SUO early-detection guidance supports offering regular prostate cancer screening every two to four years for men aged fifty to sixty-nine, with personalization based on risk and shared decision-making. The same guidance also supports baseline screening earlier, around forty-five to fifty, and earlier still for increased-risk men. That framework matters because it moves PSA away from fear and toward structured risk assessment.

The patient-friendly point is this: a man over fifty should not ask only whether his PSA is normal. He should ask what the PSA means for him.

FAMILY HISTORY CHANGES THE PLAN

A fifty-plus prostate protocol must include family history. The question should not be only, "Any prostate cancer in the family?" That is too vague. The doctor should ask who had it, how old they were, whether it was aggressive, whether it spread, whether they died from it, and whether there are related cancers in the family such as breast, ovarian, pancreatic, or certain colon cancers that could suggest inherited risk.

A father diagnosed with low-risk prostate cancer at eighty is different from a brother diagnosed with aggressive prostate cancer at fifty-two. Multiple relatives are different from one. A known genetic mutation changes the conversation even more. Family history can affect when screening starts, how often PSA is checked, whether MRI is used earlier, whether genetic testing is considered, and how aggressively abnormal results are evaluated.

A man should know his family history before the doctor needs it. If he does not know it, fifty is a good age to start asking.

THE PROSTATE SHOULD BE MEASURED WHEN SYMPTOMS EXIST

A man over fifty with urinary symptoms should not be managed for years without knowing the size and shape of his prostate. The word enlarged is not enough.

The doctor should know whether the prostate is mildly enlarged, moderately enlarged, severely enlarged, or very large. He should know whether the prostate is growing into the bladder opening. He should know whether the anatomy explains the symptoms and whether medication is likely to work.

Ultrasound is one practical way to measure the prostate and bladder. It can show the size of the gland and help assess whether prostate tissue is bulging into the bladder outlet. It can also help measure how much urine remains after the patient urinates.

This is where modern evaluation becomes different from older ways of evaluating the prostate. A finger exam may give a rough impression in selected situations, but it cannot measure the prostate accurately. It cannot show whether the gland is bulging into the bladder. It cannot tell how much urine is left behind. It cannot measure the stream. A man with urinary symptoms deserves more than a finger and a guess.

THE BLADDER MUST BE CHECKED

The 50+ Prostate Protocol is not only about the prostate. It is also about the bladder.

One of the most important questions is how much urine remains after the man urinates. Patients may feel empty and still leave urine behind. That leftover urine can suggest blockage, bladder weakness, or both. It can increase the risk of infections, stones, worsening frequency, and retention. This measurement is simple, but it changes care.

If very little urine is left behind, that is reassuring. If a large amount remains, the situation becomes more serious. A man who is leaving urine behind should not be told he is fine because he is on medication. The bladder does not care that a prescription was written.

The bladder cares whether it can empty. In BPH care, bladder safety is the central question.

THE STREAM SHOULD BE MEASURED WHEN IT MATTERS

Men describe their stream in subjective language. "It's weak.""It's not terrible.""It's slower than it used to be.""I have to wait." Those statements matter, but the stream can also be measured. A urine flow test tells us how fast the urine comes out. A very slow stream may suggest obstruction, weak bladder contraction, or both. The result is most useful when interpreted together with prostate size, prostate shape, symptoms, and urine left behind.

A man over fifty who has a weak stream, straining, stopping and starting, or incomplete emptying should not rely only on impressions. He should know whether the stream is objectively slow.

That number helps guide treatment. If the stream is strong and the bladder empties, the urgency may be more of a bladder problem. If the stream is slow and urine is left behind, prostate obstruction becomes more likely. If the stream is slow but the prostate is not very obstructive, bladder weakness or another issue may need attention.

Testing separates possibilities. That is what a protocol should do.

WHEN A CAMERA TEST IS NEEDED

Cystoscopy is a small camera test that allows the doctor to look inside the urine channel, prostate channel, bladder opening, and bladder. Not every man over fifty needs cystoscopy. It should not be automatic. But it is extremely useful in the right situations.

If a man has blood in the urine, recurrent infections, bladder stones, retention, severe symptoms, failed medication, concern for narrowing in the urine channel, or is considering a prostate procedure, cystoscopy may be the test that clarifies the anatomy. It can show whether the prostate is blocking from the inside. It can reveal a tight bladder neck, scar tissue, stones, tumors, inflammation, or changes in the bladder from long-standing obstruction.

Patients often fear cystoscopy more than they need to. In a modern office, with appropriate numbing and technique, it is usually brief and well tolerated. A camera test should not be used casually, but when the internal anatomy matters, it can prevent guessing.

WHEN BLADDER PRESSURE TESTING IS NEEDED

Some men need more than size, stream, and leftover urine measurements. They need to know whether the bladder muscle is still strong enough.

This is where bladder pressure testing comes in. Doctors call it urodynamics. The patient-friendly explanation is simple: it measures how the bladder stores urine and how well it can push urine out.

This test is not for every man with mild symptoms. But it becomes important when the patient has very high leftover urine, urinary retention, failed catheter removal attempts, symptoms that do not match prostate size, suspected weak bladder, neurologic disease, or persistent symptoms after treatment.

Before promising that a prostate procedure will fix everything, the doctor sometimes needs to know whether the bladder can still do its job. Opening the channel helps only if the bladder can push. That is why bladder testing can be so valuable in selected men.

MEDICATION SHOULD HAVE A SIX-MONTH REASSESSMENT

Many men over fifty are placed on prostate medication and then left on it for years. That should not happen without reassessment.

If medication is started, there should be a goal. Is the goal a stronger stream? Less nighttime urination? Less urgency? Better emptying? Better quality of life? Avoiding retention? The doctor and patient should know what success means.

A six-month refill should not be automatic. It should be a checkpoint.

Is the man actually better? How much better? Are side effects acceptable? Is the bladder emptying? Is the stream improved? Does the prostate anatomy suggest medication is enough? Is he still waking all night? Is he still living around bathrooms? If medication is working and the bladder is safe, continue.

If medication only helps a little and the bladder remains at risk, change the plan. Better is not fixed.

WHEN THE CONVERSATION SHOULD MOVE BEYOND MEDICATION

A fifty-plus man should move beyond a medication-only conversation when the evidence shows the medication is not enough. That may mean persistent bothersome symptoms, a very slow stream, urine left behind after urination, recurrent infections, bladder stones, retention, significant prostate tissue growing into the bladder opening, unacceptable medication side effects, or sleep that remains destroyed by nighttime urination.

Moving beyond medication does not automatically mean major surgery. It means the next conversation should be anatomy-based. Is the prostate small enough and shaped appropriately for a targeted water-vapor procedure? Is the gland larger or bulging into the bladder opening in a way that makes prostate artery embolization attractive? Is tissue removal needed? Is the bladder weak and in need of pressure testing first? Is the main issue bladder overactivity rather than obstruction?

The treatment should match the anatomy and the bladder. That is modern prostate care.

SEXUAL FUNCTION BELONGS IN THE PROTOCOL

A prostate visit over fifty should include sexual function. Many men will not bring it up unless asked. They may think it is not relevant. They may be embarrassed. They may assume the doctor is focused only on urine or PSA. But sexual function is highly relevant.

Erectile dysfunction can be a sign of vascular disease, diabetes, low testosterone, medication side effects, poor sleep, or metabolic dysfunction. Prostate medications can affect ejaculation. Prostate procedures can affect ejaculation or sexual confidence. Prostate cancer treatment can affect erections, orgasm, ejaculation, and urinary control. Testosterone therapy requires PSA monitoring.

A man over fifty should not have prostate care in one room and sexual health in another. They are connected.

A good protocol asks about erections, libido, ejaculation, orgasm, pain with ejaculation, and treatment priorities. It also asks whether preserving ejaculation matters before choosing BPH treatment.

Sexual function is not cosmetic. It is part of the man's health.

TESTOSTERONE AND THE FIFTY-PLUS PROSTATE

Many men over fifty ask about testosterone. That conversation should be welcomed, but it must be done properly. Testosterone therapy can help selected men with true testosterone deficiency, but it requires prostate awareness.

Before starting testosterone, a man should know his PSA when appropriate, his urinary baseline, his prostate history, and his risk factors. If he has significant urinary symptoms, the prostate-bladder system should be evaluated. If the PSA is elevated or rising, it should be addressed before therapy is started casually.

Testosterone is not automatic prostate cancer fuel, but it is also not a harmless supplement. Hormones are medicine. Monitoring is not optional. A fifty-plus protocol should allow men to optimize hormones safely, not recklessly.

SLEEP AND NOCTURIA

Nighttime urination deserves special attention after fifty. A man waking up three or four times a night should not be told simply that he is getting older. The cause should be evaluated. The prostate may be blocking. The bladder may be irritated. The bladder may not empty. Sleep apnea may be causing nighttime urine production. Diabetes, evening alcohol, fluid timing, leg swelling, heart function, kidney function, or medications may contribute.

Nocturia is not only a prostate symptom. It is a sleep symptom. And sleep affects everything: energy, testosterone, metabolism, weight, cardiovascular health, memory, mood, and sexual function.

A serious fifty-plus prostate protocol asks how many times the man wakes up at night and whether that pattern is worsening. No man is optimized if his bladder controls his sleep.

CONSTIPATION AND PELVIC SYMPTOMS

Constipation should be part of the fifty-plus protocol because the pelvis is a crowded space. The rectum sits behind the prostate and bladder. Chronic constipation and straining can worsen urinary urgency, pelvic pressure, incomplete emptying sensations, and pelvic floor tension. In some men, constipation is not the main problem but makes every urinary symptom worse.

A man over fifty with urinary symptoms should be asked about bowel habits. Does he strain? Does he feel incomplete bowel emptying? Do urinary symptoms worsen when constipated? Is there pelvic pressure? Treating the prostate while ignoring constipation can produce incomplete results.

The prostate, bladder, bowel, and pelvic floor live in the same neighborhood. The protocol should remember that.

RED FLAGS OVER FIFTY

Some findings should move a man more quickly into evaluation. Blood in the urine should not be ignored. Urinary retention is urgent. Recurrent urinary infections in a man need explanation. Bladder stones suggest incomplete emptying or another underlying issue. A rapidly rising PSA requires follow-up. Severe nighttime urination that damages sleep deserves attention. A very weak stream or a large amount of urine left behind after urination should not be dismissed. Bone pain or unexplained weight loss in a man with concerning prostate cancer risk requires prompt evaluation. These are not symptoms to normalize.

They are signals that the prostate, bladder, or cancer-risk pathway may need more urgent attention. A protocol helps men and doctors avoid missing those signals.

THE ANNUAL OR SEMIANNUAL PLAN

The frequency of follow-up depends on the man. A low-risk man with no symptoms and a reassuring PSA may need routine monitoring. A man on medication should be reassessed to ensure the medication still works and the bladder remains safe. A man with elevated PSA, strong family history, significant symptoms, high leftover urine, slow stream, or concerning anatomy may need closer follow-up.

The point is not that every man over fifty needs the same schedule. The point is that every man over fifty should have a plan.

What are we watching? PSA? Symptoms? Prostate size? Bladder emptying? Stream speed? Testosterone therapy? Cancer risk? Medication response? If no one can answer what is being followed, the follow-up is not meaningful.

THE MODERN UROLOGIST APPROACH

The modern fifty-plus prostate visit should not be a ritual. It should be a structured evaluation. The patient should leave understanding his urinary symptoms, prostate size if symptoms require measurement, bladder emptying, urine stream when relevant, PSA risk, family history, sexual function, hormone considerations, and next step.

If he is low risk, he should leave reassured for a reason. If medication is appropriate, he should know what it is expected to do and how success will be measured. If further testing is needed, he should know why.

If a procedure is being discussed, he should understand how the procedure matches his anatomy. If PSA is abnormal, he should understand the risk pathway. That is the difference between modern care and vague care.

DR. SHUSTERMAN'S MODERN PROSTATE TAKEAWAY

The fifty-plus prostate visit should not be casual. It should be a protocol. A man over fifty should have his urinary symptoms reviewed carefully, his PSA interpreted intelligently, his family history understood, his sexual function discussed, his bladder safety considered, and his prostate measured when symptoms or risk justify it.

Not every man needs every test. But every man deserves a structured plan.

If he has urinary symptoms, the doctor should know whether the prostate is enlarged, whether it is blocking the bladder opening, how much urine is left behind after urination, and how fast the urine comes out. If he is on medication, there should be a reassessment point. If PSA is abnormal, the risk should be clarified. If sleep is being destroyed by nighttime urination, the cause should be investigated.

The goal is not to scare men after fifty. The goal is to stop letting them drift. A modern prostate visit should answer one simple question: Are we protecting the man before the prostate becomes an emergency?

CHAPTER 30

HOW TO TALK TO YOUR UROLOGIST

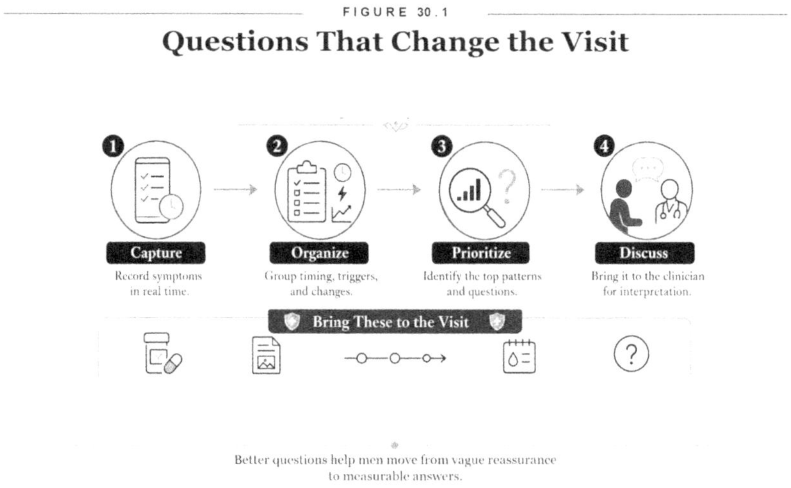

FIGURE 30.1 - QUESTIONS *That Change the Visit. Specific questions move the visit from reassurance to measurable answers.*

Most men do not know what to ask when they walk into a urology office. That is not their fault.

The prostate is confusing. The language is technical. The symptoms are personal. The decisions can be intimidating. A man may be embarrassed to talk about weak stream, urgency, waking up at night, erections, ejaculation, testosterone, or cancer fear. He may not know which details matter. He may assume the doctor will tell him everything he needs to know.

Sometimes that happens. Sometimes it does not.

A man may leave the office with only a vague phrase: "Your prostate is enlarged." He may be told, "Your PSA is a little high." He may be given medication. He may be told to come back in six months. He may be reassured that he is fine.

But fine compared to what? Fine because the PSA is stable? Fine because he can still urinate? Fine because the prostate does not feel alarming on a finger exam? Fine because medication helped a little? Fine because no one has measured what actually matters?

This is where men need to become better advocates for themselves. A man does not need to become a urologist. He does not need to memorize every medical term. He does not need to walk into the office with a stack of internet printouts. But he should know enough to ask the questions that protect him from vague care.

The most important question is simple: Is my bladder safe? That question changes the visit.

THE MAN WHO WAS TOLD HE WAS FINE

A man comes in after years of follow-up elsewhere. He has been taking medication. He has been seen regularly. He has not ignored the problem. Every visit, he was told things were stable. He was told the prostate was enlarged but not alarming. He was told to continue medication. But he still could not urinate well.

He woke up at night. His stream was weak. He sometimes felt he did not empty. He planned his life around the bathroom. Over time, these symptoms became his normal. Then he went into retention.

Suddenly he could not urinate at all. He ended up in the emergency room with a catheter. Now the conversation was no longer about mild symptoms, routine medication, or reassurance. Now it was about whether the bladder could recover. The patient's question was obvious: "How was I fine if this was happening?" That question should make every urologist uncomfortable.

A man on multiple medications who still cannot urinate well is not fine. A man waking all night is not fine. A man leaving significant urine behind after he finishes is not fine. A man with a very slow stream is not fine. A man whose bladder is being damaged every day is not fine.

The word fine should be earned. It should be based on measurement, not habit.

THE PROBLEM WITH VAGUE REASSURANCE

Reassurance has value when it is based on real information. If a man's prostate is measured, his bladder empties well, his urine stream is reasonable, his PSA is appropriate for his age and risk, and his symptoms are mild, reassurance is appropriate. That is good medicine. But reassurance without measurement can be dangerous.

"You're fine" should not mean "I did not look closely." It should not mean "your prostate feels okay by finger exam." It should not mean "you are already taking medication." It should not mean "your symptoms are common for your age." It should not mean "come back when it gets worse." Men deserve better than that. A modern urology visit should explain what is known and what is not known. If the doctor does not know how much urine is left behind after urination, then the doctor should not pretend the bladder is definitely safe. If no one has measured the urine stream, then no one knows how slow it really is. If no one has measured the prostate, then "enlarged" is not enough. If no one has evaluated whether prostate tissue is growing into the bladder opening, then the anatomy is incomplete.

A man does not need reassurance as a sedative. He needs reassurance as a conclusion.

THE MOST IMPORTANT THINGS TO KNOW

If a man has urinary symptoms, he should leave the urologist's office understanding a few basic things in plain English. He should know how large the prostate is. He should know whether part of the prostate is growing into the bladder opening and blocking the exit like a ball valve. He should know how much urine is left behind after he urinates. He should know how fast the urine comes out. He should know whether the bladder appears safe.

The medical terms matter less than the meaning. Doctors may say prostate volume, intravesical protrusion, post-void residual, and Qmax. Those terms can be useful in a medical chart. But the patient should not have to speak in abbreviations to understand his body.

He should be able to say: "My prostate is moderately enlarged." "Part of it is growing into the bladder opening." "I am leaving too much urine behind." "My urine flow is slow." "My bladder is still emptying safely." Or, "My bladder is at risk." That kind of understanding changes everything. It turns the patient from passive recipient into informed participant.

IF THE VISIT IS ONLY A FINGER EXAM

For generations, men have associated prostate care with the finger exam. That exam may still have selected uses, but it is not a modern BPH evaluation by itself.

If a man has urinary symptoms and the entire evaluation is a finger exam and a prescription, the doctor is flying blind. A finger exam cannot accurately measure prostate size. It cannot show whether prostate tissue is growing into the bladder. It cannot measure how much urine is left behind after urination. It cannot measure the speed of the stream. It cannot show whether the bladder is weakening.

That does not mean every man needs every test. It means the evaluation should match the complaint.

If the complaint is weak stream, measure the stream. If the complaint is incomplete emptying, check how much urine remains. If the complaint is waking up all night, evaluate the prostate, bladder, sleep, and metabolic contributors. If medication is not working, understand the anatomy before simply refilling the prescription.

Stone-age tools should not define modern prostate care. A man should not feel embarrassed asking for objective testing. He should not be made to feel difficult because he wants to know whether the bladder is safe. That is the purpose of seeing a modern urologist.

QUESTIONS ABOUT MEDICATION

Men often leave the office with medication without fully understanding what it does. That should not happen.

If a doctor prescribes a prostate medication, the patient should ask what the medication is supposed to accomplish. Is it relaxing the prostate opening? Is it slowly shrinking the prostate? Is it helping erections and urinary symptoms together? How soon should it work? What side effects should he watch for? How will the doctor know whether it worked?

A medication should have an endpoint. If the man is taking a prostate-relaxing pill, did the stream improve? Is he waking up less? Is urine still being left behind? If he is taking a medication that slowly shrinks the prostate, is the prostate large enough for that strategy to make sense? How does it affect PSA interpretation? If he is taking daily tadalafil, is it mainly for erections, urinary symptoms, or both?

The patient should also ask what happens if the medication only helps a little. That is critical.

A man should not stay on medication for years because it produced partial improvement. Better is not fixed. If he still urinates poorly, still wakes up all night, still leaves urine behind, or still has prostate tissue blocking the bladder opening, the plan should evolve.

Medication is a tool. It is not a lifetime excuse to avoid measurement.

QUESTIONS ABOUT PROCEDURES

If a procedure is recommended, the first question should not be, "Is it new?" The first question should be, "Why does this procedure fit my anatomy?" Every BPH procedure has a mechanism. Some relax tissue. Some pull tissue aside. Some treat tissue with water vapor. Some reduce blood supply to the prostate. Some remove tissue. Some shell out tissue. Some are better for smaller glands. Some are better for larger glands. Some are more favorable for ejaculation. Some are more definitive but more anatomy-altering.

A man should understand what the procedure actually does. Does it treat the prostate through the urine channel or through the blood supply? Does it remove tissue or shrink it? Does it address prostate tissue growing into the bladder opening? How long is recovery? Will a catheter be needed? What urinary symptoms may temporarily worsen? What sexual side effects are possible? What happens if symptoms persist? What future options remain?

These are not minor questions. They are the core of informed consent.

A man should not agree to a procedure because it sounds modern, because his friend had it, or because it was advertised well. He should agree because the mechanism matches his prostate, his bladder, and his goals.

QUESTIONS ABOUT PSA

PSA is one of the most anxiety-producing parts of prostate care, so patients need to know how to discuss it intelligently. A man should ask whether his PSA is appropriate for his age, prostate size, and risk. He should ask whether the number is stable or rising. He should ask whether infection, inflammation, urinary retention, recent procedures, ejaculation, or prostate enlargement could be affecting it. He should ask whether it should be repeated. He should ask whether an advanced blood test or MRI would help clarify the risk. He should ask whether biopsy is truly needed and why.

Most importantly, he should understand that PSA is a risk signal, not a diagnosis. An elevated PSA does not automatically mean cancer. A normal PSA does not make a man bulletproof. The number has to be interpreted. Age and life expectancy also matter.

In my practice, I use eighty as an important practical cutoff. I do not recommend routine PSA screening after age eighty in the same way I would approach a younger man, because prostate cancer screening is most useful when the man has enough life expectancy to benefit from diagnosis and treatment. Many prostate cancers grow slowly, and the harms of chasing every PSA abnormality can outweigh the benefits in older men.

That does not mean PSA can never be checked after eighty. PSA is inexpensive. In some men, it may still provide useful information. A very healthy eighty-one-year-old with excellent function, strong family history, or concerning symptoms is different from a frail eighty-eight-year-old with major medical problems. But checking PSA is not the same as automatically acting on it. After a certain age, the key question becomes whether the result would change management. A man should ask, "If my PSA is abnormal, what would we actually do with that information?" That is the mature question.

QUESTIONS ABOUT BIOPSY

If biopsy is recommended, the patient should understand why. Was the biopsy recommended because of PSA? MRI? A suspicious lesion? Family history? A prior negative biopsy with persistent concern? An advanced blood test? A combination?

The patient should ask whether MRI has been done or should be done first. He should ask whether the suspicious area will be targeted. He should ask whether systematic samples will also be taken. He should ask whether the biopsy will be performed through the rectum or through the skin between the scrotum and anus, and why that route is being chosen. He should ask how infection risk is reduced. He should ask what to expect afterward and when results will be available.

A biopsy should not feel like a mysterious event. It should be part of a risk strategy.

The patient should also understand what happens if the biopsy is negative. Will PSA be followed? Will MRI be repeated? Was the suspicious area adequately sampled? When would another biopsy be considered? A negative biopsy without a follow-up plan is incomplete.

QUESTIONS AFTER A CANCER DIAGNOSIS

If a man is diagnosed with prostate cancer, he should resist the urge to make a fear-based decision in the first five minutes. The word cancer is powerful, but the plan depends on risk.

He should ask about the Grade Group, the Gleason pattern, the number of biopsy samples involved, how much cancer was found, whether there are aggressive microscopic features, whether MRI findings match the biopsy, and whether genomic testing would help. He should ask whether the cancer is low risk, favorable intermediate risk, unfavorable intermediate risk, high risk, or metastatic. He should ask whether PSMA PET imaging is needed for staging.

He should also ask whether active surveillance is reasonable. For many low-risk prostate cancers, careful monitoring may be better than immediate treatment. For higher-risk disease, treatment may be necessary. The point is not to avoid treatment. The point is to match treatment to biology.

Do not treat the word cancer. Treat the risk.

QUESTIONS ABOUT SEXUAL FUNCTION

Sexual function should be discussed before treatment, not after. A man should ask whether a medication may affect ejaculation, libido, erections, semen volume, or fertility. Before a prostate procedure, he should ask about ejaculation preservation, erection risk, orgasm changes, catheter time, and recovery. Before prostate cancer treatment, he should ask about urinary control, erections, ejaculation, hormone therapy, penile rehabilitation, and long-term function.

The doctor should not assume sexual function does not matter because the patient is older. Men in their sixties, seventies, and even eighties may care deeply about sexual function. Some may not be currently sexually active but still want to preserve the possibility. Some may value ejaculation. Others may not. The point is that the patient should decide based on information, not assumptions.

Preserving function is not cosmetic. It is part of treating the man.

QUESTIONS ABOUT TESTOSTERONE

If a man is considering testosterone therapy, the urologist should be part of the conversation. The patient should ask whether he truly has testosterone deficiency, whether the result was confirmed, and what symptoms treatment is meant to improve. He should ask what his baseline PSA is, whether urinary symptoms need evaluation, whether prostate cancer risk has been considered, whether fertility matters, and how blood count and PSA will be monitored.

Testosterone is not automatic prostate cancer fuel, but it is also not a casual supplement. Hormones are medicine. Monitoring is not optional. A man should be cautious about any clinic that prescribes testosterone without prostate awareness, fertility discussion, blood count monitoring, and follow-up.

WHEN TO SEEK ANOTHER OPINION

A man should consider another opinion when the explanation does not make sense, when he is being rushed, when only one option is discussed, when he is still symptomatic but repeatedly told he is fine, when the doctor does not measure the bladder despite urinary symptoms, when PSA is dismissed without a plan, or when a major procedure is recommended without clear reasoning. Getting another opinion is not disrespectful. It is reasonable.

This is especially true before irreversible prostate cancer treatment, major BPH surgery, or when the patient feels the recommendation is based more on what the doctor offers than on what the patient needs. A good doctor should not be threatened by thoughtful questions or second opinions. The goal is the right plan, not the fastest decision.

THE PROBLEM WITH BEING TOO PASSIVE

Many men are passive in medical visits. They do not want to bother the doctor. They do not want to seem anxious. They do not want to talk about sex. They do not want to admit how bad the urinary symptoms are. They accept vague explanations. They take the prescription. They go home. That passivity can be costly.

A man who does not say he wakes up four times a night may not get evaluated properly. A man who does not mention sexual side effects may stay on a medication he hates. A man who does not ask whether the bladder is emptying may not know he is retaining urine. A man who does not ask what an elevated PSA means may either panic unnecessarily or ignore something important.

The patient does not need to be aggressive. He needs to be honest and prepared.

THE MODERN UROLOGIST STANDARD

A modern urologist should be able to explain the plan in ordinary language. The patient should not leave confused by abbreviations. He should not be told only that the prostate is "big." He should not be given medication without knowing what it is supposed to do. He should not be offered a procedure without understanding why that procedure fits his anatomy. He should not be told that PSA is fine or bad without understanding the reason.

Good urology is not only technical. It is explanatory.

Patients make better decisions when they understand the mechanism. What is the problem? Why is it happening? What are we measuring? What does the treatment do? How will we know if it worked? What are the risks of waiting? What are the risks of acting? Those are the questions that separate modern care from vague care.

DO NOT LEAVE UNTIL YOU UNDERSTAND THE PLAN

A man does not need to leave the office knowing everything about urology. But he should leave knowing the plan.

If he has urinary symptoms, he should know whether the prostate and bladder have been evaluated enough. If he has elevated PSA, he should know whether the next step is repeat testing, advanced blood testing, MRI, biopsy, or monitoring. If he is taking medication, he should know how success will be judged. If he is considering a procedure, he should know why that procedure fits. If he has cancer, he should know the risk group and the next decision.

If the plan is not clear, ask again. A patient has the right to understand his own body.

DR. SHUSTERMAN'S MODERN PROSTATE TAKEAWAY

A man should not need a medical degree to talk to his urologist. He should know the key questions.

Is my bladder safe? How large is my prostate? Is prostate tissue growing into the bladder opening? How much urine is left behind after I urinate? How fast does the urine come out? Is medication truly working? Is my PSA appropriate for my age, prostate size, and risk? If I am over eighty, would checking PSA change what we would actually do? If biopsy is recommended, why? If cancer is found, what is the risk group? If treatment is recommended, how will it affect urination, erections, ejaculation, and quality of life?

A vague phrase is not a plan. "You're fine" is not good enough when a man is on pills and still cannot pee well. Modern prostate care should give men answers, not just reassurance. The most important question remains simple: Is my bladder safe?

CHAPTER 31

THE FUTURE OF PROSTATE CARE

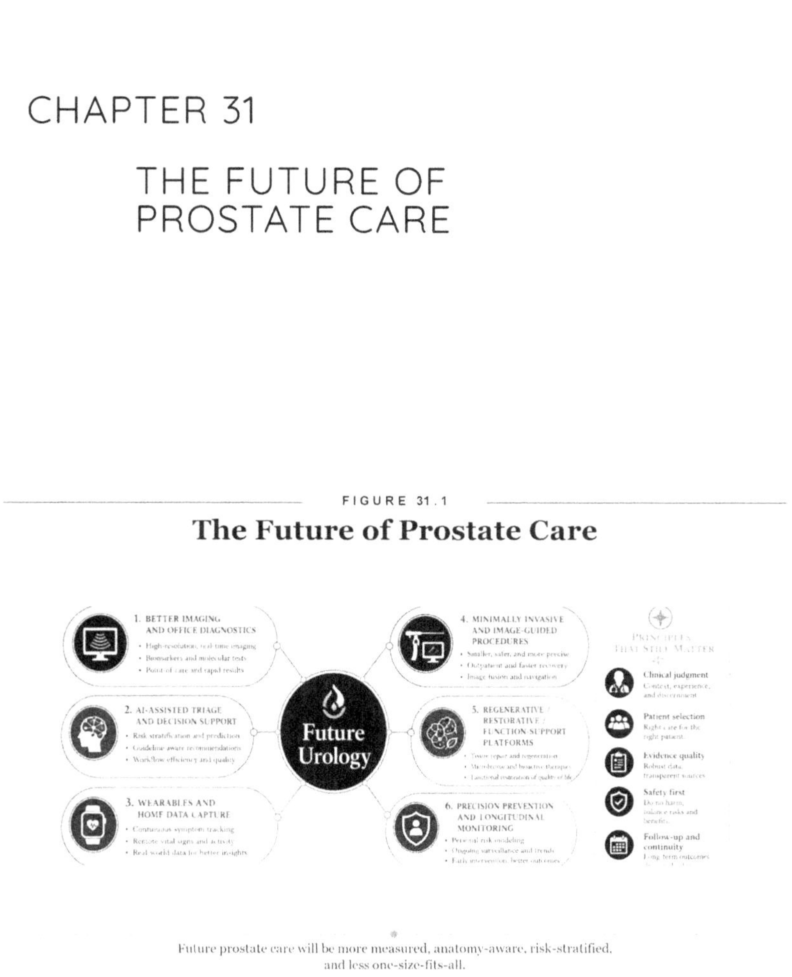

FIGURE *31.1 - The Future of Prostate Care. Future care will be more measured, anatomy-aware, and risk-stratified.*

The future of prostate care is smarter, earlier, and less destructive treatment. That is the sentence I want men to remember.

For too long, prostate care was reactive. Men waited until symptoms became severe. Doctors relied on limited tools. Patients were placed on medication and followed loosely. Procedures were delayed until the man could no longer tolerate the symptoms or until he went into retention. PSA created fear. Biopsy was often done without enough imaging. Prostate cancer treatment was too often driven by the word cancer rather than by the actual biology of the disease. That era should be ending.

Modern prostate care should not be built around fear, delay, and old habits. It should be built around measurement, imaging, risk stratification, anatomy, bladder protection, sexual function, and quality of life.

The future is not simply more treatment. It is better treatment.

A man should not have to wait until he cannot urinate before anyone measures his prostate. He should not have to take medication for years without knowing whether his bladder is safe. He should not have a biopsy without a thoughtful risk pathway. He should not have prostate cancer treated aggressively before the risk group is understood. He should not have testosterone therapy without PSA monitoring. He should not be told he is fine when he is waking up all night, urinating poorly, and living around bathrooms.

Modern prostate care should be precise enough to know when to watch, when to medicate, when to image, when to biopsy, when to treat, and when to leave the man alone. That is the future.

THE END OF STONE-AGE UROLOGY

Medicine changes slowly. Urology is no exception. Many practices still operate with habits built in an older era. A man complains of urinary symptoms. He gets a finger exam, a PSA, and a medication. If symptoms continue, the prescription is refilled. If things get worse, the dose is adjusted or another pill is added. If he eventually cannot urinate, then the conversation becomes urgent. That is not good enough anymore.

A finger exam may have had a historical role, but it cannot define modern BPH care. It cannot accurately measure prostate size. It cannot show whether prostate tissue is growing into the bladder opening. It cannot measure how much urine is left behind after urination. It cannot measure the speed of the stream. It cannot tell whether the bladder is weakening.

DRE-and-medication-only care belongs to Stone Age urology. That does not mean older doctors were foolish. They worked with the tools they had. But once better tools exist, the standard should rise. Ultrasound, bladder scans, urine flow testing, cystoscopy, MRI, advanced blood tests, PSMA PET scans, genomic testing, prostate artery embolization, focal therapy, and AI-assisted risk analysis all change what is possible.

The problem is that medical culture often lags behind technology. Even when better approaches are obvious, large systems move slowly. Training patterns persist. Institutions protect old pathways. Doctors recommend what they know. Equipment investments shape treatment habits. Guidelines evolve slowly. Patients may be offered only the options available in one office instead of the options that fit them best.

The future of prostate care requires something more aggressive than new technology. It requires a new mindset.

MEASUREMENT BEFORE REASSURANCE

The future should be built on measurement. A man with urinary symptoms should not be reassured vaguely. He should know what is happening. How large is the prostate? Is it growing into the bladder opening? Is urine left behind after he finishes? How fast does the urine come out? Is the bladder safe?

Those are not exotic questions. They are basic questions.

If the bladder empties well, the stream is reasonable, the prostate is not creating dangerous anatomy, and symptoms are mild, reassurance may be appropriate. But if the bladder is leaving urine behind, if the stream is very slow, if the prostate is physically blocking the bladder opening, or if sleep is being destroyed, reassurance without action becomes dangerous.

Modern care should not say "you're fine" unless the system has been evaluated. That does not mean every man needs every test. It means the testing should match the question. If the question is bladder emptying, check the bladder. If the question is stream strength, measure the flow. If the question is prostate anatomy, image the prostate. If the question is cancer risk, interpret PSA properly and use MRI or advanced testing when appropriate.

The future of care is not more random testing. It is the right test before the right decision.

THE PROSTATE-BLADDER SYSTEM

One of the most important shifts in modern prostate care is recognizing that BPH is not just a prostate disease. It is a prostate-bladder disease.

The prostate may create the blockage, but the bladder has to fight it. Over time, the bladder may become irritated, overactive, stretched, weakened, or unable to empty properly. If the obstruction is treated early enough, the bladder may recover well. If treatment is delayed too long, the prostate may no longer be the only problem.

This is why future BPH care should focus on bladder protection, not just symptom reduction. A medication that improves symptoms slightly but leaves the bladder retaining urine is not enough. A procedure that improves the stream but leaves the patient with terrible urgency may not feel like success. A treatment that ignores the bladder is incomplete.

The future is not just opening the channel. The future is preserving function.

That means measuring urine left behind. It means measuring the stream. It means understanding bladder strength when needed. It means not waiting for retention. It means recognizing that urgency and nighttime urination may be bladder symptoms created by years of prostate resistance.

The bladder is not a footnote. It is the organ we are trying to protect.

SMARTER PSA CARE

The future of PSA is not to abandon it. The future is to use it intelligently.

PSA is not a cancer diagnosis. It is a signal. A man's PSA has to be interpreted in context: age, prostate size, trend, family history, inflammation, infection, urinary retention, medications, MRI findings, and overall risk.

The old PSA pathway was too crude. PSA goes up, everyone panics, biopsy follows. That approach found cancers, but it also created anxiety, unnecessary biopsies, overdiagnosis, and overtreatment.

The modern pathway is more nuanced. If PSA is newly elevated, it may be repeated. If infection or retention is present, that may need to be addressed. If the prostate is very large, the PSA may be partly explained by volume. If the risk remains unclear, advanced blood tests or MRI may help. If MRI shows a suspicious lesion, biopsy can be targeted. If biopsy finds low-risk disease, surveillance may be appropriate. If higher-risk cancer is found, staging and treatment should follow.

This is the future: not ignoring PSA, not worshipping PSA, but interpreting PSA. Age also matters. I do not recommend routine PSA screening after age eighty in the same way I approach younger men. After eighty, the question becomes more practical: would this result change what we do? PSA is inexpensive, and there may be selected healthy older men where checking it still makes sense. But checking a number is not the same as automatically chasing it with biopsy or treatment.

A healthy, active eighty-one-year-old with strong risk factors is not the same as a frail eighty-eight-year-old with major medical problems. Life expectancy, health, goals, and the likely benefit of diagnosis all matter.

The future of PSA care is personalized decision-making. Not reflex.

MRI BEFORE BIOPSY

The future of prostate cancer diagnosis includes better imaging before biopsy. MRI changed the biopsy conversation because it gives us a map. PSA tells us there may be a risk. MRI helps show whether there is a suspicious area and where it is.

A man should not be rushed from PSA anxiety into blind sampling when better information is available. MRI can help decide who needs biopsy, where the biopsy should target, and how concerning the situation appears. It is especially valuable when PSA remains elevated after a prior negative biopsy, when the risk is unclear, or when targeted sampling may improve detection of meaningful cancer.

MRI is not perfect. A negative MRI does not guarantee there is no cancer. A suspicious MRI does not prove cancer. Biopsy remains the proof. But MRI makes the pathway smarter.

The future is not more biopsy. The future is smarter biopsy.

That distinction matters because prostate cancer diagnosis must balance two goals. We do not want to miss aggressive cancer. We also do not want to overdiagnose and overtreat harmless disease. MRI helps us move toward that balance.

PSMA PET AND KNOWING WHERE THE CANCER IS

For higher-risk prostate cancer, the future also includes better staging. PSMA PET scanning has changed the way physicians can look for prostate cancer outside the prostate. In selected patients, especially those with higher-risk disease, it can help identify whether cancer has spread to lymph nodes, bones, or other locations. This matters because treatment depends on location.

A cancer truly confined to the prostate may be treated with curative local therapy. A cancer that has spread needs a different strategy. A man should not undergo major local treatment for higher-risk disease without asking whether the cancer has been staged appropriately.

The future of cancer treatment starts with knowing where the cancer actually is. That may sound obvious, but for years treatment decisions were made with less precise imaging. Better staging allows better planning. It can prevent undertreatment. It can prevent overtreatment. It can identify men who need systemic therapy, radiation fields adjusted, or different combinations of care. Cancer treatment should not begin in the dark.

GENOMIC TESTING AND BIOLOGY

The future of prostate cancer care is not only imaging. It is biology.

Two cancers can look similar but behave differently. Grade, PSA, MRI, and biopsy volume are essential, but in selected cases, genomic testing can add another layer of information. These tests look at patterns of gene activity in the cancer tissue to help estimate how aggressive the cancer may be.

This can be useful when a man is deciding between active surveillance and treatment, especially in low-risk or favorable intermediate-risk disease where the decision is not obvious. The patient-friendly idea is simple: we are trying to understand not just what the cancer looks like, but how it may behave.

Genomic testing does not replace judgment. It does not decide everything by itself. But when used correctly, it can make the decision more personal and more precise. The future of prostate cancer care is not treating every cancer the same way. It is matching treatment intensity to the cancer's true risk.

FOCAL THERAPY AND PRESERVING FUNCTION

One of the most important future directions in prostate cancer treatment is focal therapy. The concept is powerful: if the cancer is visible, localized, and well mapped, why treat the entire prostate in every man? Why not treat the cancer focus while preserving more of the surrounding gland and function?

This idea will not apply to every patient. Prostate cancer can be multifocal. Some cancers are too aggressive, too widespread, or too poorly mapped for focal therapy. Follow-up after focal therapy is essential because the rest of the prostate remains. But for the right man, focal therapy represents a major philosophical shift.

It asks whether we can control cancer while preserving erections, ejaculation, urinary control, and quality of life. It moves away from the idea that every prostate cancer must be treated by removing or radiating the whole gland. This does not mean focal therapy replaces surgery or radiation.

It means the future should include more individualized options. The best cancer treatment is not only the one that controls disease. It is the one that controls disease while preserving the man as much as possible.

PAE AND THE IMAGE-GUIDED BPH FUTURE

In BPH, one of the most important modern shifts is prostate artery embolization. PAE proves that the prostate does not always have to be treated by cutting through the urine channel. It can be treated through its blood supply. By reducing blood flow to targeted areas of the prostate, the gland can shrink and soften over time.

This is especially important for larger prostates and for men whose prostate tissue is growing into the bladder opening. It is also attractive because it preserves anatomy and future options. A man may still have other treatments later if needed, but PAE can reduce the gland without directly carving through the channel. That is a different kind of thinking.

The old model was to keep men on medication as long as possible and then eventually cut or remove tissue. The modern model asks whether an image-guided vascular treatment can reduce obstruction earlier, preserve function, and protect the bladder.

PAE is not magic. It requires the right patient, the right anatomy, the right operator, and the right follow-up. But it changed the prostate conversation. It showed that BPH treatment can be less destructive and more strategic.

REZŪM AND THE MIDDLE PATH

Rezūm is another example of modern prostate care moving away from the old all-or-nothing model. For selected smaller or moderately enlarged prostates, Rezūm can treat obstructing tissue with water vapor energy. It gives men an option between indefinite medication and more aggressive tissue-removing surgery.

It is not instant. It is not right for every prostate. It requires appropriate expectations. But in properly selected men, it can treat obstruction while preserving future options. That is the point.

The future of BPH care is not one procedure replacing all others. It is a toolbox. Medication has a role. Rezūm has a role. PAE has a role. TURP, HoLEP, Aquablation, laser procedures, and other approaches have roles. The key is matching the tool to the anatomy.

The future is not procedure loyalty. It is precision selection.

AI IN PROSTATE CARE

Artificial intelligence should become a major part of prostate care, but only if it is used correctly. AI has the potential to help in many ways. It can help analyze PSA trends. It can help predict risk. It can help interpret MRI patterns. It can support prostate volume measurement and imaging segmentation. It can help evaluate biopsy risk, cancer aggressiveness, treatment outcomes, recurrence risk, and BPH progression. It can help identify men at risk of retention, men likely to fail medication, men likely to benefit from certain procedures, and men who need closer follow-up.

In the future, AI should be able to integrate the full picture: age, PSA, prostate size, family history, MRI, biopsy, urine flow, urine left behind, bladder pressure, symptoms, medication response, sexual function, hormones, metabolic health, and patient goals. That is where AI becomes powerful. But there is a warning.

If you put in bad information, you get bad results. If AI is trained on outdated assumptions, it will automate outdated care. If it is built around medication-only thinking, it will recommend medication-only thinking. If it is trained on poor data, missing bladder measurements, incomplete imaging, biased treatment pathways, or old procedural habits, it will not make care modern. It will only make old care faster.

AI should not make urology less human. It should make urology less blind.

The physician still has to ask the right questions. The patient still has to be heard. The anatomy still has to be measured. The bladder still has to be protected. AI should support judgment, not replace it. The future of AI in prostate care should be diagnostic-based, state-of-the-art, and constantly updated. Otherwise, it becomes another shiny tool delivering Stone Age recommendations.

THE END OF ONE-SIZE-FITS-ALL PROSTATE CARE

The future should end the idea that every man follows the same pathway. Not every man with urinary symptoms needs medication forever. Not every man with an elevated PSA needs immediate biopsy. Not every man with prostate cancer needs treatment. Not every man with BPH needs surgery. Not every man with ED needs only a pill. Not every man after eighty needs routine PSA screening. Not every man should be left alone because he is older.

The future is individualization. A healthy older man may still benefit from evaluation if the result would change care. A younger man with low-risk prostate cancer may avoid immediate treatment through active surveillance. A man with a moderately enlarged prostate but severe ball-valve anatomy may need treatment earlier than a man with a larger prostate growing outward. A man with a weak bladder needs a different plan than a man with strong bladder contraction. A man who values ejaculation highly may choose differently than a man who prioritizes maximum channel opening.

This is medicine. Not algorithmic laziness.

Guidelines matter. Evidence matters. But the patient in front of the doctor matters too.

MODERN UROLOGIST AND UROLONGEVITY

Modern Urologist and UroLongevity represent the direction I believe men's health should move. The prostate should not be separated from the bladder. The bladder should not be separated from sleep. Erectile dysfunction should not be separated from vascular health. Testosterone should not be separated from PSA. Weight loss should not be separated from urinary symptoms, sleep apnea, and sexual function. Cancer screening should not be separated from quality of life.

Men do not live in medical categories. They live in bodies.

A modern prostate program should integrate prostate size, bladder function, urinary symptoms, PSA risk, MRI, advanced testing, sexual function, testosterone, metabolic health, sleep, weight, and longevity. The goal is not to turn every man into a patient. The goal is to give men a strategy before the crisis.

UroLongevity is built around one idea: men should not just live longer. They should function longer.

That requires more than supplements, gadgets, and slogans. It requires measurement, medical judgment, and a serious understanding of male anatomy and aging.

THE FUTURE IS EARLIER

Earlier does not mean reckless. It means not waiting for disaster.

Do not wait until the bladder fails. Do not wait until retention. Do not wait until the catheter. Do not wait until sleep is destroyed. Do not wait until PSA has been abnormal for years. Do not wait until erectile dysfunction reveals vascular disease that could have been addressed earlier. Do not wait until testosterone is prescribed without baseline prostate safety.

Earlier means identifying the problem while there are still good options. A man with mild symptoms and safe bladder function can watch. A man with moderate symptoms and early obstruction can treat before damage occurs. A man with low-risk prostate cancer can monitor carefully. A man with high-risk disease can stage and treat properly. A man over eighty can have decisions based on whether action would truly help him, not on blind routine.

Earlier care is not more aggressive. It is more intelligent.

THE FUTURE IS LESS DESTRUCTIVE

Less destructive does not mean weaker. It means choosing the least damaging treatment that actually solves the problem.

For some men, that may be medication. For others, Rezūm. For others, PAE. For others, HoLEP, TURP, Aquablation, radiation, focal therapy, hormone therapy, or surgery. The point is not to always choose the smallest intervention. The point is to avoid unnecessary damage.

If a low-risk cancer can be safely watched, do not destroy function with unnecessary treatment. If a prostate can be treated through its blood supply, consider whether that preserves more anatomy. If a targeted tissue treatment can help a smaller gland, consider it. If a man needs definitive tissue removal, choose it for the right reason and counsel honestly.

The goal is not undertreatment. The goal is intelligent treatment. The future is less destructive because it is more precise.

THE FINAL MESSAGE

A man should not fear modern prostate care. He should fear old, vague, passive prostate care.

He should fear being told he is fine when nobody measured whether the bladder is safe. He should fear staying on pills for years while the bladder struggles. He should fear ignoring PSA because he is anxious. He should fear treating low-risk cancer too aggressively and high-risk cancer too casually. He should fear testosterone without monitoring. He should fear a procedure chosen because it was marketed well instead of because it matched his anatomy.

Modern care replaces fear with understanding. That is the whole point of this book.

The prostate is not mysterious once it is explained. The bladder is not mysterious once it is measured. PSA is not terrifying once it is interpreted. Cancer is not one disease once it is risk-stratified. Treatment is not one-size-fits-all once anatomy and biology are understood.

That future is already possible. Men just need to demand it.

DR. SHUSTERMAN'S MODERN PROSTATE TAKEAWAY

The future of prostate care is not more fear, more medication, more procedures, or more testing for its own sake. It is smarter care.

It is measuring the prostate before treating blindly. It is protecting the bladder before retention. It is using PSA as a risk signal rather than a panic button. It is using MRI before biopsy when appropriate. It is using PSMA PET and genomic testing when risk requires better information. It is considering focal therapy, PAE, Rezūm, radiation, surgery, and surveillance based on the individual man, not a default pathway. It is using AI to improve risk prediction and decision-making without allowing outdated assumptions to be automated.

It is integrating prostate, bladder, hormones, sexual function, sleep, metabolism, cancer risk, and longevity. The future is not Stone Age urology with better branding.

The future is modern, measured, and human. A modern man should not fear his prostate. He should understand it before it controls his life.

APPENDIX A: PROSTATE TERMS GLOSSARY

FIGURE A.1

Prostate Terms Map

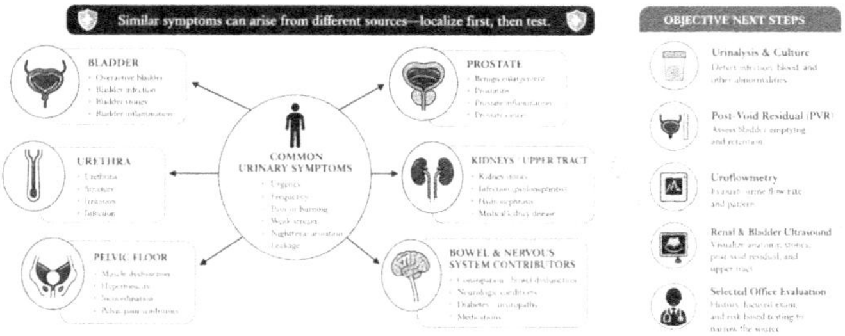

Common prostate terms become easier when they are grouped by anatomy, symptoms, tests, and treatments.

Figure A.1 - Prostate Terms Map. Grouping terms by anatomy, symptoms, tests, and treatments makes them easier.

A man should not need a medical degree to understand what his urologist is saying. This glossary is designed to translate common prostate, bladder, PSA, cancer, hormone, and sexual-function terms into plain language. It is not meant to replace a doctor's explanation. It is meant to help the patient ask better questions, understand his own results, and avoid being confused by medical shorthand. The most important rule is simple: if a word is being used in your care, you should know what it means and why it matters.

PROSTATE

The prostate is a male gland that sits under the bladder and surrounds the urine channel. It produces fluid that becomes part of semen and makes PSA, a protein used in both reproduction and prostate cancer-risk testing. Why it matters: Because the prostate surrounds the urine channel, enlargement can interfere with urination and stress the bladder. Ask your doctor: "How large is my prostate, and is it affecting my bladder?"

BLADDER

The bladder is the muscular organ that stores urine and then squeezes to empty. Why it matters: In prostate enlargement, the prostate may create the blockage, but the bladder is the organ that has to fight against it. Ask your doctor: "Is my bladder emptying safely?"

URETHRA

The urethra is the tube that carries urine from the bladder out through the penis. Why it matters: The prostate surrounds part of the urethra. If the prostate enlarges, the urethra can become compressed or distorted. Ask your doctor: "Is my urine channel being blocked by the prostate?"

BLADDER NECK

The bladder neck is the opening where urine leaves the bladder and enters the urine channel. Why it matters: A tight or blocked bladder neck can cause slow urination, straining, incomplete emptying, or retention. Ask your doctor: "Is the bladder opening tight or blocked?"

MEDIAN LOBE

The median lobe is the middle portion of the prostate that can grow upward toward the bladder opening. Why it matters: When this part grows upward, it can block urine like a ball valve. Ask your doctor: "Is the middle part of my prostate growing into the bladder opening?"

PROSTATE TISSUE GROWING INTO THE BLADDER

Doctors may call this intravesical prostatic protrusion, or IPP. The plain-English meaning is that part of the prostate is bulging into the bladder opening.

Why it matters: This can act like a ball valve. Medication may relax the prostate opening, but it usually cannot make this tissue disappear. Ask your doctor: "Is my prostate bulging into the bladder opening, and is it acting like a ball valve?"

TRANSITION ZONE

The transition zone is the part of the prostate near the urine channel where benign enlargement usually develops. Why it matters: Growth in this area can narrow or distort the urinary passage. Ask your doctor: "Is my enlargement around the urine channel?"

PERIPHERAL ZONE

The peripheral zone is the outer/back part of the prostate where many prostate cancers begin. Why it matters: Cancer in this area may not cause urinary symptoms early. Ask your doctor: "If my PSA is abnormal, does my MRI show anything suspicious in the peripheral zone?"

BPH

BPH stands for benign prostatic hyperplasia. It means noncancerous enlargement of the prostate. Why it matters: BPH is not cancer, but it can still block urine, damage sleep, cause retention, and harm bladder function. Ask your doctor: "Is my BPH mild, moderate, severe, or already affecting my bladder?"

BENIGN

Benign means not cancer. Why it matters: Benign does not mean harmless. A benign prostate can still block urine and damage the bladder. Ask your doctor: "Even though this is benign, is it still causing a dangerous blockage?"

URINARY AND BPH TERMS URINARY SYMPTOMS

Urinary symptoms include weak stream, urgency, frequency, nighttime urination, incomplete emptying, straining, and stopping and starting. Why it matters: Symptoms tell us what the patient feels, but they do not always show how serious the obstruction or bladder problem is. Ask your doctor: "Are my symptoms coming from the prostate, the bladder, or both?"

WEAK STREAM

A weak stream means urine comes out with less force than it used to. Why it matters: It may indicate prostate blockage, a weak bladder, a tight bladder opening, or narrowing in the urine channel. Ask your doctor: "Can we measure how fast my urine comes out?"

HESITANCY

Hesitancy means it takes time for urine to start. Why it matters: Urination should not feel like a negotiation. Waiting to start may suggest resistance at the outlet or poor bladder coordination. Ask your doctor: "Why does it take time for my urine to start?"

INTERMITTENCY

Intermittency means the urine stream starts and stops. Why it matters: It may suggest obstruction, bladder weakness, or both. Ask your doctor: "Is my stop-and-start stream from blockage or weak bladder muscle?"

STRAINING

Straining means pushing with the abdomen to urinate. Why it matters: The bladder should not need help from abdominal pressure to empty. Ask your doctor: "Why do I have to push to urinate?"

URGENCY

Urgency means a sudden, strong need to urinate. Why it matters: Urgency can come from overactive bladder, but it can also be the bladder reacting to prostate obstruction. Ask your doctor: "Is my bladder overactive by itself, or is it reacting to a blocked outlet?"

FREQUENCY

Frequency means urinating often during the day. Why it matters: It may occur because the bladder is irritated, because urine is left behind, or because of diabetes, fluids, caffeine, medications, or other causes. Ask your doctor: "Am I going often because my bladder does not empty?"

NOCTURIA

Nocturia means waking up at night to urinate. Why it matters: Nighttime urination damages sleep. It may be caused by prostate obstruction, bladder irritation, sleep apnea, diabetes, fluids, alcohol, medications, heart issues, kidney issues, or other causes. Ask your doctor: "Is my nighttime urination from the prostate, bladder, sleep, or another medical issue?"

INCOMPLETE EMPTYING

Incomplete emptying means the bladder does not fully empty after urination. Why it matters: A man may feel empty but still leave urine behind. Ask your doctor: "How much urine is left in my bladder after I urinate?"

URINE LEFT BEHIND AFTER URINATION

Doctors call this post-void residual, or PVR. The patient-friendly meaning is simple: urine remains in the bladder after the man thinks he is finished. Why it matters: Too much leftover urine may increase the risk of infection, stones, frequency, retention, and bladder damage. Ask your doctor: "Is the amount of urine left behind safe?"

URINARY RETENTION

Retention means the bladder cannot empty properly or cannot empty at all. Why it matters: Acute retention can require emergency catheter placement. Chronic retention may happen silently when large amounts of urine remain after urination. Ask your doctor: "Am I at risk for retention?"

CATHETER

A catheter is a tube placed into the bladder to drain urine. Why it matters: It may be needed when a man cannot urinate or when the bladder is not emptying safely. Ask your doctor: "Is this catheter temporary, and what is the plan to get me urinating again?"

TESTING TERMS URINALYSIS

A urinalysis is a basic urine test. Why it matters: It can show blood, infection, glucose, protein, and other clues. Ask your doctor: "Does my urine show infection, blood, or another reason for my symptoms?"

PSA

PSA stands for prostate-specific antigen. It is a protein made by prostate cells.

Why it matters: PSA is used as a prostate cancer-risk signal, but it is not a cancer diagnosis. PSA can also rise from benign enlargement, inflammation, infection, retention, and procedures. Ask your doctor: "What does my PSA mean for my age, prostate size, and risk?"

PROSTATE ULTRASOUND

Prostate ultrasound uses imaging to measure the prostate and evaluate its shape. Why it matters: It can show prostate size and whether tissue is growing into the bladder opening. Ask your doctor: "Can we measure my prostate instead of just saying it is enlarged?"

BLADDER SCAN

A bladder scan estimates how much urine remains in the bladder. Why it matters: It tells whether the bladder is emptying safely. Ask your doctor: "How much urine is left behind after I finish?"

URINE-FLOW TEST

A urine-flow test measures how fast urine comes out. Why it matters: A very slow stream may suggest prostate blockage, weak bladder muscle, or both. Ask your doctor: "What is my maximum speed of urination?"

MAXIMUM SPEED OF URINATION

Doctors may call this Qmax. It means the fastest speed of the urine stream during a flow test. Why it matters: A slow top speed can be a warning sign that urine is not passing freely. Ask your doctor: "Is my urine flow speed normal or too slow?"

CYSTOSCOPY

Cystoscopy is a small camera test that looks inside the urine channel, prostate channel, bladder opening, and bladder. Why it matters: It can show blockage, scar tissue, stones, tumors, inflammation, or signs of long-term obstruction. Ask your doctor: "Do we need to look inside to understand the anatomy?"

BLADDER PRESSURE TESTING

Doctors call this urodynamics. It measures how the bladder stores urine and how strongly it can push urine out. Why it matters: It helps determine whether the problem is blockage, weak bladder muscle, or both. Ask your doctor: "Is my bladder strong enough to empty if the prostate blockage is treated?"

MRI

MRI is detailed imaging of the prostate. Why it matters: It helps evaluate prostate cancer risk, identify suspicious areas, and guide biopsy decisions. Ask your doctor: "Should I have MRI before biopsy?"

MRI SCORE

Doctors often use a score from 1 to 5 to describe how suspicious a prostate MRI finding looks. Why it matters: Lower scores are usually less concerning; higher scores are more concerning. A middle score requires judgment. Ask your doctor: "What does my MRI score mean in my specific case?"

BIOPSY

A biopsy samples small pieces of prostate tissue. Why it matters: Biopsy is how prostate cancer is diagnosed and graded. Ask your doctor: "What risk signal makes biopsy necessary?"

PSMA PET SCAN

A PSMA PET scan is advanced imaging used mainly to look for prostate cancer spread in higher-risk cases. Why it matters: It can help determine whether cancer is confined to the prostate or has spread elsewhere. Ask your doctor: "Do I need PSMA PET before deciding on treatment?"

PSA AND CANCER TERMS CANCER-RISK SIGNAL

A cancer-risk signal is information that suggests cancer may be possible but does not prove it. Why it matters: PSA is a risk signal. MRI is a map. Biopsy is the proof. Ask your doctor: "Is this a signal, a map, or proof?"

GLEASON SCORE

The Gleason score describes how aggressive prostate cancer looks under the microscope. Why it matters: Gleason 3+3 is different from 4+3, even though both use similar numbers. Ask your doctor: "What is my Gleason score, and what does it mean?"

GRADE GROUP

Grade Group is a newer, simpler way to describe prostate cancer aggressiveness. Why it matters: Grade Group 1 is usually the lowest-risk category. Grade Group 5 is the highest. Ask your doctor: "What is my Grade Group?"

LOW-RISK PROSTATE CANCER

Low-risk prostate cancer is cancer that appears unlikely to harm the man quickly. Why it matters: Many low-risk cancers can be monitored with active surveillance instead of treated immediately. Ask your doctor: "Am I a candidate for active surveillance?"

ACTIVE SURVEILLANCE

Active surveillance means carefully monitoring low-risk prostate cancer instead of treating it immediately. Why it matters: It helps avoid unnecessary surgery or radiation in men whose cancer may never harm them. Ask your doctor: "What is the surveillance plan, and what would make us switch to treatment?"

FAVORABLE INTERMEDIATE-RISK CANCER

This is a middle category where some men may still be candidates for surveillance, depending on details. Why it matters: Not every intermediate-risk cancer behaves the same way. Ask your doctor: "Is my intermediate-risk cancer favorable or unfavorable?"

UNFAVORABLE INTERMEDIATE-RISK CANCER

This is a more concerning category that usually pushes more strongly toward treatment. Why it matters: Gleason 4+3 disease is generally more concerning than 3+4. Ask your doctor: "How much pattern 4 cancer do I have?"

HIGH-RISK CANCER

High-risk prostate cancer has features suggesting a greater chance of growth, spread, or recurrence. Why it matters: It usually requires staging and more serious treatment planning. Ask your doctor: "Do I need PSMA PET or other staging before treatment?"

METASTATIC PROSTATE CANCER

Metastatic means cancer has spread beyond the prostate. Why it matters: Treatment becomes systemic, not just local. Ask your doctor:

"Where has the cancer spread, and what treatment controls the whole disease?"

BPH TREATMENT TERMS ALPHA BLOCKER

An alpha blocker is a medication that relaxes muscle around the prostate opening and bladder neck. Why it matters: It may improve urination quickly, but it does not shrink the prostate or remove tissue. Possible side effects: Dizziness, lightheadedness, blood pressure effects, ejaculation changes. Ask your doctor: "Is this medication relaxing the outlet, and how will we know if it is enough?"

PROSTATE-SHRINKING MEDICATION

Finasteride and dutasteride are examples. They can slowly shrink selected enlarged prostates by affecting DHT, a hormone involved in prostate growth. Why it matters: They can help selected men with larger glands, but they take time and change PSA interpretation.

Possible side effects: Decreased libido, erectile changes, ejaculation changes, breast tenderness, mood changes in some men. Ask your doctor: "Is my prostate large enough for this medication to make sense?"

DAILY TADALAFIL

Tadalafil is commonly known by the brand name Cialis. It can help erections and may improve urinary symptoms in selected men. Why it matters: It is useful when erectile dysfunction and mild or moderate urinary symptoms overlap, but it is not an anatomy fix.

Possible side effects: Headache, flushing, heartburn, nasal congestion, back or muscle aches. It should not be used with nitrates. Ask your doctor: "Is this mainly for erections, urinary symptoms, or both?"

REZŪM

Rezūm uses water vapor energy to treat selected enlarged prostate tissue. Why it matters: It can help men move beyond medication without traditional surgery, especially when the prostate size and anatomy fit. Ask your doctor: "Does my prostate anatomy fit Rezūm, and what recovery should I expect?"

PAE

PAE stands for prostate artery embolization. It treats the prostate through its blood supply. Why it matters: It can be especially important for larger prostates and prostates growing into the bladder opening. Ask your doctor: "Am I a candidate for PAE based on my prostate size and shape?"

UROLIFT

UroLift uses implants to pull prostate tissue aside. Why it matters: It may help selected men with smaller, favorable anatomy but does not shrink or remove tissue. Ask your doctor: "Is my prostate shape truly right for UroLift?"

AQUABLATION

Aquablation uses a robotic waterjet to remove prostate tissue. Why it matters: It can improve obstruction in selected men but should be considered carefully, especially when bladder irritation symptoms are already prominent. Ask your doctor: "Will this improve only flow, or also my urgency and nighttime urination?"

TURP

TURP is a traditional procedure that shaves out obstructing prostate tissue through the urine channel. Why it matters: It can be effective but is more anatomy-altering and commonly affects ejaculation. Ask your doctor: "Why is TURP the best choice for my anatomy?"

HOLEP

HoLEP is a laser procedure that shells out obstructing prostate tissue. Why it matters: It can be powerful for large glands in experienced hands but commonly changes ejaculation. Ask your doctor: "What are the sexual and recovery tradeoffs?"

SEXUAL FUNCTION AND HORMONE TERMS

ERECTILE DYSFUNCTION

Erectile dysfunction means difficulty getting or keeping an erection firm enough for sex. Why it matters: ED can be a vascular warning sign and may overlap with prostate, hormone, sleep, metabolic, and medication issues. Ask your doctor: "Is my ED a sign of a broader vascular or metabolic problem?"

LIBIDO

Libido means sexual desire. Why it matters: Low libido may relate to testosterone, sleep, stress, relationship factors, medication, depression, or general health. Ask your doctor: "Should my testosterone or other health factors be checked?"

RETROGRADE EJACULATION

Retrograde ejaculation means semen goes backward into the bladder instead of out through the penis. Why it matters: It can occur with some prostate medications and procedures. It is usually not dangerous but may bother men and can affect fertility. Ask your doctor: "Could this medication or procedure change ejaculation?"

DRY ORGASM

Dry orgasm means orgasm occurs with little or no semen coming out. Why it matters: It may occur after prostate procedures, prostate cancer surgery, or certain medications. Ask your doctor: "Will this treatment affect ejaculation or orgasm?"

TESTOSTERONE

Testosterone is the main male hormone involved in libido, energy, muscle, mood, sexual function, bone health, and other systems. Why it matters: Low testosterone can affect quality of life, but testosterone therapy requires prostate monitoring. Ask your doctor: "What is my PSA before starting testosterone, and how will it be monitored?"

FREE TESTOSTERONE

Free testosterone is the portion of testosterone more available to tissues. Why it matters: Total testosterone alone may not tell the full story. Ask your doctor: "Is my free testosterone low, or only the total number?"

SHBG

SHBG stands for sex hormone binding globulin. It is a protein that binds testosterone. Why it matters: High or low SHBG can affect how much testosterone is available. Ask your doctor: "Is SHBG affecting my testosterone interpretation?"

ESTRADIOL

Estradiol is a form of estrogen present in men. Why it matters: Men need some estradiol, but imbalance may affect libido, mood, breast tenderness, and other symptoms. Ask your doctor: "Is estradiol relevant to my symptoms or testosterone therapy?"

DHT

DHT is a stronger androgen made from testosterone. Why it matters: It is involved in prostate growth, hair biology, and sexual biology. Ask your doctor: "Is DHT relevant to my prostate medication or hormone plan?"

SIGNATURE BOOK TERMS PROSTATE-BLADDER CONNECTION

This means the prostate and bladder must be understood together. Why it matters: The prostate may create the blockage, but the bladder is the organ that gets damaged. Ask your doctor: "Is my prostate affecting my bladder?"

BETTER IS NOT FIXED

This means partial improvement is not always enough. Why it matters: A man may feel somewhat better while still leaving urine behind or having a dangerously slow stream. Ask your doctor: "Am I truly fixed, or just slightly improved?"

STONE AGE UROLOGY

This refers to outdated care that relies too heavily on finger exam, vague reassurance, and medication refills without objective measurement. Why it matters: Modern care should measure the prostate, bladder emptying, urine flow, and PSA risk intelligently. Ask your doctor: "Are we measuring the problem or guessing?"

PROSTATE SIZE GAUGE

A practical way to understand prostate size. Why it matters: "Enlarged" is too vague. Men should know whether the prostate is mildly, moderately, severely, or very enlarged. Ask your doctor: "Where am I on the prostate size gauge?"

AGE-25 URINE FLOW TEST

A patient self-check: compare your current urination to how you urinated at age twenty-five. Why it matters: Men often normalize gradual decline. Ask yourself: "How different is my urination from when I was younger?"

MECHANISM FIRST

This means every treatment should explain how it works. Why it matters: A treatment without a mechanism is marketing, not medicine. Ask your doctor: "What is the mechanism of this treatment?"

ENDPOINT SECOND

This means every treatment should have a measurable goal. Why it matters: If no one knows what should improve, no one knows whether treatment worked. Ask your doctor: "How will we know if this worked?"

MAGIC IS NOT A MECHANISM OF ACTION

This is the book's rule for supplements, devices, procedures, and hormone claims. Why it matters: Claims should be judged by mechanism, evidence, endpoints, and safety. Ask your doctor: "What evidence shows this improves the problem I actually have?"

UROLONGEVITY

UroLongevity means integrating prostate, bladder, sexual function, hormones, sleep, metabolism, cancer risk, and healthspan. Why it matters: Men do not age in separate departments. Ask your doctor: "How does this prostate issue connect to my broader health?"

FINAL GLOSSARY TAKEAWAY

The prostate should not be explained in code. A man should understand his own care in ordinary language. He should know what is being measured, what the result means, and what question the treatment is supposed to answer. If a term matters to your diagnosis, it should be explained.

If a number matters to your plan, you should know what it means. If a treatment is recommended, you should understand its mechanism and endpoint. The goal is not to speak like a doctor. The goal is to make decisions like an informed patient.

APPENDIX B: THE PROSTATE SIZE GAUGE

"Your prostate is enlarged" is not enough information. A man should know where he actually stands.

The Prostate Size Gauge is a practical way to understand prostate size in plain language. It does not replace a full urology evaluation, and it does not decide treatment by itself. But it gives men a framework.

The key point is this: prostate size matters, but size is not the story. Shape, direction of growth, bladder emptying, urine-flow speed, symptoms, PSA, and bladder safety all matter.

A small prostate can still cause problems if it grows in the wrong direction. A larger prostate may be less dangerous if it grows outward and the bladder empties well. The prostate must be understood as part of the prostate-bladder system.

THE BASIC GAUGE

A normal young prostate is often around 20 grams or less. As men age, the prostate can grow. Doctors may measure prostate size in grams or cubic centimeters. For patient understanding, those numbers are close enough that they can usually be discussed similarly.

A prostate measured at 50 cubic centimeters is often discussed as roughly 50 grams. The exact unit matters less than the category.

20 GRAMS OR LESS: SMALL OR NORMAL

A prostate around 20 grams or less is usually considered small or normal-sized. This does not guarantee that the man has no urinary issue. A man with a small prostate can still have urinary symptoms from bladder dysfunction, pelvic floor tension, infection, inflammation, urethral narrowing, tight bladder neck, diabetes, sleep problems, medication effects, or other causes.

If a man has severe urinary symptoms with a small prostate, the doctor should not automatically blame BPH. A small prostate should push the evaluation toward other possible causes.

Patient meaning: The prostate is probably not very enlarged. If symptoms are significant, the doctor should look carefully for bladder, pelvic floor, urethral, infection, sleep, metabolic, or neurologic causes. Ask your doctor: "My prostate is small, so what else could be causing my symptoms?"

20 TO 40 GRAMS: MILD ENLARGEMENT

A prostate between 20 and 40 grams is mildly enlarged. Many men in this range can be managed with observation, lifestyle changes, or medication if symptoms are mild and the bladder is emptying well.

But mild enlargement does not always mean mild disease. If prostate tissue is growing upward into the bladder opening, even a prostate in this range can cause meaningful blockage. The gland may not be huge, but it may be growing in a strategically bad direction.

This is the "ball-valve" problem. Part of the prostate bulges into the bladder opening and interferes with urine leaving the bladder.

Patient meaning: The prostate is mildly enlarged, but the shape matters. The doctor should determine whether the bladder empties safely and whether the prostate is growing into the bladder opening. Ask your doctor: "Is this mild enlargement actually blocking the bladder opening?"

40 TO 60 GRAMS: MODERATE ENLARGEMENT

A prostate between 40 and 60 grams is moderately enlarged. This is where prostate size becomes more clinically important. Medication may still help some men, especially when the bladder empties well and symptoms are not severe. But the evaluation should become more serious if the man has a weak stream, nighttime urination, urgency, urine left behind after urination, or prostate tissue growing into the bladder opening.

A moderate prostate can create a major quality-of-life problem. The patient may be told it is "not that big," but that may miss the point. The prostate does not have to be enormous to obstruct.

Patient meaning: This is not a tiny prostate anymore. Symptoms, bladder emptying, urine-flow speed, and prostate shape should guide the plan. Ask your doctor: "Is my bladder still emptying safely, or is this moderate enlargement already causing obstruction?"

60 TO 100 GRAMS: SEVERE ENLARGEMENT

A prostate between 60 and 100 grams is severely enlarged. At this size, medication alone may become less convincing, especially if the patient remains symptomatic. A prostate-relaxing pill can reduce muscle tightness around the prostate opening, but it does not make a large gland small. A prostate-shrinking pill may help selected men over time, but it works slowly and may not be enough if the bladder is already struggling.

Men in this range should have a real discussion about anatomy and bladder safety. The question is not simply whether the patient can tolerate symptoms. The question is whether the prostate is forcing the bladder to work too hard.

Patient meaning: The prostate is large enough that careful planning is needed. If symptoms persist or urine is left behind, medication may not be enough. Ask your doctor: "Is this prostate size putting my bladder at risk?"

OVER 100 GRAMS: VERY LARGE PROSTATE

A prostate over 100 grams is very large. This does not automatically mean the man needs immediate surgery, but it does mean the conversation should be strategic. A very large prostate deserves modern evaluation. The doctor should understand how the prostate is shaped, whether it is growing into the bladder opening, whether urine is left behind, how fast urine comes out, and whether the bladder still appears strong.

Very large prostates often require a discussion beyond simple medication. Options may include prostate artery embolization, HoLEP, simple prostatectomy, or other treatments depending on the man's anatomy, bladder function, medical condition, sexual priorities, and goals.

Patient meaning: The prostate is very large and should not be managed vaguely. A modern treatment discussion is appropriate if symptoms, bladder emptying, or quality of life are affected. Ask your doctor: "What are the best large-prostate options for my anatomy?"

SIZE IS NOT EVERYTHING

The Prostate Size Gauge is useful, but it is not enough by itself. Two men can both have a 50-gram prostate and have different problems.

One man may have a prostate that grows outward and causes little blockage. Another may have a prostate that grows upward into the bladder opening and blocks the exit like a ball valve. The size may be the same, but the effect on urination can be different.

This is why every man should ask not only how large the prostate is, but what the prostate is doing to the bladder. The most important questions are: Is the prostate enlarged?

Is it growing into the bladder opening? How much urine is left behind after urination? How fast does the urine come out?

Is the bladder safe? A prostate size number without bladder information is incomplete.

THE BALL-VALVE PROSTATE

One of the most important prostate patterns is when tissue grows into the bladder opening. Doctors may call this intravesical prostatic protrusion, or IPP. The patient-friendly explanation is simpler: the prostate is bulging into the bladder outlet and can block urine like a ball valve.

This matters because medication may not work well enough. A pill can relax muscle. It cannot reliably remove tissue sitting in the wrong place. A moderately enlarged prostate with a ball-valve shape can sometimes behave more seriously than a larger prostate that grows outward. Ask your doctor: "Is part of my prostate growing into the bladder opening?"

BLADDER EMPTYING

A man may feel empty and still leave urine behind. That is why measuring leftover urine after urination matters. If little urine remains, that is reassuring. If a significant amount remains, the bladder is not emptying normally.

Leftover urine may suggest prostate blockage, weak bladder muscle, or both. It can increase the risk of infections, bladder stones, frequency, urgency, and retention. Ask your doctor: "How much urine is left in my bladder after I urinate?"

URINE-FLOW SPEED

The speed of urination is also important. A man may say his stream is weak, but a urine-flow test can measure how slow it really is. Doctors may call the top speed Qmax, but the patient only needs to understand the plain-English meaning: how fast the urine comes out.

A slow stream may suggest prostate blockage, weak bladder muscle, or both. Ask your doctor: "Is my maximum urine-flow speed normal or too slow?"

PSA AND PROSTATE SIZE

Prostate size also helps interpret PSA. PSA is made by prostate cells. A larger prostate may produce more PSA because there is more prostate tissue. That does not mean a high PSA is automatically harmless, and it does not mean a large prostate protects a man from cancer. But prostate size gives important context.

A PSA result should be interpreted with age, prostate size, PSA trend, inflammation, infection, retention, family history, MRI findings, and overall risk. Ask your doctor: "Does my prostate size help explain my PSA?"

PROCEDURE CHOICE AND PROSTATE SIZE

Different BPH treatments fit different prostate sizes and shapes. A smaller or moderate prostate may be considered for certain minimally invasive treatments if the anatomy fits. A larger prostate may require a different strategy. A prostate that grows into the bladder opening may need a treatment that addresses that specific shape. A weak bladder may require additional testing before choosing a procedure.

The best treatment is not the newest or most advertised. The best treatment is the one that fits the prostate, protects the bladder, and respects the man's goals. Ask your doctor: "Which treatment fits my prostate size, prostate shape, bladder function, and sexual priorities?"

PROSTATE SIZE GAUGE SUMMARY

Small or normal prostate: 20 grams or less Mild enlargement: 20 to 40 grams Moderate enlargement: 40 to 60 grams Severe enlargement: 60 to 100 grams Very large prostate: over 100 grams These categories are a guide, not a complete diagnosis. A man should know the number, but he should not stop there.

FINAL TAKEAWAY

"Enlarged prostate" is too vague. A man should know where he falls on the Prostate Size Gauge. He should also know whether the prostate is growing into the bladder opening, how much urine is left behind after urination, how fast urine comes out, and whether the bladder is safe.

Size matters. Shape matters. Bladder emptying matters.

Urine-flow speed matters. Symptoms matter. PSA context matters. The prostate should be measured, not guessed.

APPENDIX C: URINARY SYMPTOM SCORE GUIDE

Aurinary symptom score helps turn a man's experience into something that can be tracked. Men often describe urinary symptoms vaguely. They say the stream is weak, they go too often, or they wake up at night. That information matters, but it can be hard to compare from visit to visit. A symptom score gives the patient and doctor a common language.

The most common score used in prostate care is the International Prostate Symptom Score, often called the IPSS. It is based on seven urinary symptom questions and one quality-of-life question. Each symptom question is scored from 0 to 5, and the total symptom score ranges from 0 to 35. Scores are generally grouped as mild, moderate, or severe. But the score is only a starting point.

A symptom score tells us what the man feels. It does not measure prostate size. It does not show whether the prostate is growing into the bladder opening. It does not tell how much urine is left behind after urination. It does not measure how fast the urine comes out. It does not prove the bladder is safe. That is why this appendix should be read with one rule in mind: A symptom score is useful, but it is not the whole diagnosis.

HOW THE SCORE WORKS

The symptom score asks about seven urinary issues: incomplete emptying, frequency, stopping and starting, urgency, weak stream, straining, and nighttime urination. Each symptom is scored based on how often it happens. A score of 0 means it does not happen. Higher numbers mean it happens more often. When the seven symptom scores are added together, the result gives a general severity category.

A total score of 0 to 7 is usually considered mild. A score of 8 to 19 is considered moderate. A score of 20 to 35 is considered severe.

The score also includes a quality-of-life question. That question is important because two men with the same score may feel very differently about their symptoms. One man may tolerate them. Another may feel that urinary symptoms are ruining his sleep, confidence, travel, and daily life.

The number matters. The man's experience matters too.

MILD SYMPTOMS

A mild score generally means the patient has relatively few urinary complaints. That can be reassuring, but it does not always mean the urinary system is normal. A man with mild symptoms may still have a concerning PSA pattern, a family history of prostate cancer, blood in the urine, infection, or another issue that deserves attention. He may also be underreporting symptoms because he has adapted to them.

If symptoms are truly mild, the bladder empties well, the urine stream is reasonable, and there are no red flags, observation may be appropriate. The patient-friendly meaning is simple: mild symptoms often allow time, but they do not eliminate the need for judgment.

MODERATE SYMPTOMS

Moderate symptoms are where many men get stuck. The word moderate can sound acceptable. It may make the patient and doctor think the problem is not serious. But a moderate score can still represent a major quality-of-life issue.

A man with a moderate score may wake up several times at night. He may have urgency. He may stop and start. He may feel he does not empty. He may have a weak stream. He may plan his day around bathrooms.

On paper, he is moderate. In real life, he may be miserable.

Moderate symptoms also do not tell us whether the bladder is safe. A man can have a moderate score and still leave too much urine behind. He can have a moderate score and still have prostate tissue blocking the bladder opening. He can have a moderate score and still have a very slow stream.

This is why the doctor should not say, "It is only moderate," without checking the rest of the system. Moderate does not mean harmless.

SEVERE SYMPTOMS

A severe score usually means urinary symptoms are significantly affecting the patient's life. The man may wake repeatedly, strain, have urgency, have a very weak stream, feel incomplete emptying, and experience major disruption. Severe symptoms deserve serious evaluation.

But even severe symptoms do not automatically identify the cause. The prostate may be blocking. The bladder may be overactive. The bladder may be weak. Infection, stones, constipation, pelvic floor dysfunction, diabetes, sleep apnea, medications, or other issues may contribute. A severe score tells us the man is suffering.

It does not tell us the mechanism. The next step is to measure and evaluate.

INCOMPLETE EMPTYING

This symptom asks whether the man feels that the bladder is not empty after urination. This is one of the most important symptoms, but it can be misleading. A man may feel incomplete emptying because urine is truly left behind. He may also feel that way because the bladder is irritated or because pelvic floor tension creates a sensation of pressure.

The only way to know whether urine is left behind is to measure it. A bladder scan or ultrasound can check how much urine remains after the man urinates. Ask your doctor: "Do I only feel like I am not emptying, or is urine actually being left behind?"

FREQUENCY

Frequency means urinating often during the day. The symptom score usually asks how often the man has to urinate again less than two hours after finishing. This can happen because the bladder is irritated, because the prostate is blocking, because urine is left behind, because of excess fluids, caffeine, alcohol, diabetes, medications, or other causes.

A man who urinates frequently may not be making too much urine. He may simply never be emptying well. Ask your doctor: "Am I going often because my bladder is irritated, or because it does not empty?"

STOPPING AND STARTING

This symptom refers to a urine stream that starts, stops, and starts again. This can be a sign of prostate blockage, poor bladder contraction, or poor coordination between the bladder and the outlet.

A healthy stream should not usually feel like a stop-and-start process. If this symptom is common, the urine stream should often be measured. Ask your doctor: "Is my stop-and-start stream from blockage, weak bladder muscle, or both?"

URGENCY

Urgency means the sudden need to urinate. This is often one of the most disruptive symptoms because it makes the bladder feel unpredictable. Men with urgency may avoid travel, long meetings, restaurants, golf, concerts, and social situations because they are worried they may not reach a bathroom in time.

Urgency can come from overactive bladder, but it can also be the bladder reacting to prostate obstruction. Before calming the bladder with medication, the doctor should know whether the bladder empties safely. Ask your doctor: "Is my urgency a bladder problem by itself, or is the bladder reacting to a blocked prostate?"

WEAK STREAM

Weak stream means urine comes out with less force. Men often know this symptom well. They may say the stream is not what it used to be. The best comparison is not to other older men. The best comparison is to the man's own younger baseline.

A weak stream can come from prostate blockage, a tight bladder opening, narrowing in the urine channel, weak bladder muscle, or several factors together. A urine-flow test can measure the maximum speed of urination. Ask your doctor: "How fast does my urine come out, and is that speed normal?"

STRAINING

Straining means the man has to push to urinate. The bladder should not need help from the abdominal muscles to empty. Straining may suggest obstruction, weak bladder muscle, or poor coordination. A man who strains may still get urine out, but that does not mean the system is healthy. Ask your doctor: "Why do I have to push to urinate?"

NIGHTTIME URINATION

Nighttime urination means waking up from sleep to urinate. Doctors call this nocturia, but the plain-English meaning matters more. Waking once occasionally may not be a major problem. Waking several times every night can damage sleep and quality of life.

Nighttime urination can be caused by prostate blockage, overactive bladder, urine left behind, sleep apnea, diabetes, evening fluids, alcohol, leg swelling, heart issues, kidney issues, medications, or other factors. It should not automatically be blamed on age. Ask your doctor: "Is my nighttime urination from the prostate, bladder, sleep, or another medical issue?"

QUALITY OF LIFE QUESTION

The quality-of-life question asks how the man would feel if he had to live with his current urinary condition for the rest of his life. This may be the most important question on the entire form.

A man may have a moderate symptom score, but if he is deeply unhappy, the treatment conversation should be serious. Another man may have a similar score but feel minimally bothered. The doctor still needs to check safety, but patient preference matters.

Quality of life is not cosmetic. Sleep, confidence, travel, work, sex, and daily comfort matter. Ask yourself: "If my urination stayed like this forever, would I be okay with that?"

WHY THE SCORE CAN BE MISLEADING

The urinary symptom score is useful, but it can mislead if used alone. Some men underreport. They have adapted to poor urination and think it is normal. Some overreport because anxiety makes symptoms feel more threatening. Some symptoms come from the bladder, not the prostate. Some come from sleep problems, constipation, infection, or diabetes.

The score also does not measure danger. A man can have moderate symptoms and a very unsafe bladder. Another man can have severe urgency but a bladder that empties well.

The score should trigger better questions. It should not replace evaluation.

HOW TO USE THE SCORE CORRECTLY

The symptom score is best used to track change. If a man starts medication, the score can show whether symptoms improved. If he has a procedure, the score can help measure recovery. If symptoms worsen over time, the score can document progression.

But every score should be interpreted with the rest of the evaluation. A good prostate visit should connect the symptom score to prostate size, prostate shape, urine left behind, urine-flow speed, PSA risk, and bladder safety. That is how the score becomes useful.

WHEN TO SEEK EVALUATION

A man should seek evaluation if urinary symptoms are new, worsening, bothersome, affecting sleep, or interfering with life. He should also seek care if he has blood in the urine, recurrent infections, urinary retention, bladder stones, fever with urinary symptoms, pelvic pain, rapidly worsening stream, or a rising PSA.

A symptom score of 8 or higher is often considered at least moderate, and many scoring forms advise discussion with a physician when symptoms reach that range. But the number should not be the only reason to seek care. A man with a lower score but red flags still needs evaluation. Do not wait for the score to become severe if the bladder may already be at risk.

FINAL TAKEAWAY

A urinary symptom score is a useful tool. It helps measure what the man feels and track whether symptoms improve or worsen over time. But it does not measure the prostate. It does not measure the bladder. It does not measure the stream. It does not diagnose cancer. It does not prove the bladder is safe.

Use the score. Do not worship the score. The right question is not only, "Is my score mild, moderate, or severe?" The better question is: "Do my symptoms match what the prostate and bladder are doing?"

APPENDIX D: PSA RISK SIGNAL GUIDE

PSA is one of the most useful and most misunderstood blood tests in men's health. It can help detect important prostate cancer earlier, but it can also create fear when interpreted poorly. It can lead to smart evaluation, but it can also lead to unnecessary anxiety, biopsy, or treatment if doctors and patients forget what PSA actually is.

The central rule is simple: PSA is a risk signal, not a diagnosis. A PSA result should start a thoughtful conversation. It should not automatically create panic. It should not be ignored. It should not be treated like a yes-or-no cancer test. The question is not only, "Is my PSA high?" The better question is: "What does my PSA mean for my age, prostate size, trend, symptoms, family history, and risk?"

WHAT PSA IS

PSA stands for prostate-specific antigen. It is a protein made by prostate cells. PSA is mostly known as a blood test used in prostate cancer screening, but PSA also has a normal biological role in semen. The prostate produces PSA as part of its reproductive function.

Because PSA is made by prostate cells, prostate cancer can raise PSA. But cancer is not the only reason PSA rises. That is why PSA is a signal.

It tells us the prostate deserves attention. It does not tell us the final diagnosis.

WHY PSA CAN BE ELEVATED

A PSA can rise for several reasons. It may rise because of prostate cancer. It may also rise because of benign prostate enlargement, inflammation, infection, urinary retention, recent instrumentation, catheterization, recent prostate procedures, or irritation.

A larger prostate may produce more PSA because there is more prostate tissue. A man with prostatitis or urinary infection may have a temporary PSA rise. A man who recently could not urinate may also have a PSA elevation related to retention and prostate stress.

This is why a single PSA number should not be interpreted in isolation. A high PSA does not automatically mean cancer. A normal PSA does not guarantee there is no cancer. Context matters.

PSA IS NOT A CANCER DIAGNOSIS

A man should never hear "your PSA is elevated" and assume he has prostate cancer. He may need repeat testing. He may need his prostate size measured. He may need urine testing. He may need an advanced blood test. He may need MRI. He may need biopsy. But the PSA itself is not the diagnosis.

The diagnosis of prostate cancer requires tissue. That means biopsy. The useful phrase is:

PSA is the signal. MRI is the map. Biopsy is the proof. Each step has a purpose.

REPEAT TESTING

If PSA is newly elevated, repeating the test can be appropriate. PSA can fluctuate. Infection, inflammation, ejaculation, vigorous cycling, urinary retention, or recent procedures may affect the result. A repeat PSA can confirm whether the elevation is persistent or temporary.

AUA/SUO early-detection guidance recommends repeating a newly elevated PSA before moving to secondary biomarkers, imaging, or biopsy. That does not mean ignoring the result. It means confirming the signal before escalating.

A repeated PSA that returns to baseline is reassuring. A repeated PSA that remains elevated or continues rising deserves further evaluation.

AGE MATTERS

A PSA result should be interpreted by age. A PSA that may be less concerning in an older man with a large prostate may be more concerning in a younger man with a small prostate. A man under sixty with a PSA around or above 2.5 deserves attention, especially if the PSA is rising, the prostate is not large, or risk factors are present. In men over sixty, the traditional cutoff of 4 may be more relevant, but it still should not be used blindly.

The number matters. But the pattern matters more. A man should ask: "Is my PSA appropriate for my age?"

TREND MATTERS

A single PSA is a snapshot. Several PSA tests over time create a story.

A PSA that is stable over many years is different from one that is rising quickly. A PSA that rises during infection is different from one that continues to rise after inflammation resolves. A PSA that rises in a man on prostate-shrinking medication may be especially important.

Trend should not be the only reason to biopsy, but it is an important part of the picture. A man should ask: "How does this PSA compare with my prior PSA results?"

PROSTATE SIZE MATTERS

The prostate makes PSA. A larger prostate may produce more PSA because there is more prostate tissue. That does not mean cancer is impossible. A man can have both a large benign prostate and prostate cancer. But prostate size gives important context.

A PSA of 4 in a very large prostate may mean something different from a PSA of 4 in a small prostate. This is why prostate size should be part of PSA interpretation. A man should ask: "Does my prostate size help explain my PSA?"

INFECTION, INFLAMMATION, AND RETENTION MATTER

PSA can rise from prostate inflammation, urinary infection, and urinary retention. If a man has burning, fever, pelvic pain, abnormal urine testing, or recent retention, the PSA should be interpreted carefully. The doctor may treat the infection or inflammation and repeat the PSA later. But inflammation should not become a permanent excuse.

If the PSA remains elevated, continues rising, or does not fit the clinical picture, further evaluation may be needed. A man should ask: "Could infection, inflammation, or retention be affecting my PSA, and when should we recheck it?"

FAMILY HISTORY MATTERS

Family history can change PSA interpretation. A man whose father or brother had aggressive prostate cancer should not be treated the same as a man with no family history. Multiple affected relatives, early-age diagnosis, metastatic prostate cancer in the family, or related cancers such as breast, ovarian, or pancreatic cancer may raise concern for inherited risk.

A man should know his family history. He should ask: "Does my family history change how we interpret this PSA?"

RACE, ANCESTRY, AND GENETIC RISK

Some men are at higher risk for prostate cancer and aggressive disease, including men of African ancestry and men with certain inherited mutations such as BRCA2. Risk does not mean diagnosis. It means the threshold for attention may be different.

A man with higher baseline risk may need earlier PSA discussion, closer monitoring, or a lower threshold for MRI or advanced testing. A man should ask: "Am I in a higher-risk group?"

ADVANCED BLOOD TESTS

Advanced blood tests can sometimes help clarify risk when PSA is abnormal. One example is IsoPSA. Other tests may also be used depending on the practice and patient. These tests are designed to refine risk and help decide whether MRI or biopsy is appropriate.

They do not replace judgment. They help sharpen it. A man should ask: "Would an advanced blood test help decide whether I need MRI or biopsy?"

MRI

MRI can help evaluate prostate cancer risk before biopsy. A prostate MRI may show suspicious areas that need targeted biopsy. It may also be reassuring in selected men, especially when PSA is only mildly elevated and other risk factors are low.

MRI is not perfect. A negative MRI does not guarantee there is no cancer. A suspicious MRI does not prove cancer. But MRI can make the biopsy decision smarter. A man should ask: "Should I have prostate MRI before biopsy?"

BIOPSY

Biopsy is how prostate cancer is diagnosed. PSA does not diagnose cancer. MRI does not diagnose cancer. Advanced blood tests do not diagnose cancer. They estimate risk. If the risk is high enough, biopsy may be needed.

A biopsy should answer a real question. It should not be done reflexively, and it should not be avoided when the risk is meaningful. A man should ask: "What risk signal makes biopsy necessary?"

LOW-RISK CANCER DOES NOT MEAN AUTOMATIC TREATMENT

This is one of the most important points in modern prostate care. The old problem with PSA screening was not simply that PSA gave information. The old problem was that medicine often overreacted to the information. Too many men were biopsied reflexively. Too many low-risk cancers were treated aggressively. Too many men had surgery or radiation for cancers that may never have harmed them.

Modern urology is different. Many low-risk prostate cancers are now managed with active surveillance. That means careful monitoring rather than immediate treatment.

Checking PSA does not mean automatic biopsy. Biopsy does not mean automatic treatment. Low-grade prostate cancer does not mean automatic surgery or radiation.

The modern answer to overtreatment is not ignorance. The modern answer is smarter interpretation.

UROLOGY EVALUATION VERSUS PRIMARY-CARE SCREENING RULES

Primary-care screening guidelines are written for broad populations. Urology is different.

A urologist evaluates the individual man in front of him. Is he healthy? Is he active? Does he have meaningful life expectancy? Is he high risk? Is his PSA rising? Is the prostate large enough to explain the PSA? Would MRI clarify the risk? Would biopsy even be appropriate? If low-risk cancer is found, would it be treated or monitored? Those questions matter.

A population guideline may discourage routine screening in older men because of the historical risks of overdiagnosis and overtreatment. That concern is real. But applying age cutoffs too rigidly can be too blunt.

PSA is inexpensive and gives information. The danger is not the number. The danger is acting on the number without judgment. A man should ask: "Are we making this decision based on my individual risk, health, and goals?"

AGE 70 AND PSA

Some primary-care population recommendations discourage routine PSA screening after age seventy. From a urology perspective, that can be too simplistic.

A healthy seventy-two-year-old who exercises, works, travels, has excellent function, and may live fifteen more years is not the same as a frail seventy-two-year-old with severe medical problems. Age matters, but age alone should not replace judgment. The real question is not whether PSA can be checked.

The real question is: "What would we do with the result?" If the answer is that the result would guide monitoring, MRI, reassurance, or selective evaluation, checking PSA may be reasonable. If the result would not change management, then checking may be unnecessary.

AGE 80 AND PSA

After age eighty, routine PSA screening should not be treated the same way as in younger men. The ten-year life expectancy issue becomes central. Many prostate cancers grow slowly. If a man is unlikely to benefit from diagnosis or treatment, routine screening may create more confusion than value. But PSA should not be forbidden after eighty.

A healthy, active eighty-one-year-old with meaningful life expectancy, concerning symptoms, strong family history, or a reason that the result would change management is different from a frail eighty-eight-year-old with multiple serious medical problems. Checking PSA after eighty is not the same as automatically doing a biopsy or treating cancer.

In many older men, PSA may guide observation, reassurance, symptom evaluation, or selective imaging rather than aggressive intervention. A man should ask: "If my PSA is abnormal, would we actually do anything differently?"

PUBLIC CASES AND AGE-BASED SCREENING

Public cases of advanced prostate cancer in older men have raised important questions about age-based screening. We should be careful with individual cases because we usually do not know the full private medical history. It is not appropriate to claim certainty from headlines. But the broader lesson is fair.

If PSA is not checked at all because a man crossed an age cutoff, the opportunity for earlier detection may be lost. That does not mean every older man should automatically be biopsied. It does not mean every low-risk cancer should be treated. It means that refusing to look can also carry risk.

The solution is not automatic treatment. The solution is intelligent evaluation.

WHAT PSA CAN AND CANNOT TELL YOU

PSA can tell you that the prostate deserves attention. It can help identify men who may need repeat testing, advanced blood tests, MRI, biopsy, or closer follow-up. PSA cannot tell you by itself whether you have cancer.

It cannot tell you whether cancer is aggressive. It cannot tell you whether treatment is needed. It cannot replace MRI, biopsy, pathology, staging, or clinical judgment.

PSA is a starting point. Not the story.

QUESTIONS TO ASK ABOUT PSA

A man should ask his doctor: What is my PSA? What was my prior PSA? Is this PSA appropriate for my age?

Does my prostate size explain the number? Could infection, inflammation, or retention be affecting it? Should we repeat it?

Do I need an advanced blood test? Do I need MRI? Do I need biopsy?

If cancer is found, would we treat it or monitor it? If I am older, would this result change management? These questions make PSA useful rather than terrifying.

FINAL TAKEAWAY

PSA is not the enemy. Poor interpretation is the enemy.

The old problem was not that PSA gave information. The old problem was that medicine often overreacted to the information. Modern urology should do better.

PSA should be checked and interpreted intelligently when it fits the man's age, risk, health, and goals. Abnormal PSA should be confirmed and evaluated thoughtfully. MRI and advanced tests can refine risk. Biopsy should be done when justified. Low-risk cancer can often be monitored. Higher-risk cancer should not be missed.

Checking PSA does not mean automatic biopsy. Biopsy does not mean automatic treatment. Low-grade cancer does not mean automatic surgery or radiation.

The goal is not to fear PSA. The goal is to use it wisely.

APPENDIX E: PROSTATE CANCER RISK GROUPS

The word cancer creates fear. The risk group creates the plan.

That is the most important idea in prostate cancer decision-making. A man should never hear only, "You have prostate cancer," and then rush into treatment without understanding what kind of cancer was found.

Prostate cancer exists on a spectrum. Some prostate cancers are low-risk and may never harm the patient. Others are aggressive and require timely treatment. Some can be monitored carefully. Some need radiation, focal therapy, hormone therapy, surgery, or a combination of treatments. Some are confined to the prostate. Others have spread outside it. This appendix is designed to help patients understand the language of prostate cancer risk in plain English.

GRADE GROUP

Grade Group is a modern way to describe how aggressive prostate cancer looks under the microscope. It is based on the older Gleason score system, but it is easier for patients to understand. Grade Group 1 is the least aggressive. Grade Group 5 is the most aggressive. A patient should always ask: "What is my Grade Group?" That question is often more useful than simply asking whether cancer was found.

GLEASON SCORE

The Gleason score is the older grading system used to describe prostate cancer aggressiveness. The pathologist looks at the biopsy tissue and identifies the most common cancer pattern and the next most common pattern. These two patterns are added together. That is why patients may hear numbers like: Gleason 3+3Gleason 3+4Gleason 4+3Gleason 4+4Gleason 4+5 The order matters.

Gleason 3+4 is not the same as Gleason 4+3, even though both add up to 7. In 3+4, the less aggressive pattern is dominant. In 4+3, the more aggressive pattern is dominant. A man should ask: "Is this 3+4 or 4+3?" That difference can change the treatment discussion.

GRADE GROUP 1

Grade Group 1 usually corresponds to Gleason 3+3, also called Gleason 6. This is generally the lowest-risk prostate cancer category commonly diagnosed on biopsy.

Many men with Grade Group 1 disease may be candidates for active surveillance rather than immediate treatment. Active surveillance means careful monitoring with PSA, MRI when appropriate, repeat biopsy when needed, and clinical follow-up. It is not ignoring cancer. It is watching a low-risk cancer carefully so the man can avoid unnecessary treatment unless the cancer changes.

Patient meaning: This may be low-risk cancer that does not need immediate surgery or radiation. Ask your doctor: "Am I a candidate for active surveillance?"

GRADE GROUP 2

Grade Group 2 usually corresponds to Gleason 3+4. This means the cancer is mostly pattern 3, with some pattern 4. Pattern 4 is more concerning than pattern 3, so Grade Group 2 needs a more nuanced discussion than Grade Group 1.

Some men with low-volume Grade Group 2 disease may still be considered for active surveillance, especially if the amount of pattern 4 is small, PSA is not high, MRI is reassuring, and genomic testing is favorable. Other men may be better served with treatment.

Patient meaning: This is not the lowest-risk category, but it may still be favorable depending on the amount and pattern of cancer. Ask your doctor: "How much pattern 4 is present, and is active surveillance still reasonable?"

GRADE GROUP 3

Grade Group 3 usually corresponds to Gleason 4+3. This is different from 3+4.

In Grade Group 3, the more concerning pattern is dominant. This often moves the patient into a more serious treatment discussion.

A man with 4+3 disease should not think, "It is just a 7." The order of the numbers matters. Dominant pattern 4 disease behaves more aggressively than 3+4 disease. Patient meaning: This is usually more concerning and often pushes toward treatment rather than surveillance. Ask your doctor: "Does this behave more like unfavorable intermediate-risk disease?"

GRADE GROUP 4

Grade Group 4 usually corresponds to Gleason 8. This is a high-grade prostate cancer category.

High-grade cancer has a greater chance of growth, spread, and recurrence. A man with Grade Group 4 disease usually needs staging and a serious treatment discussion. Patient meaning: This is high-risk biology and should not be managed casually. Ask your doctor: "Do I need PSMA PET or other staging before treatment?"

GRADE GROUP 5

Grade Group 5 usually corresponds to Gleason 9 or 10. This is the highest-grade category.

A man with Grade Group 5 disease needs careful staging and a treatment plan designed for aggressive cancer. This may include radiation, hormone therapy, surgery in selected cases, systemic therapy, or a combination depending on stage and overall health. Patient meaning: This is aggressive prostate cancer and requires timely, expert management. Ask your doctor: "Has the cancer spread, and what is the full treatment strategy?"

LOW-RISK PROSTATE CANCER

Low-risk prostate cancer generally means the cancer appears unlikely to grow or spread quickly. Many low-risk cancers are Grade Group 1, with a relatively low PSA and limited disease on biopsy. The key modern point is that low-risk cancer often does not need immediate treatment.

Active surveillance is often preferred because it can help avoid unnecessary side effects from surgery or radiation. Patient meaning: Low-risk does not mean "nothing." It means the cancer may be safely monitored. Ask your doctor: "What would make us move from surveillance to treatment?"

FAVORABLE INTERMEDIATE-RISK PROSTATE CANCER

Favorable intermediate-risk cancer is a middle category. It may include some Grade Group 2 disease or other features that are not as low-risk as Grade Group 1 but are still not clearly aggressive.

Some men in this group may be considered for active surveillance if the cancer volume is low, PSA density is low, MRI is reassuring, and the amount of pattern 4 is small. Other men may choose or need treatment. Patient meaning: This is a gray-zone category where individual details matter. Ask your doctor: "What makes my intermediate-risk cancer favorable, and what makes it concerning?"

UNFAVORABLE INTERMEDIATE-RISK PROSTATE CANCER

Unfavorable intermediate-risk cancer is more concerning. This may include Grade Group 3 disease, more extensive cancer, higher PSA, or other features that suggest the cancer is more likely to progress. Men in this category are usually pushed more strongly toward treatment rather than surveillance.

Patient meaning: This is generally not the same as low-risk cancer and usually needs active treatment discussion. Ask your doctor: "What are my treatment options, and do I need additional imaging?"

HIGH-RISK PROSTATE CANCER

High-risk prostate cancer has features that suggest a greater chance of spread or recurrence. This may involve high Grade Group, high PSA, more advanced local findings, or concerning imaging.

High-risk cancer needs staging. In many men, PSMA PET imaging may be considered to look for spread outside the prostate. Patient meaning: Before choosing treatment, doctors need to know whether the cancer is truly confined to the prostate. Ask your doctor: "Has this cancer been fully staged?"

METASTATIC PROSTATE CANCER

Metastatic prostate cancer means the cancer has spread beyond the prostate. It may spread to lymph nodes, bones, or other areas. Once cancer is metastatic, treatment becomes systemic, meaning it must treat the whole body, not just the prostate.

Hormone therapy is often central. Additional medications, radiation, chemotherapy, targeted therapy, radiopharmaceuticals, or clinical trials may be considered depending on the case. Patient meaning: This is no longer only a local prostate problem. Ask your doctor: "What treatments control the disease throughout the body?"

CANCER VOLUME

Cancer volume refers to how much cancer was found. A man with one tiny biopsy sample showing low-grade cancer is not the same as a man with cancer in many biopsy samples. The number of positive biopsy cores and the amount of cancer in each core matter.

Patient meaning: How much cancer was found helps define risk. Ask your doctor: "How many biopsy samples were positive, and how much cancer was in each?"

PSA LEVEL

PSA helps define risk, but it does not act alone. A higher PSA may increase concern, but PSA must be interpreted with prostate size, infection, inflammation, urinary retention, MRI, biopsy results, family history, and age. Patient meaning: PSA is one piece of the risk puzzle. Ask your doctor: "Does my PSA fit the cancer found, or is something else contributing?"

MRI FINDINGS

MRI can show suspicious areas in the prostate and help determine whether cancer appears confined or more extensive. A suspicious MRI finding does not prove cancer, but it can guide biopsy and treatment planning. Patient meaning: MRI helps show where the cancer may be and whether the biopsy findings match the imaging. Ask your doctor: "Does my MRI match the biopsy result?"

PSMA PET

PSMA PET is advanced imaging used mainly in higher-risk prostate cancer. It can help detect whether cancer has spread to lymph nodes, bones, or other areas. Patient meaning: PSMA PET can help determine whether treatment should focus only on the prostate or include the rest of the body. Ask your doctor: "Do I need PSMA PET before choosing treatment?"

GENOMIC TESTING

Genomic testing looks at gene activity in the cancer tissue. It may help estimate how aggressive the cancer is, especially when the decision between surveillance and treatment is uncertain. Patient meaning: Genomic testing can sometimes clarify whether a cancer that looks borderline behaves more quietly or more aggressively. Ask your doctor: "Would genomic testing help decide whether I need treatment?"

CRIBRIFORM AND INTRADUCTAL FEATURES

These are microscopic features that the pathologist may see. They can suggest more aggressive cancer behavior. Patient meaning: Even if the Gleason score seems moderate, these features may make the cancer more concerning. Ask your doctor: "Did the pathology report mention cribriform or intraductal cancer?"

ACTIVE SURVEILLANCE

Active surveillance means monitoring prostate cancer carefully instead of treating it immediately. It may include PSA tests, MRI, repeat biopsy, and clinical follow-up.

Patient meaning: This is not ignoring cancer. It is structured monitoring for selected lower-risk cancers. Ask your doctor: "What is the exact surveillance schedule?"

WATCHFUL WAITING

Watchful waiting is different from active surveillance. It is usually less intensive and often used in older or frailer men where treatment may not improve life expectancy or quality of life. Patient meaning: The goal may be to avoid treatment unless symptoms develop. Ask your doctor: "Are we doing active surveillance or watchful waiting?"

TREATMENT DECISION

The treatment decision depends on risk group, age, health, life expectancy, urinary function, sexual priorities, cancer location, cancer volume, imaging, and patient preference. A man should not choose treatment based only on fear. Patient meaning: The word cancer is not enough to choose surgery, radiation, focal therapy, or surveillance. Ask your doctor: "What plan matches my cancer risk and my life goals?"

RISK GROUP SUMMARY

Low risk: Often active surveillance. Favorable intermediate risk:

Surveillance or treatment may both be reasonable depending on details.

Unfavorable intermediate risk: Usually treatment discussion. High risk: Staging and serious treatment planning. Metastatic: Systemic treatment strategy.

FINAL TAKEAWAY

A prostate cancer diagnosis is not the end of the conversation. It is the beginning of risk classification. The key facts are Grade Group, Gleason pattern, PSA, amount of cancer, MRI findings, staging, genomic risk when appropriate, and whether the cancer is low risk, intermediate risk, high risk, or metastatic.

Do not treat the word cancer. Treat the biology. The question is not only: "Do I have prostate cancer?" The better question is: "What kind of prostate cancer do I have, and what plan matches the risk?"

APPENDIX F: MRI, BIOPSY, AND PSMA PET DECISION GUIDE

Prostate cancer evaluation should happen in steps. A man should not hear that his PSA is elevated and assume he automatically has cancer. He also should not hear that his MRI is suspicious and assume the diagnosis is already proven. Each test has a role.

The simplest way to understand the pathway is this: PSA is the signal. MRI is the map. Biopsy is the proof.

PSMA PET helps stage higher-risk cancer. Those four ideas help patients understand why tests are ordered and what each one can and cannot tell us.

PSA: THE SIGNAL

PSA is a prostate-made protein measured in the blood. It can rise because of prostate cancer, but it can also rise because of benign prostate enlargement, inflammation, infection, urinary retention, recent procedures, catheterization, or irritation.

An elevated PSA should not create panic, but it should start a thoughtful risk evaluation. Current AUA/SUO early-detection guidance states that clinicians should use PSA as the first screening test and should repeat a newly elevated PSA before moving to secondary biomarkers, imaging, or biopsy.

The patient-friendly meaning is simple: if the PSA is newly abnormal, confirm the signal and interpret it in context. Ask your doctor: "Is this PSA truly abnormal for me, and should we repeat it before moving forward?"

MRI: THE MAP

A prostate MRI gives detailed imaging of the prostate. It can show suspicious areas that may need biopsy. It can help estimate prostate size. It can identify where a lesion is located. It can help guide biopsy targeting. It is especially useful when PSA is elevated, when a prior biopsy was negative but concern remains, or when the doctor wants a better map before sampling tissue.

MRI does not diagnose prostate cancer by itself. A suspicious MRI means there may be an area that needs to be sampled. A negative MRI lowers concern in many men but does not guarantee that no cancer exists. The patient-friendly meaning is: MRI helps show where to look. Ask your doctor: "What does the MRI show, and does it change whether I need biopsy?"

MRI SCORE

Prostate MRI reports often use a suspicion score called PI-RADS. Patients do not need to memorize every detail, but the general idea matters. A lower score is usually less suspicious. A higher score is more suspicious. A middle score is the gray zone.

A clearly suspicious MRI finding usually makes biopsy more likely if the man is healthy enough for the diagnosis to matter. A borderline finding requires judgment. A reassuring MRI may support monitoring in selected men, especially if the PSA pattern, prostate size, and risk factors are also reassuring.

The MRI score should not be interpreted alone. The man's age, PSA trend, prostate size, family history, prior biopsy history, and overall risk all matter. Ask your doctor: "What does this MRI score mean in my specific case?"

BIOPSY: THE PROOF

A prostate biopsy samples tissue from the prostate. The tissue is then examined under a microscope by a pathologist. This is how prostate cancer is diagnosed and graded.

PSA cannot prove cancer. MRI cannot prove cancer. Advanced blood tests cannot prove cancer. They estimate risk and help decide whether biopsy is needed. Biopsy provides the proof.

The biopsy also tells us what kind of cancer is present if cancer is found. It helps determine Grade Group, Gleason pattern, how much cancer was sampled, and whether the cancer appears low risk or more aggressive. Ask your doctor: "What risk signal makes biopsy necessary, and what will the biopsy answer?"

TARGETED BIOPSY

If MRI shows a suspicious area, the biopsy can target that area. This is different from a purely systematic biopsy, where samples are taken from standard regions of the prostate without a specific MRI target.

In many modern evaluations, doctors may combine targeted samples of the suspicious MRI area with systematic samples from the rest of the prostate. The goal is to reduce the chance of missing meaningful cancer. Ask your doctor: "Will the MRI lesion be targeted during biopsy?"

SYSTEMATIC BIOPSY

A systematic biopsy samples the prostate in a planned pattern. This can find cancers that are not clearly visible on MRI. MRI-targeted biopsy is important when a lesion is visible, but systematic sampling may still be useful depending on the patient and the doctor's approach.

The key is to understand the plan. Ask your doctor: "Are you doing targeted biopsy, systematic biopsy, or both?"

TRANSRECTAL BIOPSY

A transrectal biopsy samples the prostate through the rectal wall under ultrasound guidance. This has been the traditional biopsy route for many years. It can be fast, accurate, and well tolerated when performed carefully with a strong infection-prevention protocol.

The main concern is infection risk because the needle passes through the rectal wall. Antibiotic planning matters. Ask your doctor: "How do you reduce infection risk with this biopsy route?"

TRANSPERINEAL BIOPSY

A transperineal biopsy samples the prostate through the skin between the scrotum and anus. This approach has gained popularity because it may reduce infection risk by avoiding passage through the rectal wall. It can also be useful for certain anterior or difficult-to-reach lesions.

AUA/SUO guidance notes that cancer detection rates between transrectal and transperineal biopsy routes are not significantly different overall, while transperineal biopsy may have lower infection risk in some analyses and may be valuable in men at higher infection risk or with anterior lesions. The patient-friendly meaning is: both routes can be appropriate, but the route should be chosen based on patient risk, anatomy, doctor experience, comfort, and safety. Ask your doctor: "Why are you recommending this biopsy route for me?"

INFECTION PREVENTION

Biopsy infection risk should be taken seriously. Different practices use different protocols. Some use antibiotics. Some use rectal swabs to check for resistant bacteria. Some choose transperineal biopsy in higher-risk patients. Some use enhanced prophylaxis. The details depend on the patient and the practice.

A man should know the plan before biopsy. Fever, chills, severe pain, worsening urinary symptoms, or feeling very ill after biopsy should prompt urgent medical attention. Ask your doctor: "What should I do if I develop fever after biopsy?"

NEGATIVE BIOPSY

A negative biopsy means cancer was not found in the sampled tissue. That is reassuring, but it does not always end the story. If PSA remains concerning, continues rising, or does not match the prostate size and MRI findings, follow-up is still needed.

AUA/SUO guidance notes that PSA alone should not be used as the sole reason to repeat biopsy after a prior negative biopsy; repeat-biopsy decisions should consider the broader risk picture. The patient-friendly meaning is: a negative biopsy lowers concern, but persistent risk still needs a plan. Ask your doctor: "What is the follow-up plan after this negative biopsy?"

POSITIVE BIOPSY

A positive biopsy means prostate cancer was found. The next question is not simply whether cancer exists. The next question is what kind of cancer exists.

The biopsy should report the Grade Group, Gleason score, number of positive samples, amount of cancer in each sample, and any concerning microscopic features. These details help determine whether the cancer is low risk, intermediate risk, high risk, or more advanced. Ask your doctor: "What is my Grade Group, and what risk group does this place me in?"

LOW-RISK CANCER AFTER BIOPSY

Low-risk prostate cancer often does not need immediate treatment. Many men with low-risk disease can be managed with active surveillance, which means careful monitoring rather than immediate surgery or radiation.

This is one reason PSA evaluation should not be feared. The old problem was that low-risk cancers were often overtreated. Modern care should not automatically treat low-grade cancer. Ask your doctor: "Is active surveillance appropriate for me?"

HIGHER-RISK CANCER AFTER BIOPSY

If the biopsy shows higher-risk cancer, the next step may include additional staging. This is where imaging such as PSMA PET may become important.

Higher-risk cancer should not be assumed to be confined to the prostate until staging is considered. Treatment planning depends on whether disease is localized, in lymph nodes, in bones, or elsewhere. Ask your doctor: "Do I need staging before choosing treatment?"

PSMA PET: STAGING HIGHER-RISK CANCER

PSMA PET is an advanced scan that helps detect prostate cancer outside the prostate. It is not needed for every man with low-risk cancer. It is more important when the cancer appears higher risk or when doctors need to know whether disease has spread. Reports on guideline use note PSMA PET indications in NCCN-style pathways for initial risk stratification in localized prostate cancer and other settings, and major urology/nuclear medicine organizations have incorporated PSMA PET into prostate cancer evaluation when clinically appropriate.

The patient-friendly meaning is: PSMA PET helps determine where the cancer is. Ask your doctor: "Is my cancer high enough risk to justify PSMA PET?"

WHAT EACH TEST CAN AND CANNOT DO

PSA can suggest risk, but it does not diagnose cancer. MRI can show suspicious areas, but it does not prove cancer. Biopsy can prove cancer and grade it.

PSMA PET can help stage higher-risk cancer, but it is not needed for every low-risk case. Each test answers a different question. The mistake is expecting one test to answer everything.

PRACTICAL DECISION PATHWAY

If PSA is newly elevated, repeat it when appropriate and interpret it in context. If PSA remains concerning, consider prostate size, age, family history, inflammation, retention, advanced blood testing, and MRI. If MRI shows a suspicious lesion or the overall risk remains meaningful, biopsy may be appropriate.

If biopsy shows low-risk cancer, active surveillance may be the right plan. If biopsy shows higher-risk cancer, staging with PSMA PET or other imaging may be needed. If cancer is localized, treatment options depend on risk group and patient goals. If cancer has spread, systemic treatment becomes part of the plan.

FINAL TAKEAWAY

Prostate cancer evaluation is a sequence. Do not panic over one PSA. Do not treat MRI as proof.

Do not biopsy without a reason. Do not treat low-risk cancer automatically. Do not treat high-risk cancer without staging.

The modern pathway is smarter: PSA is the signal. MRI is the map. Biopsy is the proof.

PSMA PET helps show where higher-risk cancer has gone. A man should understand which step he is in and what question that step is supposed to answer.

APPENDIX G: BPH MEDICATION GUIDE

BPH medications can be useful. They can improve urinary symptoms, help the stream, reduce urgency, decrease nighttime urination in selected men, and delay or avoid procedures in properly chosen patients. But medication has limits.

A pill cannot replace diagnosis. A pill cannot always protect the bladder. A pill cannot make every large prostate small. A pill cannot remove a ball-valve prostate blockage at the bladder opening. A pill cannot prove the bladder is emptying safely. The goal of this appendix is to help patients understand what BPH medications do, what they do not do, and when medication is no longer enough.

THE MAIN RULE

Medication should have three things: A mechanism. A goal. A reassessment plan.

A man should know what the medication is supposed to do. He should know how success will be measured. He should know what happens if the medication only helps a little. If no one can explain the mechanism or the endpoint, the medication plan is incomplete.

PROSTATE-RELAXING PILLS

These medications are commonly called alpha blockers. Examples include tamsulosin, alfuzosin, silodosin, doxazosin, and terazosin. Patients often know tamsulosin by the brand name Flomax.

These medications relax muscle around the prostate opening and bladder neck. When that area relaxes, urine may pass more easily.

They often work relatively quickly. Some men notice improvement within days. Others need a few weeks.

WHAT PROSTATE-RELAXING PILLS CAN DO

They may help the stream start more easily. They may reduce straining. They may improve the urine stream.

They may reduce some urinary symptoms. They may help men who have a tight prostate opening or bladder neck.

WHAT PROSTATE-RELAXING PILLS CANNOT DO

They do not shrink the prostate. They do not remove tissue. They do not make a very large prostate small.

They do not remove the middle part of the prostate if it is growing into the bladder opening. They do not prove the bladder is emptying safely. This is the key concept: A prostate-relaxing pill may help the doorway open more easily, but it does not remove furniture blocking the doorway. If prostate tissue is physically bulging into the bladder opening like a ball valve, a relaxing pill may only partially help.

COMMON SIDE EFFECTS OF PROSTATE-RELAXING PILLS

Possible side effects include dizziness, lightheadedness, blood pressure changes, fatigue, nasal congestion, and ejaculation changes. Some men notice reduced semen volume or dry orgasm.

Some men develop retrograde ejaculation, where semen goes backward into the bladder instead of out through the penis. This is usually not dangerous, but it can bother men and can affect fertility. Men at risk of falls, men taking blood pressure medications, and sexually active men should discuss side effects before starting.

ASK YOUR DOCTOR

"What is this medication supposed to relax?" "How quickly should I notice improvement?" "How will we know if it worked?" "Could this medication affect ejaculation?" "Is my bladder emptying safely while I take this?"

PROSTATE-SHRINKING PILLS

These medications are called 5-alpha reductase inhibitors. The main examples are finasteride and dutasteride.

They work by reducing the conversion of testosterone into DHT, a stronger hormone involved in prostate growth. By lowering DHT activity, these medications can slowly shrink selected enlarged prostates.

These medications are not quick-relief pills. They usually take months.

WHAT PROSTATE-SHRINKING PILLS CAN DO

They may slowly reduce prostate size in selected men. They may improve symptoms over time. They may reduce the risk of urinary retention in selected men.

They may reduce the chance of needing BPH surgery in selected men. They are most useful when the prostate is large enough that shrinking it makes sense.

WHAT PROSTATE-SHRINKING PILLS CANNOT DO

They do not work immediately. They do not reliably solve severe obstruction quickly. They do not always help men with smaller prostates.

They do not always fix a ball-valve blockage at the bladder opening. They do not remove the need for PSA monitoring. They do not replace prostate measurement or bladder evaluation.

PSA AND PROSTATE-SHRINKING PILLS

Finasteride and dutasteride can lower PSA. That matters.

A man taking one of these medications must tell every doctor who interprets his PSA. The number may look lower than it otherwise would. A rising PSA while taking these medications may be especially important. A man should not take these medications without understanding how PSA will be monitored.

COMMON SIDE EFFECTS OF PROSTATE-SHRINKING PILLS

Possible side effects include decreased libido, erectile difficulties, ejaculation changes, breast tenderness, mood changes, and concerns about persistent sexual side effects in a subset of men. Not every man gets these side effects. But patients should know they can occur.

ASK YOUR DOCTOR

"Is my prostate large enough for this medication to make sense?" "How long before we know if it works?" "How will this medication affect my PSA?" "What sexual side effects should I watch for?" "What happens if my symptoms are still bothersome after several months?"

DAILY TADALAFIL

Tadalafil is commonly known by the brand name Cialis. At a daily low dose, usually 5 mg, it may help urinary symptoms in selected men and can also help erectile dysfunction. AUA BPH guidance supports discussing daily tadalafil 5 mg as a treatment option for urinary symptoms attributed to BPH. Updated AUA materials have also become more open to selected tadalafil combination approaches in appropriate patients. () Tadalafil is often most attractive when a man has both erectile dysfunction and mild or moderate urinary symptoms.

WHAT DAILY TADALAFIL CAN DO

It can improve erections in many men. It can improve urinary symptoms in selected men. It can support sexual confidence. It can be useful when ED and BPH symptoms overlap.

WHAT DAILY TADALAFIL CANNOT DO

It does not shrink a large prostate. It does not remove prostate tissue. It does not make a ball-valve blockage disappear.

It does not prove the bladder is emptying safely. It is usually ED-first and BPH-second. That means it is excellent for selected men with erectile dysfunction and urinary symptoms, but it should not be treated as the strongest option for serious prostate obstruction.

IMPORTANT SAFETY WARNING

Tadalafil should not be used with nitrates. This combination can cause a dangerous drop in blood pressure. Men with significant heart disease, unstable chest pain, complex blood pressure medications, or multiple cardiovascular risks should discuss safety carefully.

COMMON SIDE EFFECTS OF TADALAFIL

Possible side effects include headache, flushing, nasal congestion, heartburn, back discomfort, muscle aches, and lightheadedness. Most men tolerate it well, but it is still a medication and should be used responsibly.

ASK YOUR DOCTOR

"Is this mainly for erections, urinary symptoms, or both?" "Is my bladder emptying safely?" "Can I take this with my other medications?" "Am I taking nitrates or blood pressure medications that make this unsafe?" "What happens if it helps erections but not urination?"

COMBINATION MEDICATION THERAPY

Some men take more than one BPH medication. A common combination is a prostate-relaxing pill plus a prostate-shrinking pill. This may make sense in selected men because one medication works more quickly by relaxing the outlet, while the other may slowly shrink a larger prostate over time. Daily tadalafil may also be combined with selected BPH medications in certain situations, but combination treatment should be supervised because of blood pressure, side effects, and patient selection.

WHEN COMBINATION THERAPY MAKES SENSE

Combination therapy may be reasonable when: The prostate is large. Symptoms are bothersome. The bladder is still safe.

The patient understands the side effects. There is a clear reassessment plan.

WHEN COMBINATION THERAPY IS NOT ENOUGH

If a man takes multiple medications and still cannot urinate well, the medication plan may have reached its limit. A man on two medications who still wakes up all night, has a slow stream, leaves urine behind, or has prostate tissue blocking the bladder opening should not be told he is fine. He may be undertreated.

MEDICATION FAILURE

Medication failure does not always mean the medication did nothing. It may mean the medication did not do enough. A medication may fail because symptoms remain bothersome, urine is still left behind, the stream remains very slow, nighttime urination continues, side effects are unacceptable, or the prostate anatomy is too mechanical for a pill to fix. The endpoint is not "some improvement." The endpoint is meaningful improvement and bladder protection.

SIGNS MEDICATION MAY NOT BE ENOUGH

Medication may not be enough if: The stream remains weak. The man still wakes up repeatedly at night. Urgency remains severe.

The bladder leaves urine behind. The prostate is growing into the bladder opening. There are recurrent infections.

There are bladder stones. The patient has had urinary retention. Side effects are unacceptable. The man's life is still controlled by bathrooms.

THE REFILL VISIT

A refill visit should be a checkpoint. It should not be automatic. The doctor should ask whether the medication is truly working, whether symptoms improved enough, whether side effects matter, whether urine is still being left behind, and whether the bladder is safe.

If the man is doing well, continue. If he is only slightly better, reassess. Better is not fixed.

MEDICATION QUESTIONS EVERY MAN SHOULD ASK

"What is this medication supposed to do?" "Does it relax, shrink, or support erections?" "How soon should it work?" "What side effects matter?" "How will we measure success?" "Is my bladder emptying safely?" "How fast does my urine come out?" "How much urine is left behind?" "Is my prostate growing into the bladder opening?" "What happens if this medication is not enough?"

FINAL TAKEAWAY

BPH medications are useful when they match the problem. Prostate-relaxing pills can help the outlet relax. Prostate-shrinking pills can slowly reduce selected larger prostates.

Daily tadalafil can help erectile dysfunction and urinary symptoms in selected men. But medication has limits. A pill cannot remove a ball-valve blockage at the bladder opening.

A pill cannot always protect a bladder that is leaving urine behind. A pill cannot replace prostate measurement, urine-flow testing, bladder-emptying measurement, or intelligent follow-up. Medication should have a mechanism, a goal, and a reassessment plan. If the man is better but not fixed, the plan needs to evolve.

APPENDIX H: BPH PROCEDURE COMPARISON

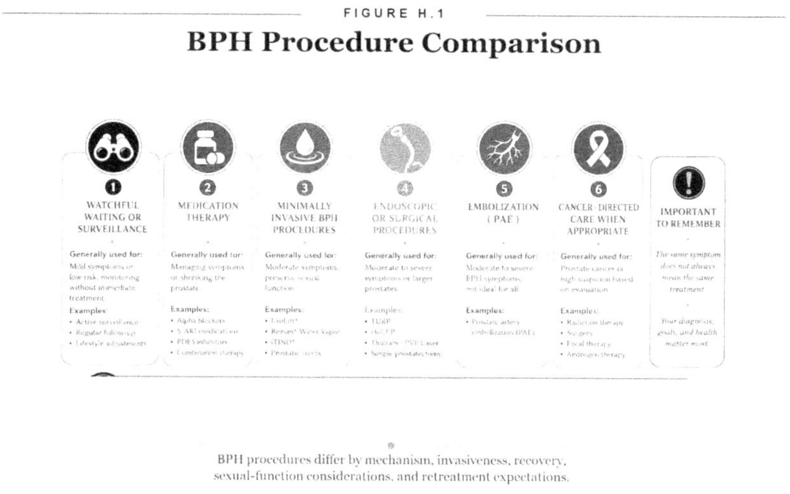

Figure H.1 - BPH Procedure Comparison. Procedures differ by mechanism, recovery, sexual considerations, and durability.

MY PREFERRED PROCEDURE HIERARCHY

In my practice, I do not view all BPH procedures as equal. All have roles, but they are not equal in invasiveness, recovery, catheter expectations, urinary-channel disruption, or postoperative symptom burden.

For many properly selected men with prostate enlargement, especially men with larger glands or prostate tissue growing into the bladder opening, PAE is the option I evaluate first. PAE treats the prostate through the blood vessels rather than through the penis and urinary channel. It is image-guided, anatomy-preserving, and often avoids a postoperative urinary catheter.

My next favored procedure is Rezūm. Rezūm is quick to perform and can work well for selected smaller or moderately enlarged prostates. The main tradeoff is recovery: most men need a temporary catheter, often about seven days in my practice, and may have one to three months of urinary irritation before the final improvement becomes clear.

UroLift, Aquablation, TURP, HoLEP, GreenLight laser, and simple prostatectomy remain part of the overall BPH landscape, but I use them much more selectively. They may be appropriate when the anatomy demands them, but they are not my first-line favorites when PAE or Rezūm can solve the problem with less unnecessary disruption.

There is no single best BPH procedure for every man. That is the most important point. The best procedure is the one that fits the prostate, protects the bladder, respects sexual priorities, and makes sense for the patient's age, health, anatomy, symptoms, and goals.

A man should not choose a procedure because it is advertised heavily, because a friend had it, because it sounds high-tech, or because it is the only option one office happens to offer. The right question is: "What does this procedure actually do, and does that mechanism match my problem?" This appendix compares the major BPH procedures in plain language.

REZŪM WHAT IT DOES

Rezūm uses water vapor energy to treat selected enlarged prostate tissue. The treated tissue gradually shrinks and opens the urine channel over time.

BEST-FIT ANATOMY

Rezūm often fits smaller or moderately enlarged prostates when the obstructing tissue can be treated efficiently. It may also treat selected cases where the middle part of the prostate pushes upward into the bladder opening, but recovery may be slower when that anatomy is more significant.

RECOVERY CONCEPT

Recovery is not always instant. Symptoms can temporarily worsen because the prostate swells and becomes inflamed before it improves.

A temporary catheter may be needed. Improvement often occurs gradually over weeks to months.

SEXUAL CONSIDERATIONS

Rezūm is generally considered more favorable for preserving sexual function than many tissue-removing operations, but no procedure has zero risk. Men should ask specifically about ejaculation, erections, orgasm, and recovery expectations.

FUTURE OPTIONS

Rezūm generally preserves future treatment options. If symptoms persist or return, other treatments may still be possible.

KEY CAUTION

Rezūm is not magic and not instant. It works best when the prostate size and shape fit the treatment.

ASK YOUR DOCTOR

"Does my prostate size and shape make me a good Rezūm candidate?"

PAE WHAT IT DOES

PAE stands for prostate artery embolization. It treats the prostate through its blood supply. Tiny particles are placed into selected arteries feeding the prostate, reducing blood flow so the gland can shrink and soften over time.

BEST-FIT ANATOMY

PAE is especially important for larger prostates and for prostates growing into the bladder opening. It may also be considered in some moderately enlarged prostates when the shape is especially obstructive.

RECOVERY CONCEPT

PAE does not carve open the urine channel immediately. Improvement can be gradual as the prostate responds over weeks to months. Some men have pelvic discomfort, urinary irritation, or temporary symptom changes during recovery.

SEXUAL CONSIDERATIONS

PAE is often attractive for men who want to preserve anatomy and sexual function. Because it does not cut through the urine channel, it may have advantages for ejaculation preservation in selected men. No procedure should be described as zero-risk.

FUTURE OPTIONS

PAE preserves many future options. Men may still have Rezūm, TURP, HoLEP, or other treatments later if needed.

KEY CAUTION

PAE requires an experienced interventional radiologist. The quality of the operator matters.

ASK YOUR DOCTOR

"Am I a good PAE candidate based on my prostate size, prostate shape, and bladder function?"

BLADDER BOTOX WHAT IT DOES

Bladder Botox treats bladder overactivity, not prostate blockage. It is injected into the bladder muscle to reduce urgency, frequency, and urge leakage in selected patients.

BEST-FIT ANATOMY

Bladder Botox may be appropriate when urgency and frequency persist even after obstruction has been evaluated or treated, and when the bladder empties safely.

RECOVERY CONCEPT

The procedure is usually done through a small camera. Improvement may take days to weeks.

SEXUAL CONSIDERATIONS

Bladder Botox does not directly treat erections or ejaculation.

FUTURE OPTIONS

It can be repeated if effective.

KEY CAUTION

Bladder Botox can worsen emptying in some men. It should be used carefully if urine is already being left behind.

ASK YOUR DOCTOR

"Is my bladder emptying safely enough for Botox?"

NEUROMODULATION WHAT IT DOES

Neuromodulation uses nerve stimulation to improve bladder control. Examples include tibial nerve stimulation and sacral neuromodulation.

BEST-FIT ANATOMY

It may help selected men with persistent urgency, frequency, or urge leakage after prostate obstruction and bladder-emptying issues have been evaluated.

RECOVERY CONCEPT

Recovery depends on the type of neuromodulation. Some treatments are office-based; others involve an implanted device.

SEXUAL CONSIDERATIONS

Neuromodulation is mainly a bladder treatment and does not directly treat prostate obstruction or erectile dysfunction.

FUTURE OPTIONS

Other bladder or prostate treatments may still be possible depending on the case.

KEY CAUTION

Neuromodulation should not be used to ignore a blocked prostate or unsafe bladder emptying.

ASK YOUR DOCTOR

"Are my symptoms truly bladder signaling symptoms, or is the prostate still blocking?"

HOW TO COMPARE PROCEDURES

When comparing BPH procedures, do not ask only which one is newest or least invasive. Ask what the procedure actually does. Does it relax tissue?

Pull tissue aside? Shrink tissue? Reduce blood supply?

Remove tissue? Treat bladder overactivity? Stimulate bladder nerves? Each mechanism fits a different problem.

THE CORE COMPARISON QUESTIONS

A man should ask: "How large is my prostate?" "Is the prostate growing into the bladder opening?" "How much urine is left behind after I urinate?" "How fast does my urine come out?" "Does my bladder still seem strong?" "Which procedure fits my anatomy?" "How will this affect ejaculation?" "What is recovery like?" "Will I need a catheter?" "What symptoms may persist?" "What future options remain?"

PROCEDURE SELECTION BY CONCEPT

Medication fits early symptoms and safe bladder emptying. Rezūm fits selected smaller or moderate prostates. PAE fits many larger prostates and prostates growing into the bladder opening.

UroLift fits selected smaller, favorable anatomy. Aquablation, TURP, HoLEP, laser procedures, and simple prostatectomy fit selected men who need tissue removal. Bladder Botox and neuromodulation fit selected bladder problems, not untreated prostate blockage.

FINAL TAKEAWAY

BPH treatment should not be procedure-driven. It should be anatomy-driven. The best procedure is not the newest, loudest, most advertised, or most available procedure.

The best procedure is the one whose mechanism matches the patient's prostate, bladder, symptoms, sexual priorities, recovery goals, and future options. A man should not ask only: "What procedure do you do?" He should ask: "Why is this the right procedure for my prostate, my bladder, and my life?"

APPENDIX I: QUESTIONS TO ASK YOUR UROLOGIST

FIGURE I.1

Visit Question Set

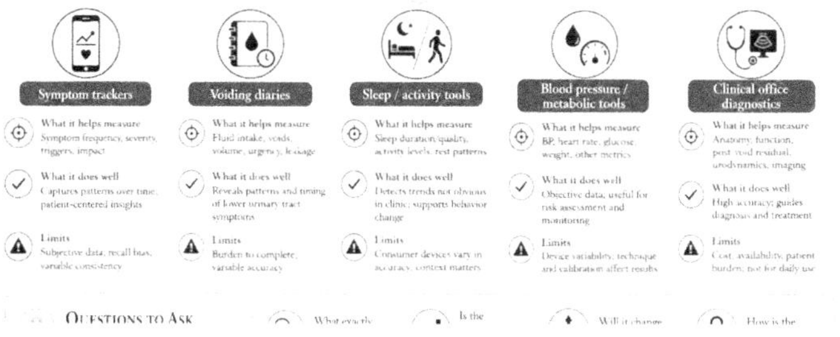

A prepared visit turns anxiety into specific clinical questions.

Figure I.1 - Visit Question Set. Prepared questions help men use the visit well.

A good urology visit should not leave a man confused. You do not need to speak like a doctor. You do not need to memorize every abbreviation. You do not need to know every procedure. But you should leave the office understanding what problem is being treated, what has been measured, what the plan is, and how the doctor will know whether that plan worked.

This appendix is designed as a patient self-advocacy guide. The most important question is: Is my bladder safe? Everything else builds from there.

THE MOST IMPORTANT QUESTION IS MY BLADDER SAFE?

This is the central BPH question. The prostate may be enlarged, but the bladder is the organ that can be damaged over time. If the bladder is emptying well, the conversation is different. If urine is being left behind, the stream is very slow, infections are recurring, stones are forming, or retention has occurred, the situation is more serious. Ask: "Is my bladder emptying safely, or is the prostate putting my bladder at risk?"

QUESTIONS ABOUT URINARY SYMPTOMS WHY AM I PEEING DIFFERENTLY?

Do not accept "it is just age" as a complete answer. A weak stream, urgency, frequency, nighttime urination, and incomplete emptying may come from prostate enlargement, bladder dysfunction, infection, inflammation, diabetes, sleep apnea, constipation, medications, pelvic floor tension, or several causes together. Ask: "What do you think is causing my urinary symptoms?"

IS THIS FROM THE PROSTATE, THE BLADDER, OR BOTH?

Many men assume every urinary problem is prostate-related. That is not always true. The bladder can be overactive, weak, irritated, or reacting to prostate blockage. Ask: "Are my symptoms mainly prostate-driven, bladder-driven, or mixed?"

IS NIGHTTIME URINATION DAMAGING MY SLEEP?

Waking up several times per night is not a minor issue. It can affect energy, testosterone, metabolism, mood, cardiovascular health, and sexual function. Ask: "Is my nighttime urination from prostate blockage, bladder irritation, sleep apnea, diabetes, fluids, alcohol, or another issue?"

QUESTIONS ABOUT PROSTATE SIZE AND SHAPE HOW LARGE IS MY PROSTATE?

"Enlarged" is too vague. You should know whether the prostate is mildly enlarged, moderately enlarged, severely enlarged, or very large. Ask: "What is my prostate size in grams or cubic centimeters?"

WHERE AM I ON THE PROSTATE SIZE GAUGE?

A practical guide: 20 grams or less is small or normal. 20 to 40 grams is mild enlargement. 40 to 60 grams is moderate enlargement. 60 to 100 grams is severe enlargement. Over 100 grams is very large. Ask: "Where do I fall on the prostate size gauge?"

IS PART OF MY PROSTATE GROWING INTO THE BLADDER OPENING?

This is one of the most important questions. Doctors may call this IPP or median-lobe enlargement. The plain-English issue is whether prostate tissue is bulging into the bladder opening and blocking urine like a ball valve. Ask: "Is the prostate growing into the bladder opening?"

IS THIS A BALL-VALVE TYPE BLOCKAGE?

A prostate does not have to be enormous to cause trouble. A moderately enlarged prostate growing in the wrong direction can be very obstructive. Ask: "Is my prostate acting like a ball valve?"

QUESTIONS ABOUT BLADDER EMPTYING HOW MUCH URINE IS LEFT BEHIND AFTER I URINATE?

Doctors call this post-void residual. The plain-English meaning is how much urine remains after you think you are finished. Ask: "How much urine is left in my bladder after I urinate?"

IS THE AMOUNT LEFT BEHIND SAFE?

A small amount may be acceptable. A large amount may increase risk of infection, stones, frequency, urgency, retention, and bladder damage. Ask: "Is this amount of leftover urine concerning?"

IS MY LEFTOVER URINE INCREASING OVER TIME?

Trend matters. Ask: "Is my bladder emptying getting worse compared with prior visits?"

QUESTIONS ABOUT URINE FLOW HOW FAST DOES MY URINE COME OUT?

Doctors may call this Qmax. Patients should think of it as the maximum speed of urination. Ask: "What is my maximum urine-flow speed?"

IS MY STREAM SLOW BECAUSE OF BLOCKAGE OR WEAK BLADDER MUSCLE?

A slow stream can come from prostate blockage, weak bladder muscle, or both. Ask: "Is my slow stream from obstruction, bladder weakness, or both?"

WAS THE FLOW TEST RELIABLE?

A urine-flow test is more useful if enough urine is passed during the test. Ask: "Did I urinate enough during the test for the result to be meaningful?"

QUESTIONS ABOUT MEDICATION WHAT DOES THIS MEDICATION ACTUALLY DO?

Some medications relax the prostate opening. Some slowly shrink selected enlarged prostates. Daily tadalafil can help erections and urinary symptoms in selected men. Ask: "Does this medication relax, shrink, or help erections and urinary symptoms?"

HOW WILL WE KNOW IF THE MEDICATION WORKED?

A medication should have an endpoint. Ask: "Are we judging success by symptoms, urine-flow speed, urine left behind, sleep, or quality of life?"

WHAT ARE THE SIDE EFFECTS?

Prostate medications may affect blood pressure, dizziness, libido, erections, ejaculation, semen volume, and PSA interpretation. Ask: "What sexual, blood pressure, or PSA-related side effects should I know about?"

WHAT HAPPENS IF THE MEDICATION ONLY HELPS A LITTLE?

Partial improvement is not always enough. Ask: "If I am better but not fixed, what is the next step?"

QUESTIONS ABOUT PROCEDURES WHY DOES THIS PROCEDURE FIT MY ANATOMY?

Do not choose a procedure only because it is advertised, new, robotic, or available in one office. Ask: "Why is this the best procedure for my prostate size, prostate shape, bladder function, and goals?"

WHAT DOES THE PROCEDURE ACTUALLY DO?

Different procedures work differently. Some pull tissue aside. Some treat tissue with water vapor. Some reduce blood supply. Some remove tissue. Some treat bladder overactivity. Ask: "Does this procedure pull, shrink, embolize, heat, remove, or relax tissue?"

DOES THIS PROCEDURE GO THROUGH THE URINARY CHANNEL?

This matters. Most BPH procedures are performed through the penis and urinary channel. PAE is different because it treats the prostate through the blood vessels. Ask: "Is this procedure done through the urinary channel or through the blood vessels?"

AM I A CANDIDATE FOR PAE?

PAE is often an important option for larger prostates, prostates growing into the bladder opening, and men who want a less disruptive, anatomy-preserving approach. Ask: "Should I consider prostate artery embolization?"

AM I A CANDIDATE FOR REZŪM?

Rezūm may be a strong option for selected smaller or moderately enlarged prostates. Ask: "Does my prostate size and shape fit Rezūm?"

WILL I NEED A CATHETER?

Catheter expectations should be discussed before the procedure. Ask: "Will I need a catheter after this treatment, and for how long?"

WHAT SYMPTOMS MAY TEMPORARILY WORSEN?

Some procedures can cause burning, urgency, frequency, slower urination, or irritation during recovery. Ask: "What should I expect during the first weeks or months after treatment?"

WHAT FUTURE OPTIONS REMAIN?

A good prostate plan should think beyond the next month. Ask: "If this treatment is not enough, what options would still be available?"

QUESTIONS ABOUT PSA WHAT DOES MY PSA MEAN FOR ME?

PSA is not a cancer diagnosis. It is a risk signal. Ask: "Is my PSA appropriate for my age, prostate size, trend, and risk?"

SHOULD WE REPEAT THE PSA?

A newly elevated PSA may need confirmation before moving to imaging or biopsy. Ask: "Should we repeat this PSA before deciding the next step?"

COULD SOMETHING BENIGN BE RAISING MY PSA?

Benign enlargement, inflammation, infection, urinary retention, catheterization, and procedures can raise PSA. Ask: "Could infection, inflammation, retention, or prostate size explain this PSA?"

DO I NEED MRI BEFORE BIOPSY?

MRI can help map the prostate and identify suspicious areas. Ask: "Should I have prostate MRI before biopsy?"

DOES CHECKING PSA MEAN I NEED BIOPSY?

No. PSA gives information. It does not automatically commit a man to biopsy. Ask: "What would make biopsy necessary?"

IF CANCER IS FOUND, DOES THAT MEAN TREATMENT?

No. Many low-risk prostate cancers can be monitored with active surveillance. Ask: "If cancer is low-risk, would we monitor it instead of treating it?"

IF I AM OLDER, WOULD PSA CHANGE MANAGEMENT?

This is especially important after age eighty. Ask: "If my PSA is abnormal, would we actually do anything differently?"

QUESTIONS ABOUT BIOPSY WHY DO I NEED A BIOPSY?

Biopsy should answer a real risk question. Ask: "What specific finding makes biopsy necessary?"

WILL THE BIOPSY TARGET AN MRI LESION?

If MRI shows a suspicious area, the biopsy should usually account for it. Ask: "Will you target the suspicious area seen on MRI?"

WHAT BIOPSY ROUTE ARE YOU USING?

Biopsy may be transrectal or transperineal. The right approach depends on patient risk, anatomy, physician experience, infection prevention, and comfort. Ask: "Why are you recommending this biopsy route for me?"

HOW DO YOU REDUCE INFECTION RISK?

This should always be discussed. Ask: "What is your infection-prevention protocol?"

WHAT HAPPENS IF THE BIOPSY IS NEGATIVE?

A negative biopsy is reassuring, but persistent risk may still need follow-up. Ask: "If the biopsy is negative, what is our follow-up plan?"

QUESTIONS AFTER A PROSTATE CANCER DIAGNOSIS WHAT IS MY GRADE GROUP?

Grade Group helps describe how aggressive the cancer appears. Ask: "What is my Grade Group?"

WHAT IS MY GLEASON SCORE?

The difference between 3+4 and 4+3 matters. Ask: "Is this 3+4 or 4+3?"

HOW MUCH CANCER WAS FOUND?

Cancer volume matters. Ask: "How many biopsy samples were positive, and how much cancer was in each?"

WHAT RISK GROUP AM I IN?

Treatment depends on whether the cancer is low risk, favorable intermediate risk, unfavorable intermediate risk, high risk, or metastatic. Ask: "What risk group does this cancer fall into?"

IS ACTIVE SURVEILLANCE REASONABLE?

Low-risk cancer often does not need immediate treatment. Ask: "Can this cancer be monitored safely?"

DO I NEED PSMA PET?

Higher-risk cancer may need staging to look for spread. Ask: "Do I need PSMA PET before deciding treatment?"

SHOULD GENOMIC TESTING BE CONSIDERED?

Genomic testing may help in selected borderline cases. Ask: "Would genomic testing help decide between surveillance and treatment?"

QUESTIONS ABOUT SEXUAL FUNCTION WILL THIS MEDICATION AFFECT EJACULATION?

Many prostate medications can affect semen volume or ejaculation. Ask: "Could this medication cause dry orgasm or retrograde ejaculation?"

WILL THIS PROCEDURE AFFECT ERECTIONS OR EJACULATION?

This should be discussed before treatment. Ask: "What are the risks to erections, ejaculation, orgasm, and sexual confidence?"

IF I HAVE PROSTATE CANCER TREATMENT, WHAT HAPPENS SEXUALLY?

Surgery, radiation, focal therapy, and hormone therapy have different sexual side-effect profiles. Ask: "How will this treatment affect erections, ejaculation, orgasm, and recovery?"

SHOULD I HAVE A SEXUAL-FUNCTION PLAN AFTER TREATMENT?

This may include tadalafil, sildenafil, injections, vacuum devices, pelvic floor therapy, testosterone evaluation, or other strategies. Ask: "What is the plan to preserve or recover sexual function?"

QUESTIONS ABOUT TESTOSTERONE DO I TRULY HAVE LOW TESTOSTERONE?

Symptoms and labs both matter. Ask: "Was my testosterone checked properly, and do my symptoms fit?"

WHAT IS MY PSA BEFORE STARTING TESTOSTERONE?

Testosterone therapy requires prostate awareness. Ask: "What is my baseline PSA, and how will we monitor it?"

WILL TESTOSTERONE AFFECT FERTILITY?

Testosterone therapy can reduce sperm production. Ask: "Do I need fertility preservation before testosterone therapy?"

WHAT HAPPENS IF PSA RISES WHILE I AM ON TESTOSTERONE?

PSA movement should be evaluated, not ignored. Ask: "If my PSA rises, what is the plan?"

QUESTIONS ABOUT SUPPLEMENTS WHAT PROBLEM IS THIS SUPPLEMENT SUPPOSED TO TREAT?

"Prostate health" is not specific enough. Ask: "Is this supposed to improve symptoms, urine flow, PSA, inflammation, or cancer risk?"

WHAT IS THE MECHANISM?

A supplement should not rely on vague marketing language. Ask: "How is this supposed to work?"

WHAT ENDPOINT IMPROVES?

A real claim should connect to a measurable result. Ask: "Does this improve symptoms, urine-flow speed, urine left behind, prostate size, or cancer outcomes?"

IS THIS DELAYING REAL EVALUATION?

This is the most important supplement question. Ask yourself: "Am I taking this instead of finding out what is wrong?"

QUESTIONS ABOUT LONGEVITY AND UROLONGEVITY HOW DOES MY PROSTATE CONNECT TO MY OVERALL HEALTH?

Prostate care overlaps with bladder function, sleep, sexual function, testosterone, metabolic health, and cancer risk. Ask: "How does this prostate issue fit into my broader health?"

IS MY SLEEP BEING DAMAGED BY URINATION?

Waking at night is a longevity issue. Ask: "Is my bladder controlling my sleep?"

IS ED A VASCULAR WARNING SIGN?

Erectile dysfunction may reveal blood vessel, metabolic, hormone, or cardiovascular problems. Ask: "Should we evaluate my heart, blood sugar, cholesterol, testosterone, and sleep?"

WHEN TO SEEK ANOTHER OPINION

Consider another opinion if: You are told you are fine but still cannot urinate well. You are on medication but no one has checked your bladder emptying. A procedure is recommended without explaining why it fits your anatomy.

Your PSA is dismissed without a plan. You are rushed into prostate cancer treatment without understanding the risk group. Sexual side effects are not discussed.

Only one treatment option is presented. You feel confused after the visit. A second opinion is not disrespectful. It is part of informed care.

FINAL TAKEAWAY

A man should not leave the urologist's office with vague reassurance. He should understand the problem, the measurements, the plan, and the endpoint. The most important question remains:

Is my bladder safe? The second most important question is: What are we doing to prove it?

APPENDIX J: TESTOSTERONE SAFETY CHECKLIST

Testosterone can be powerful medicine. For the right man, it can improve libido, energy, mood, muscle, motivation, sexual function, body composition, and quality of life. But testosterone should not be treated like a casual wellness product. It is a hormone therapy that affects the whole man.

That means it requires a real diagnosis, a real plan, and real monitoring. The central rule is simple:

Hormones are medicine. Monitoring is not optional. This checklist is designed to help men start testosterone therapy safely, ask better questions, and understand what should be checked before and during treatment.

CONFIRM THE DIAGNOSIS

A man should not start testosterone only because he feels tired. Fatigue, low libido, erectile dysfunction, weight gain, depressed mood, poor sleep, and low motivation can come from many causes. Testosterone deficiency may be one of them, but sleep apnea, diabetes, depression, medications, obesity, alcohol, stress, thyroid disease, poor conditioning, and cardiovascular disease can all create similar symptoms.

A testosterone diagnosis should include symptoms and bloodwork. The AUA guideline uses a total testosterone level below 300 ng/dL as a reasonable cutoff supporting the diagnosis of low testosterone, but the number should be interpreted with the patient's symptoms and clinical picture. Ask your doctor: "Do my symptoms and lab results both support testosterone deficiency?"

CHECK TESTOSTERONE CORRECTLY

Testosterone should usually be checked in the morning, when levels are typically highest. If the result is low, it is often repeated to confirm the diagnosis. Depending on the patient, the doctor may also check free testosterone, sex hormone binding globulin, luteinizing hormone, prolactin, thyroid function, and other labs to understand why testosterone is low. Ask your doctor: "Was my testosterone checked at the right time, and should it be repeated?"

TOTAL TESTOSTERONE

Total testosterone measures the total amount of testosterone in the blood. It is useful, but it may not tell the story. Some testosterone is bound tightly to proteins and is less available to tissues. Ask your doctor: "What is my total testosterone, and does it fit my symptoms?"

FREE TESTOSTERONE

Free testosterone is the portion more available to tissues. Some men have a total testosterone that looks borderline but a low free testosterone because of high binding protein. Others may have a low total number but enough free testosterone that symptoms require a broader explanation. Ask your doctor: "Should we check free testosterone?"

SHBG

SHBG stands for sex hormone binding globulin. It binds testosterone in the blood.

High SHBG may reduce available testosterone. Low SHBG may make total testosterone harder to interpret. Ask your doctor: "Is SHBG affecting my testosterone interpretation?"

LH AND FSH

LH and FSH are pituitary hormones that signal the testicles. They help determine whether low testosterone is coming from the testicles themselves or from the brain's signaling system. Ask your doctor: "Is my low testosterone primary testicular failure or a signaling problem?"

PROLACTIN

Prolactin is a pituitary hormone. If testosterone is low, especially with low or abnormal pituitary signaling, prolactin may be checked to look for pituitary causes. Ask your doctor: "Do I need prolactin or pituitary evaluation?"

BASELINE PSA

A man should know his PSA before starting testosterone when age and risk make PSA relevant. The AUA testosterone guideline states that PSA should be measured in men over 40 before starting testosterone therapy to help exclude a prostate cancer diagnosis.

This does not mean testosterone is automatic prostate cancer fuel. It means the prostate should not be ignored. Ask your doctor: "What is my baseline PSA before starting testosterone?"

PROSTATE HISTORY

Before testosterone therapy, the doctor should ask about prostate history. Has the man had prostate cancer? A biopsy? MRI? Elevated PSA? Prostatitis? BPH? Urinary retention? Prostate procedures? Family history of prostate cancer? The answer changes monitoring and risk discussion. Ask your doctor: "Does my prostate history change whether testosterone is appropriate?"

URINARY SYMPTOMS

Testosterone should not be started in a vacuum if the man has significant urinary symptoms. If he has a weak stream, nighttime urination, urgency, incomplete emptying, retention history, or a very enlarged prostate, the prostate-bladder system should be evaluated. Testosterone may not automatically worsen urinary symptoms in every man, but untreated urinary obstruction should still be taken seriously. Ask your doctor: "Do my urinary symptoms need evaluation before testosterone therapy?"

PROSTATE CANCER HISTORY

Men with prior prostate cancer require individualized counseling. The AUA guideline states that men with a history of prostate cancer should be told there is inadequate evidence to quantify the risk-benefit ratio of testosterone therapy.

That does not mean testosterone is always impossible. It means the decision must be individualized based on the original cancer risk, treatment, PSA stability, symptoms, life expectancy, and patient goals. Ask your doctor: "Given my prostate cancer history, what are the risks and what monitoring would be required?"

ACTIVE SURVEILLANCE

Testosterone therapy in men on active surveillance for prostate cancer requires special caution. It may be considered only in selected men after careful discussion, low-risk disease characterization, informed consent, and close monitoring. This should never be casual. Ask your doctor: "If I am on active surveillance, how would testosterone change my monitoring plan?"

ADVANCED OR METASTATIC PROSTATE CANCER

Men with active advanced or metastatic prostate cancer generally should not receive testosterone therapy because testosterone signaling can stimulate many advanced prostate cancers. The Endocrine Society guideline recommends against testosterone therapy in men with breast or prostate cancer, prostate nodule or induration, high PSA without urologic evaluation, elevated hematocrit, untreated severe sleep apnea, and men planning fertility in the near term, among other contraindications. Ask your doctor: "Is there any prostate cancer reason testosterone is unsafe for me?"

FERTILITY GOALS

Testosterone therapy can suppress sperm production. This is one of the biggest things men are not told clearly enough. A man can feel better sexually on testosterone while his fertility worsens. If a man wants children now or may want children in the future, this must be discussed before starting.

The Endocrine Society recommends against testosterone therapy in men planning fertility in the near term. Ask your doctor: "Could testosterone reduce my sperm production, and do I need fertility preservation?"

SEMEN ANALYSIS

If fertility matters, a semen analysis may be appropriate before treatment. This gives a baseline sperm count and helps guide whether testosterone therapy, alternative medications, or fertility-preserving strategies should be considered. Ask your doctor: "Should I check a semen analysis before starting?"

ALTERNATIVES WHEN FERTILITY MATTERS

Some men who want to preserve fertility may be candidates for alternatives that stimulate the body's own testosterone production rather than replacing testosterone directly. Options may include medications such as clomiphene or other approaches depending on the patient. Some men may use hCG under specialist supervision to help support testicular function. These approaches are not right for everyone. Ask your doctor: "Are there fertility-preserving alternatives to testosterone replacement?"

BASELINE BLOOD COUNT

Testosterone can raise red blood cell levels. This is called erythrocytosis or polycythemia. If the blood becomes too concentrated, risk may increase. That is why hemoglobin and hematocrit should be checked before treatment and monitored during therapy. AUA guidance recommends measuring hemoglobin and hematocrit before offering testosterone therapy and informing patients about the increased risk of polycythemia. Ask your doctor: "What is my hematocrit before starting testosterone?"

HEMATOCRIT MONITORING

Hematocrit should be monitored during therapy. If it rises too high, the doctor may lower the dose, change the delivery method, pause therapy, evaluate sleep apnea, recommend blood donation or therapeutic phlebotomy in selected cases, or investigate other causes. Ask your doctor: "How often will we monitor my hematocrit, and what level would make us change treatment?"

SLEEP APNEA

Untreated severe obstructive sleep apnea is a major concern before testosterone therapy. Sleep apnea can worsen fatigue, low testosterone symptoms, cardiovascular risk, nighttime urination, blood pressure, and red blood cell elevation. Testosterone may worsen sleep apnea in some men or complicate the picture.

The Endocrine Society recommends against testosterone therapy in men with untreated severe obstructive sleep apnea. Ask your doctor: "Do I need sleep apnea evaluation before starting testosterone?"

CARDIOVASCULAR RISK

Testosterone therapy should be considered in the context of cardiovascular health. A man with unstable heart disease, recent major cardiovascular events, uncontrolled risk factors, or complex medical history needs a careful discussion. Testosterone should not be used as a shortcut around proper cardiovascular evaluation. Ask your doctor: "Is my heart and vascular risk appropriate for testosterone therapy?"

BLOOD PRESSURE

Blood pressure should be known and managed. Testosterone therapy may interact indirectly with weight, fluid balance, sleep apnea, red blood cell levels, and cardiovascular risk. Ask your doctor: "Is my blood pressure controlled?"

LIPIDS AND METABOLIC HEALTH

Cholesterol, triglycerides, blood sugar, insulin resistance, weight, waist circumference, and liver health all matter in men considering testosterone therapy. Low testosterone may overlap with metabolic syndrome, obesity, diabetes, and poor sleep. Ask your doctor: "Are we treating testosterone alone, or also the metabolic issues driving low testosterone?"

LIVER AND KIDNEY FUNCTION

Baseline chemistry labs can help assess overall health and medication safety. Testosterone therapy should be part of a broader medical plan, not isolated from the rest of the body. Ask your doctor: "Are my liver and kidney labs appropriate?"

ESTRADIOL

Some testosterone converts to estradiol, a form of estrogen. Men need some estradiol, but imbalance can cause symptoms such as breast tenderness, mood changes, libido issues, fluid retention, or other concerns. Estradiol should be checked when clinically relevant, especially if symptoms suggest imbalance. Ask your doctor: "Should estradiol be monitored based on my symptoms?"

DHT

DHT is a stronger androgen made from testosterone. It is involved in prostate biology, hair biology, and sexual function. DHT is not always measured, but it may be relevant in selected men, especially when discussing prostate growth, hair loss, or medications that affect DHT. Ask your doctor: "Is DHT relevant to my prostate or hair concerns?"

DELIVERY METHOD

Testosterone can be given in several ways. Common options include injections, gels, patches, pellets, and auto-injectors. Each has advantages and tradeoffs.

Injections are flexible but may create peaks and troughs depending on dose and schedule. Gels can be steady but require daily application and precautions to avoid transfer to others. Pellets last for months but require insertion. Auto-injectors can be convenient but may be expensive. Ask your doctor: "Which delivery method fits my life, labs, risk profile, and follow-up reliability?"

DOSE AND TARGET

More is not always better. The goal is not to chase the highest testosterone number. The goal is to improve symptoms safely while keeping labs in an appropriate range. A man who feels well at a reasonable level does not need to be pushed into excessive dosing. Ask your doctor: "What testosterone range are we targeting and why?"

FOLLOW-UP TIMING

Follow-up should be scheduled before therapy starts. The doctor should monitor symptoms, testosterone levels, hematocrit, PSA when appropriate, side effects, blood pressure, fertility concerns, and overall response. The Endocrine Society recommends monitoring testosterone therapy with a standardized plan including symptoms, adverse effects, compliance, serum testosterone, hematocrit, and prostate cancer risk during the first year after starting therapy. Ask your doctor: "When is my first follow-up after starting?"

WHEN TO PAUSE OR RE-EVALUATE

Testosterone therapy should be paused or reassessed if concerning issues arise. Reasons may include a concerning PSA rise, elevated hematocrit, severe side effects, worsening untreated sleep apnea, fertility concerns, new prostate cancer diagnosis, major cardiovascular event, or lack of benefit despite adequate levels. Ask your doctor: "What findings would make us pause or change therapy?"

ONLINE TESTOSTERONE CLINICS

Some online clinics prescribe testosterone too casually. A safe program should include diagnosis, symptom review, confirmatory labs when appropriate, PSA evaluation, blood count monitoring, fertility discussion, sleep apnea screening, cardiovascular risk review, and follow-up. If a clinic offers testosterone without monitoring, that is a warning sign. Ask yourself: "Is this medical care or hormone sales?"

MINIMUM SAFETY CHECKLIST BEFORE STARTING

Before testosterone therapy, a man should know: Whether he truly has testosterone deficiency. His symptoms and goals. His baseline testosterone level.

Whether free testosterone and SHBG matter. His PSA when age and risk make it appropriate. His prostate history.

His urinary symptoms. His family history of prostate cancer. His fertility goals.

His baseline hematocrit. Whether sleep apnea is suspected. His cardiovascular risk.

His blood pressure. His metabolic health. His follow-up plan.

MONITORING CHECKLIST DURING THERAPY

During testosterone therapy, monitor: Symptoms and benefit. Testosterone level. Hematocrit.

PSA when appropriate. Urinary symptoms. Estradiol when clinically relevant.

Blood pressure. Side effects. Fertility goals if relevant.

Sleep apnea status. Cardiovascular and metabolic health.

FINAL TAKEAWAY

Testosterone therapy can help the right man. But it should not be casual.

Before starting, confirm the diagnosis. Check the prostate when appropriate. Know the PSA. Review urinary symptoms. Discuss fertility. Check blood count. Consider sleep apnea. Review heart and metabolic risk. Choose the right delivery method. Monitor regularly. Testosterone is not automatic prostate cancer fuel.

It is also not a harmless wellness supplement. Hormones are medicine. Monitoring is not optional.

APPENDIX K: ED AND BPH MEDICATION GUIDE

Erectile dysfunction and urinary symptoms often travel together. A man may come to the urologist because erections are less reliable, but then mention he also wakes up at night to urinate. Another man may come in for a weak stream and later admit that sexual confidence has declined. A third man may be taking a prostate medication that helps urination but changes ejaculation. Another may be taking ED medication without knowing that erectile dysfunction can be a warning sign for vascular disease. These issues should not be separated too rigidly.

The prostate, bladder, erections, blood vessels, testosterone, sleep, metabolic health, and medications all overlap. This guide explains the main medication issues men should understand when ED and BPH symptoms exist together.

DAILY TADALAFIL

Tadalafil is commonly known by the brand name Cialis. It is best known as an erectile dysfunction medication, but at a low daily dose it can also improve urinary symptoms in selected men with BPH.

Daily tadalafil is often attractive because it can support erections and may also improve urinary comfort.

WHAT IT CAN DO

Daily tadalafil may help erections. It may improve sexual confidence.

It may allow more spontaneity because the medication is taken daily rather than only before sex. It may improve urinary symptoms in selected men. It may be useful when erectile dysfunction and mild or moderate urinary symptoms overlap. AUA BPH guidance states that daily tadalafil 5 mg should be discussed as a treatment option for men with urinary symptoms attributed to BPH, whether or not ED is also present.

WHAT IT CANNOT DO

Daily tadalafil does not shrink a large prostate. It does not remove prostate tissue. It does not make a ball-valve blockage at the bladder opening disappear.

It does not prove the bladder is emptying safely. It is not a substitute for prostate measurement, bladder-emptying evaluation, or urine-flow testing when urinary symptoms are significant.

ASK YOUR DOCTOR

"Is tadalafil being prescribed mainly for erections, urinary symptoms, or both?" "Is my bladder emptying safely?" "Do I have prostate anatomy that a pill cannot fix?"

AS-NEEDED ED MEDICATION

Some ED medications are taken before sexual activity. Sildenafil, commonly known by the brand name Viagra, is one example. Tadalafil can also be used as needed at different doses, though daily tadalafil is often preferred when urinary symptoms and ED overlap. As-needed ED medication can be useful when the main goal is improving erections for sexual activity.

WHAT IT CAN DO

It may improve erection firmness. It may improve reliability. It may reduce performance anxiety when used correctly. It may be useful when the man does not need daily medication.

WHAT IT CANNOT DO

It does not treat significant prostate blockage. It does not improve bladder emptying in a reliable way. It does not replace cardiovascular, metabolic, hormonal, or prostate evaluation.

ASK YOUR DOCTOR

"Is my ED medication treating the symptom only, or are we also evaluating why ED is happening?"

DAILY TADALAFIL PLUS AS-NEEDED SILDENAFIL

Some men ask whether they can take daily tadalafil and still use sildenafil before sex. In selected patients, under physician supervision, combination strategies may sometimes be used. But this should not be done casually.

These medications affect blood vessel relaxation and blood pressure. The patient's heart history, blood pressure, medication list, nitrate use, alpha blocker use, and overall cardiovascular risk must be reviewed. A man should not combine ED medications on his own using leftover pills, online prescriptions, or advice from friends.

ASK YOUR DOCTOR

"Is it safe for me to combine daily tadalafil with an as-needed ED medication?" "What dose and timing are safe?" "What blood pressure or heart risks matter in my case?"

NITRATE WARNING

This is the most important safety warning in ED medication. Men taking nitrates should not take PDE5 inhibitors such as tadalafil, sildenafil, vardenafil, or avanafil. Nitrates are often used for chest pain or certain heart conditions.

Combining nitrates with ED medication can cause a dangerous drop in blood pressure. The European Association of Urology states that concomitant use of PDE5 inhibitors with organic nitrates or nitric oxide donors is an absolute contraindication because it can cause unpredictable blood-pressure drops.

COMMON NITRATE FORMS

Nitroglycerin tablets. Nitroglycerin sprays. Nitroglycerin patches.

Long-acting nitrate pills. Some recreational "poppers" also contain nitrate-like compounds and are dangerous with ED medications.

ASK YOUR DOCTOR

"Am I taking any nitrate medication?" "If I get chest pain, what should I do if I have taken ED medication?"

ALPHA BLOCKERS AND ED MEDICATION

Alpha blockers are common prostate medications. They relax muscle around the prostate opening and bladder neck. Examples include tamsulosin, alfuzosin, silodosin, doxazosin, and terazosin.

ED medications can also lower blood pressure in some men. When combined with alpha blockers, blood pressure effects may become more important.

This does not mean the combination is always impossible. It means it should be supervised carefully.

Some guideline recommendations have evolved over time, and evidence around combination therapy is nuanced. Older AUA guideline material advised against routine daily tadalafil plus alpha blocker for BPH symptom treatment because added symptom benefit was not clearly superior to either medication alone, while later updates and clinical practice discussions have become more open to selected combination use in appropriate men.

ASK YOUR DOCTOR

"Can I safely take tadalafil or sildenafil with my prostate medication?" "Should the doses be separated?" "Could this make me dizzy or lower my blood pressure?"

ED AS A VASCULAR WARNING SIGN

Erectile dysfunction can be a warning sign of broader vascular health problems. The penis depends on blood flow. If the blood vessels are not working well, erections may become unreliable before a man develops more obvious heart or vascular symptoms.

A man with new or worsening ED should not receive only a prescription. He should also be evaluated for cardiovascular and metabolic risk factors when appropriate.

IMPORTANT HEALTH ISSUES TO CONSIDER

Blood pressure. Cholesterol. Diabetes or insulin resistance.

Smoking. Weight. Sleep apnea.

Low testosterone. Medication side effects. Depression, stress, or anxiety.

Cardiovascular disease. The AUA erectile dysfunction guideline describes ED care as requiring clinical evaluation and shared decision-making, not just automatic treatment with one medication.

ASK YOUR DOCTOR

"Could my ED be a warning sign of vascular disease?" "Should we check blood pressure, cholesterol, blood sugar, testosterone, and sleep apnea risk?"

TESTOSTERONE AND ED MEDICATION

Testosterone and ED medications are not the same thing. Tadalafil and sildenafil support the erection pathway.

Testosterone affects libido, energy, mood, muscle, and sexual desire. It may also affect erectile function in some men, especially when testosterone is truly low. A man with low libido, fatigue, poor morning erections, loss of muscle, weight gain, or poor response to ED medications may need testosterone evaluation. But testosterone therapy requires prostate monitoring, blood-count monitoring, fertility discussion, and follow-up.

ASK YOUR DOCTOR

"Should my testosterone be checked?" "If testosterone is low, how will we monitor PSA and blood count?" "Do I still want fertility, and could testosterone affect sperm production?"

ED MEDICATION AFTER BPH PROCEDURES

Some men use ED medication after BPH procedures to support confidence and sexual function. This does not necessarily mean the procedure caused ED. In many cases, the medication is used to support erections during a period of anxiety, recovery, inflammation, catheter experience, or temporary urinary changes.

After PAE or Rezūm, for example, many men are focused on urinary recovery but still want sexual confidence preserved. Daily tadalafil may be useful in selected men.

ASK YOUR DOCTOR

"Should I use tadalafil during recovery?" "Is this for urinary symptoms, erections, or confidence?" "When can I resume sexual activity?"

ED MEDICATION AFTER PROSTATE CANCER TREATMENT

After radical prostatectomy, radiation, or focal therapy, men may need a sexual recovery plan. ED medication may be part of that plan, but it may not be enough by itself. Some men need vacuum devices, penile injections, pelvic floor therapy, testosterone evaluation when appropriate, or other strategies.

After radical prostatectomy, erections may take time to recover, especially if the erection nerves were stretched, bruised, or injured. After radiation, erectile function may decline gradually over time.

ASK YOUR DOCTOR

"What is my sexual recovery plan after prostate cancer treatment?" "If pills do not work, what are the next options?"

COMMON SIDE EFFECTS OF ED MEDICATIONS

Possible side effects include headache, flushing, nasal congestion, heartburn, dizziness, back discomfort, and muscle aches. Rare but serious side effects can include prolonged erection, sudden vision changes, or sudden hearing changes. Men should seek urgent medical care for an erection lasting more than four hours.

ASK YOUR DOCTOR

"What side effects should I expect?" "What side effects require urgent care?"

WHEN ED MEDICATION IS NOT ENOUGH

ED medication may not be enough if the man has severe vascular disease, advanced diabetes-related nerve or blood vessel damage, major low testosterone, severe pelvic nerve injury after cancer treatment, medication side effects, untreated sleep apnea, depression, or severe performance anxiety. Failure of ED pills should not be treated as personal failure. It means the next step should be evaluated.

OTHER POSSIBLE OPTIONS

Dose adjustment. Different ED medication. Daily tadalafil strategy.

Testosterone evaluation. Vacuum erection device. Penile injection therapy.

Intraurethral medication. Penile implant in selected men. Cardiovascular and metabolic evaluation. Pelvic floor therapy in selected men.

ASK YOUR DOCTOR

"If pills are not enough, what is the next step?"

ED AND BPH MEDICATION SAFETY QUESTIONS

A man taking ED or BPH medication should ask: Am I taking nitrates? Am I taking alpha blockers? Am I on blood pressure medication?

Do I have heart disease? Is sexual activity safe for me? Is my ED new or worsening?

Could ED be a vascular warning sign? Do I have low testosterone symptoms? Is my bladder emptying safely?

Is this medication treating the prostate, erections, or both? Could this medication affect ejaculation? Could this medication make me dizzy? What should I do if it does not work?

FINAL TAKEAWAY

ED and BPH medications can be helpful when used correctly. Daily tadalafil can help erections and urinary symptoms in selected men.

As-needed ED medication can support sexual function. Alpha blockers can relax the prostate opening. But none of these medications should replace proper evaluation.

ED may be a vascular warning sign. Urinary symptoms may reflect prostate blockage, bladder dysfunction, or both. Tadalafil does not remove a large prostate.

Sildenafil does not protect the bladder. Alpha blockers can affect ejaculation and blood pressure. Nitrates and ED medications are a dangerous combination.

The safest approach is simple: Treat erections, but evaluate the man. Treat urinary symptoms, but protect the bladder. Use medication intelligently, not blindly.

APPENDIX L: SUPPLEMENTS EVIDENCE FILTER

A prostate supplement should not get a free pass because it sounds natural. That is the purpose of this appendix.

Men are surrounded by products that claim to support prostate health, improve flow, reduce nighttime urination, balance PSA, lower inflammation, improve vitality, or protect the prostate naturally. Some of these products may be harmless for some men. Some may be expensive but ineffective. Some may interact with medications. Some may create false confidence. Some may delay real evaluation.

The most important question is not whether the label sounds good. The most important question is whether the product solves the problem the man actually has.

A man with prostate tissue blocking the bladder opening does not need vague prostate support. He needs to know whether the bladder is safe. A man leaving urine behind after urination does not need marketing language. He needs measurement. A man with a rising PSA does not need a supplement to "support PSA health." He needs intelligent risk evaluation.

Supplements should be judged by the same logic used for every other treatment in this book: Mechanism first. Endpoint second. Marketing last.

QUESTION 1: WHAT PROBLEM AM I TRYING TO TREAT?

Before taking any prostate supplement, define the problem. Is the goal to improve a weak stream? Reduce nighttime urination? Lower urgency? Treat inflammation? Reduce prostate size? Improve PSA? Prevent cancer? Improve sexual function? Support general health? Those are not the same problems.

A supplement that claims to support prostate health may not tell you which problem it actually treats. That is the warning sign. If the problem is vague, the outcome will be vague.

A man should not take a supplement because the word prostate is printed on the bottle. He should know what symptom, measurement, or risk factor the product is supposed to improve. Ask: “What specific problem is this supposed to treat?”

QUESTION 2: WHAT IS THE MECHANISM?

Mechanism means how something works. A prostate-relaxing medication relaxes muscle around the prostate opening. A prostate-shrinking medication lowers DHT activity and can shrink selected larger glands over time. PAE reduces blood flow to the prostate so the gland can shrink and soften. Rezūm uses water vapor energy to treat tissue. Those mechanisms are understandable.

A supplement should also be able to explain its mechanism. Does it affect hormones? Inflammation? Smooth muscle? Blood flow? Oxidative stress? Prostate cell growth? Bladder signaling? The immune system? If the explanation is only “supports prostate health,” that is not a mechanism.

Magic is not a mechanism of action. Ask: “How is this supposed to work?”

QUESTION 3: WHAT ENDPOINT IMPROVES?

An endpoint is the measurable result. For urinary symptoms, meaningful endpoints may include fewer nighttime trips to the bathroom, better symptom score, faster urine flow, less urine left behind after urination, smaller prostate size, fewer infections, lower retention risk, or better quality of life.

For cancer prevention, the endpoint should be actual cancer outcomes, not vague antioxidant theory. For PSA claims, the endpoint should clarify whether the supplement changes cancer risk, inflammation, prostate size, or simply creates confusion.

A supplement should not be judged only by whether it sounds plausible. It should be judged by what improves. Ask: "What measurable result should improve if this works?"

QUESTION 4: DOES IT IMPROVE URINARY SYMPTOMS?

Many prostate supplements are marketed for urinary symptoms. The most common claim is that they help men urinate better. That should lead to a practical question: how much better?

Does the man wake up less often? Does the stream improve? Does urgency improve? Does the bladder empty better? Does the symptom score improve more than placebo?

Saw palmetto is the classic example. It has been used for years for urinary symptoms from benign prostate enlargement. But NCCIH summarizes that a 2023 review of 27 studies found saw palmetto alone provides little or no benefit for BPH symptoms. Ask: "Does this supplement actually improve urinary symptoms in good studies?"

QUESTION 5: DOES IT IMPROVE URINE FLOW?

A man may feel that he is urinating better, but the stream should be measurable when symptoms matter. If a supplement claims to improve flow, ask whether it improves the maximum speed of urination. Does urine come out faster in real testing, or is the claim based only on subjective feeling?

A man with a very slow stream should not rely on a supplement without objective evaluation. Ask: "Does this improve the measured speed of urination?"

QUESTION 6: DOES IT REDUCE URINE LEFT BEHIND?

This is one of the most important questions. A man may feel somewhat better but still leave too much urine in the bladder after urination. That leftover urine can increase the risk of infections, bladder stones, urgency, frequency, and retention. If a supplement does not reduce urine left behind, it may not be protecting the bladder. Ask: "Does this help the bladder empty, or only make me feel slightly better?"

QUESTION 7: DOES IT SHRINK THE PROSTATE?

If a supplement claims to shrink the prostate, ask for proof. Does prostate volume decrease? By how much? Over what period? In what type of patients? Was the result compared with placebo? Was the study large enough and long enough to matter?

A prostate-shrinking claim should not be accepted because the label mentions DHT, hormones, or natural ingredients. If the prostate is physically enlarged and obstructing the bladder opening, the treatment has to be strong enough to matter. Ask: "Does this actually shrink prostate size in measurable studies?"

QUESTION 8: DOES IT TREAT THE BALL-VALVE PROBLEM?

This is crucial. Some men have prostate tissue growing upward into the bladder opening. This can block urine like a ball valve. A supplement is very unlikely to make that anatomy disappear. Even medications can struggle with this pattern because relaxing muscle does not remove tissue sitting in the wrong place.

A man with this anatomy should not rely on supplements. Ask: "Is my prostate growing into the bladder opening, and would this supplement do anything about that?"

QUESTION 9: DOES IT REDUCE RETENTION RISK?

Urinary retention means the bladder cannot empty. If a supplement claims to protect prostate health, ask whether it reduces the risk of retention. Does it reduce emergency catheter placement? Does it reduce progression to surgery? Does it protect bladder function? These are meaningful outcomes.

Feeling slightly better is not the same as avoiding retention. Ask: "Does this reduce the chance of retention or needing a catheter?"

QUESTION 10: DOES IT REDUCE PROSTATE CANCER RISK?

Cancer-prevention claims deserve strict scrutiny. The supplement industry often uses antioxidant language to suggest cancer protection. But a theory is not proof. High-dose isolated supplements can behave differently from nutrients in food.

Selenium and vitamin E are cautionary examples. The National Cancer Institute's SELECT materials report no prostate cancer prevention benefit from selenium or vitamin E supplementation, and later findings raised concern that vitamin E may increase prostate cancer risk. A man should not take a supplement for prostate cancer prevention unless the claim is supported by meaningful human outcomes. Ask: "Does this reduce actual prostate cancer risk, or is it only a theory?"

QUESTION 11: COULD IT AFFECT PSA INTERPRETATION?

Some products claim to support healthy PSA. That phrase can be dangerous if it is not defined.

Does the supplement lower PSA without reducing cancer risk? Does it reduce inflammation? Does it change prostate size? Does it mask a signal? Does it do nothing at all? A man with a rising PSA should not use supplements to avoid evaluation. Ask: "If my PSA changes while taking this, how will we interpret it?"

QUESTION 12: IS IT DELAYING REAL EVALUATION?

This may be the most important question in the entire appendix. The biggest danger of a prostate supplement may not be direct toxicity. The biggest danger may be delay.

A man wakes up at night. He buys a supplement. The stream remains weak. He buys another bottle. He feels slightly better or hopes it is working. Months pass. Years pass. Nobody measures the prostate. Nobody checks how much urine is left behind. Nobody measures the stream. Nobody evaluates PSA.

Then he presents with retention, infection, stones, or advanced disease. The supplement may have made him feel proactive while the real problem progressed. Ask yourself: "Am I taking this instead of finding out what is wrong?"

QUESTION 13: IS IT SAFE WITH MY MEDICATIONS?

Supplements can interact with medications. Some may affect bleeding risk. Some may interact with blood pressure medications, blood thinners, diabetes medications, hormone therapies, anesthesia, or prostate medications. Some may affect liver metabolism. A man should not assume a supplement is safe because it is natural.

Natural does not mean risk-free. Ask your doctor: "Could this interact with my medications or procedures?"

QUESTION 14: IS PRODUCT QUALITY RELIABLE?

Dietary supplements are not regulated like prescription drugs. The FDA explains that under the Dietary Supplement Health and Education Act, the FDA is not authorized to approve dietary supplements for safety and effectiveness before they are marketed, and in many cases companies can sell supplements without notifying the FDA.

This means product quality matters. The label may not always tell the story. Dose, purity, contamination, active ingredient concentration, and manufacturing quality can vary. Ask: "Is this product third-party tested, and do I trust the manufacturer?"

QUESTION 15: IS THIS A FOOD STRATEGY OR A PILL STRATEGY?

Healthy food and high-dose supplements are not the same thing. A diet rich in vegetables, fiber, protein, healthy fats, and minimally processed foods can support metabolic health, weight, inflammation, cardiovascular function, and overall longevity. That can help the environment in which the prostate, bladder, and sexual system function.

A concentrated supplement pill is different. It is an intervention and should be judged like one. A tomato is food.

A pill claiming to prevent prostate cancer is a medical claim. Ask: "Am I improving my health, or am I relying on a capsule to replace medical evaluation?"

QUESTION 16: WHAT IS THE COST?

Cost matters. Some men spend hundreds or thousands of dollars on supplements over years without ever measuring the prostate, checking bladder emptying, or properly evaluating PSA. That is not smart prevention.

If the supplement has uncertain benefit, no clear endpoint, and is delaying diagnosis, the cost is not only financial. The cost may be lost time. Ask: "Is this money better spent on proper evaluation?"

QUESTION 17: WHAT WOULD MAKE ME STOP?

Before starting a supplement, decide what would make you stop. If symptoms do not improve, how long will you continue? If the stream worsens, will you seek evaluation? If PSA rises, will you stop delaying and get worked up? If urine is left behind, will you move beyond supplements?

A supplement should not become a permanent belief system. Ask: "What is my stop rule?"

THE FIVE-PART SUPPLEMENT FILTER

Before taking a prostate supplement, apply this five-part filter: First, define the problem. Second, explain the mechanism. Third, identify the endpoint.

Fourth, check safety and interactions. Fifth, make sure it is not delaying real evaluation. If a supplement cannot pass that filter, it should not be central to the plan.

EXAMPLE: SAW PALMETTO

Saw palmetto is commonly marketed for BPH symptoms. The claim is that it supports urinary function or prostate health. Some proposed mechanisms include hormonal or anti-inflammatory effects.

But the endpoint is the problem. High-quality evidence has not shown strong enough benefit to make it a substitute for real BPH care. NCCIH notes that saw palmetto alone provides little or no benefit for BPH symptoms based on a 2023 review.

A man with mild symptoms and a safe evaluation may choose to try it with realistic expectations. A man with severe symptoms, slow flow, urine left behind, a prostate growing into the bladder opening, retention, infections, stones, or rising PSA should not use saw palmetto as a substitute for care.

EXAMPLE: VITAMIN E AND SELENIUM

Vitamin E and selenium were once promoted for prostate cancer prevention. The theory sounded plausible. But the SELECT trial did not show prevention benefit, and later findings raised concern about increased prostate cancer risk with vitamin E supplementation.

This is why theory is not enough. The body is more complicated than supplement marketing.

EXAMPLE: "PROSTATE FORMULA" BLENDS

Many products combine multiple ingredients. That may look impressive, but it can make the product harder to judge. If symptoms improve, which ingredient helped? If side effects occur, which ingredient caused them? Was the product tested as a combination, or is the label just a collection of prostate buzzwords?

Long labels can create the illusion of science. They are not the same as evidence.

WHEN SUPPLEMENTS MAY BE REASONABLE

Supplements may be reasonable when a man has been properly evaluated, symptoms are mild, the bladder empties safely, PSA risk is being followed appropriately, there are no concerning red flags, the product is low risk, and the patient understands the uncertainty. Supplements may also be reasonable when correcting a true deficiency. But supplements should be adjuncts, not substitutes. They should not replace evaluation of urinary symptoms, bladder safety, prostate size, urine flow, PSA risk, or cancer concern.

WHEN SUPPLEMENTS ARE NOT REASONABLE

Supplements are not reasonable as the main plan when a man has severe urinary symptoms, retention, a very slow stream, urine left behind, recurrent infections, bladder stones, blood in the urine, rapidly rising PSA, abnormal MRI, high-risk family history, or symptoms suggesting infection or cancer concern. In those cases, the man needs evaluation. Not a bottle.

FINAL TAKEAWAY

Supplements are not automatically bad. But they should be judged like every other treatment. What is the problem?

What is the mechanism? What endpoint improves? Is it safe?

Is it delaying real evaluation? A prostate supplement does not have GPS. It does not know whether a man has benign enlargement, prostate tissue blocking the bladder opening, bladder dysfunction, prostatitis, retention, or prostate cancer risk. The biggest danger is often not the pill itself.

The biggest danger is delay. Mechanism first. Endpoint second.

Marketing last. Magic is not a mechanism of action.

APPENDIX M: UROLONGEVITY LAB AND HEALTHSPAN CHECKLIST

A man's prostate should not be evaluated in isolation. The prostate sits inside a larger male health system. Urinary function, bladder emptying, sleep, sexual function, testosterone, metabolic health, cardiovascular risk, body composition, inflammation, and cancer screening all overlap. That is the idea behind UroLongevity.

The goal is not simply to live longer. The goal is to function longer.

A man may have normal basic labs but still wake up all night to urinate. He may have good muscle but poor erections. He may take testosterone but have no PSA monitoring. He may track his sleep but never measure how much urine is left behind after he urinates. He may focus on supplements while ignoring blood pressure, insulin resistance, or prostate cancer risk.

A complete men's health evaluation should connect the dots. This checklist is not meant to say every man needs every test. Testing should be individualized based on age, symptoms, risk, medical history, medications, goals, and physician judgment. But it gives men a framework for what a serious male healthspan evaluation may include.

PSA

PSA is a prostate-made protein used as a prostate cancer-risk signal. It should be interpreted based on age, trend, prostate size, inflammation, infection, urinary retention, family history, and overall risk.

PSA is not a cancer diagnosis. It is information. Ask your doctor: "What does my PSA mean for my age, prostate size, trend, and risk?"

PROSTATE SIZE

Prostate size helps explain urinary symptoms and PSA. A man should know whether his prostate is small, mildly enlarged, moderately enlarged, severely enlarged, or very large. Ask your doctor: "Where am I on the Prostate Size Gauge?"

PROSTATE SHAPE

Size is not everything. A moderately enlarged prostate that grows into the bladder opening may create more trouble than a larger prostate that grows outward. This is the ball-valve prostate problem. Ask your doctor: "Is my prostate growing into the bladder opening?"

BLADDER EMPTYING

A man may feel empty and still leave urine behind. Checking how much urine remains after urination helps determine whether the bladder is safe. Ask your doctor: "How much urine is left in my bladder after I urinate?"

URINE-FLOW SPEED

The speed of urination matters. A slow stream may suggest prostate blockage, weak bladder muscle, or both. Ask your doctor: "How fast does my urine come out?"

URINALYSIS

A urine test can show blood, infection, glucose, protein, and other clues. It is simple, but it can reveal important information. Ask your doctor: "Does my urine show blood, infection, sugar, protein, or another abnormality?"

TOTAL TESTOSTERONE

Total testosterone measures the total amount of testosterone in the blood. It helps evaluate libido, energy, mood, muscle, sexual function, and symptoms of testosterone deficiency. Ask your doctor: "Is my testosterone low enough to explain my symptoms?"

FREE TESTOSTERONE

Free testosterone is the portion more available to tissues. Some men have a total testosterone number that does not tell the story. Free testosterone can help clarify the picture. Ask your doctor: "Should we check free testosterone?"

SHBG

SHBG stands for sex hormone binding globulin. It affects how much testosterone is available to the body. High or low SHBG can change how testosterone results are interpreted. Ask your doctor: "Is SHBG affecting my testosterone interpretation?"

ESTRADIOL

Estradiol is a form of estrogen present in men. Men need some estradiol, but imbalance can affect libido, mood, breast tenderness, fluid retention, and hormone symptoms. Ask your doctor: "Is estradiol relevant to my symptoms or testosterone therapy?"

DHT

DHT is a stronger androgen made from testosterone. It is involved in prostate biology, hair biology, and sexual function. It may matter when discussing prostate growth, hair loss, and medications that affect DHT. Ask your doctor: "Is DHT relevant to my prostate or hormone plan?"

CBC

CBC stands for complete blood count. It measures red blood cells, white blood cells, hemoglobin, hematocrit, and platelets. It is especially important for men on testosterone because testosterone can raise hematocrit. Ask your doctor: "Is my hematocrit safe, especially if I am on testosterone?"

CMP

CMP stands for comprehensive metabolic panel. It gives information about kidney function, liver function, electrolytes, blood sugar, and overall metabolic status. Ask your doctor: "Are my kidney, liver, electrolyte, and metabolic markers normal?"

KIDNEY FUNCTION

Kidney function matters in prostate care because severe urinary obstruction can sometimes affect the upper urinary tract. It also matters for medication safety and overall health. Ask your doctor: "Is my kidney function normal, and could urinary obstruction be affecting it?"

LIVER FUNCTION

Liver function matters for medication metabolism, hormone therapy, alcohol effects, metabolic health, and overall safety. Ask your doctor: "Are my liver markers normal?"

FASTING GLUCOSE

Fasting glucose helps assess blood sugar. High blood sugar can cause frequent urination, worsen vascular health, damage nerves, and contribute to erectile dysfunction. Ask your doctor: "Could blood sugar be contributing to urinary frequency or ED?"

HEMOGLOBIN A1C

A1c estimates average blood sugar over several months. It is useful for detecting diabetes or prediabetes. Ask your doctor: "Is diabetes or prediabetes affecting my urinary or sexual function?"

FASTING INSULIN

Fasting insulin can help identify insulin resistance before blood sugar becomes obviously abnormal. Insulin resistance is tied to weight gain, inflammation, metabolic syndrome, cardiovascular risk, and possibly urinary symptoms. Ask your doctor: "Do I have insulin resistance even if my glucose is still normal?"

LIPID PANEL

A lipid panel measures cholesterol and triglycerides. This matters because erectile dysfunction can be an early sign of vascular disease. Cholesterol and vascular health are directly relevant to erections, heart risk, and longevity. Ask your doctor: "Could my cholesterol be affecting erections or vascular health?"

BLOOD PRESSURE

Blood pressure is one of the most important longevity markers. High blood pressure affects the heart, brain, kidneys, erections, and overall vascular health. Ask your doctor: "Is my blood pressure controlled, and could it be affecting erections or kidney health?"

BODY COMPOSITION

Weight alone is not enough. Body composition looks at fat mass, muscle mass, and visceral fat. A man may weigh the same but have different metabolic health depending on muscle and fat distribution. Ask your doctor: "Am I losing fat, preserving muscle, and improving metabolic health?"

WAIST CIRCUMFERENCE

Waist size helps estimate visceral fat and metabolic risk. A growing waistline often tracks with insulin resistance, lower testosterone, sleep apnea, erectile dysfunction, and inflammation. Ask your doctor: "Is abdominal fat contributing to my hormone, urinary, or sexual symptoms?"

THYROID FUNCTION

Thyroid problems can affect energy, weight, mood, heart rhythm, sexual function, and metabolism. Thyroid testing may be useful when symptoms overlap with fatigue, weight changes, mood changes, or low libido. Ask your doctor: "Could thyroid function be contributing to my symptoms?"

VITAMIN D

Vitamin D matters for bone health, immune function, and general health. Low vitamin D is common. It should be corrected when appropriate, but it should not be treated as a cure-all. Ask your doctor: "Is my vitamin D low, and does it need correction?"

VITAMIN B12

B12 is important for nerve function, blood cells, and energy. Low B12 can contribute to fatigue, neuropathy, cognitive symptoms, and anemia. Ask your doctor: "Could B12 deficiency be contributing to fatigue or nerve symptoms?"

INFLAMMATION MARKERS

Inflammation markers may be useful in selected men, especially when looking at cardiovascular risk, metabolic disease, autoimmune issues, or chronic inflammatory states. Inflammation should not become a vague marketing term. If it is measured, the doctor should explain what the result means. Ask your doctor: "What kind of inflammation are we measuring, and what would we do with the result?"

SLEEP ASSESSMENT

Sleep is central to male health. Poor sleep can worsen testosterone, weight, insulin resistance, blood pressure, mood, memory, erections, and urinary symptoms. Nighttime urination can also destroy sleep. A man who wakes up several times per night to urinate needs evaluation. Ask your doctor: "Is my sleep being disrupted by my bladder, sleep apnea, or both?"

SLEEP APNEA SCREENING

Sleep apnea can cause fatigue, low testosterone symptoms, high blood pressure, erectile dysfunction, nighttime urination, and cardiovascular risk. It should be considered in men who snore, wake unrefreshed, have daytime fatigue, high blood pressure, obesity, or nighttime urination. Ask your doctor: "Should I be evaluated for sleep apnea?"

ERECTILE FUNCTION ASSESSMENT

Erections are a health signal. ED can reveal vascular disease, diabetes, low testosterone, medication effects, sleep problems, depression, pelvic surgery effects, or prostate treatment side effects. Ask your doctor: "Is my ED a warning sign of a broader health problem?"

LIBIDO ASSESSMENT

Low libido may come from low testosterone, sleep problems, stress, depression, medication, relationship issues, chronic illness, or hormonal imbalance. It should not be dismissed. Ask your doctor: "Is my low libido hormonal, psychological, medication-related, or part of a broader health issue?"

EJACULATION AND ORGASM ASSESSMENT

Prostate medications, BPH procedures, pelvic floor dysfunction, prostatitis, and prostate cancer treatments can affect ejaculation and orgasm. Men should be asked about this directly. Ask your doctor: "Could my medication or treatment affect ejaculation or orgasm?"

FERTILITY GOALS

Men should be asked whether they still want children before testosterone therapy, prostate procedures, or prostate cancer treatment. Testosterone therapy can reduce sperm production. Prostate procedures can affect ejaculation. Prostate cancer surgery eliminates normal ejaculation. Ask your doctor: "Do I need fertility testing or sperm banking before treatment?"

CONSTIPATION AND BOWEL HABITS

Constipation can worsen urinary urgency, pelvic pressure, incomplete emptying sensations, pelvic floor tension, and prostatitis-like symptoms. The bowel is part of the pelvic health picture. Ask your doctor: "Could constipation be worsening my urinary or pelvic symptoms?"

ALCOHOL INTAKE

Alcohol can worsen nighttime urination, sleep quality, erections, blood pressure, weight, liver health, and hormone balance. A man should be honest about intake. Ask your doctor: "Could alcohol be worsening my sleep, urinary symptoms, or erections?"

CAFFEINE AND BLADDER IRRITANTS

Caffeine can worsen urgency, frequency, and bladder sensitivity in some men. Spicy foods, carbonated drinks, acidic drinks, and artificial sweeteners may also irritate the bladder in selected patients. Ask your doctor: "Could bladder irritants be making my urgency worse?"

MEDICATION REVIEW

Many medications can affect urination, erections, libido, ejaculation, blood pressure, sleep, or hormones. A medication review is essential. Ask your doctor: "Could any of my medications be affecting urination or sexual function?"

SUPPLEMENT REVIEW

Supplements may interact with medications, affect bleeding risk, create false confidence, or delay proper evaluation. A man should bring the actual supplement list or bottles to the visit. Ask your doctor: "Are any of my supplements unsafe, unnecessary, or interfering with my care?"

CARDIOVASCULAR RISK

Heart and vascular health are central to male longevity. ED, low energy, poor exercise tolerance, high blood pressure, abnormal cholesterol, diabetes, smoking, and family history should prompt cardiovascular risk evaluation. Ask your doctor: "Do I need cardiology evaluation or cardiovascular risk testing?"

CANCER SCREENING BEYOND THE PROSTATE

A longevity plan should include age-appropriate cancer screening beyond PSA. This may include colon cancer screening, skin checks, lung cancer screening in eligible smokers or former smokers, and other screening based on risk. Ask your doctor: "Am I up to date on age-appropriate cancer screening?"

UROLONGEVITY VISIT GOALS

A UroLongevity evaluation should answer practical questions. Is the prostate safe? Is the bladder safe?

Is PSA being interpreted intelligently? Is testosterone appropriate and monitored? Is ED a vascular warning sign?

Is sleep being destroyed by urination or sleep apnea? Is weight or insulin resistance driving symptoms? Is metabolic health improving or worsening?

Is sexual function being preserved? Is the patient functioning better, not just living longer?

CORE UROLONGEVITY CHECKLIST

A complete evaluation may include: PSA. Urinalysis. Prostate size when indicated.

Bladder-emptying measurement when indicated. Urine-flow testing when indicated. Total testosterone.

Free testosterone. SHBG. Estradiol when relevant.

DHT when relevant. CBC. CMP.

Lipid panel. A1c. Fasting glucose.

Fasting insulin when appropriate. Thyroid testing when appropriate. Vitamin D.

B12. Blood pressure. Body composition.

Sleep assessment. ED assessment. Fertility goals.

Constipation review. Medication review. Supplement review.

Cardiovascular risk review. Age-appropriate cancer screening review.

FINAL TAKEAWAY

UroLongevity is not about ordering every test on every man. It is about refusing to treat men as disconnected body parts. The prostate affects the bladder.

The bladder affects sleep. Sleep affects testosterone. Testosterone affects sexual function, energy, and body composition.

Erectile dysfunction can reveal vascular disease. Metabolic health affects urinary symptoms, erections, inflammation, and longevity. PSA affects cancer-risk strategy.

A man's health is one system. The goal is not just to live longer. The goal is to function longer.

APPENDIX N: VISIT PREPARATION SHEET

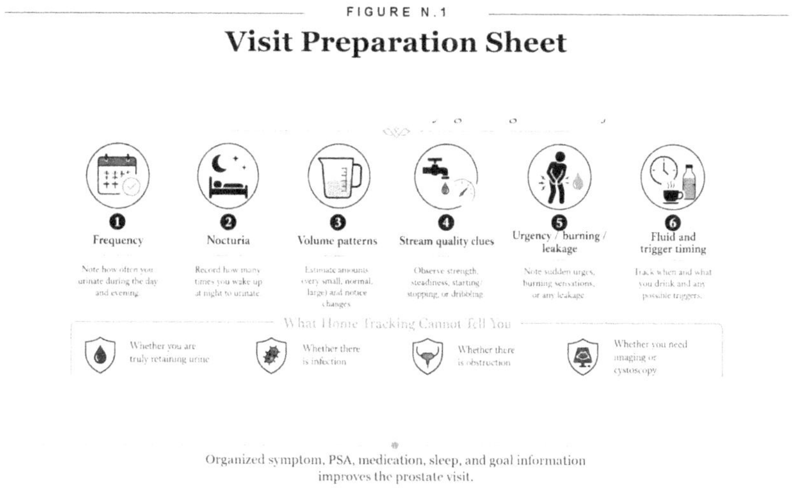

Figure N.1 - Visit Preparation Sheet. Organized information improves the prostate visit.

Bring this sheet to your urology visit or use it to organize your thoughts before the appointment.

URINARY SYMPTOMS PROSTATE AND BLADDER HISTORY PSA AND CANCER RISK SEXUAL FUNCTION AND HORMONES MEDICATIONS AND SUPPLEMENTS BOWEL, SLEEP, AND LIFESTYLE YOUR MAIN GOALS QUESTIONS TO ASK AT THE VISIT FINAL REMINDER

CLOSING AUTHOR'S NOTE

Men are often told to accept prostate problems as part of aging. I disagree.

Aging is real. Prostate enlargement is common. Urinary changes are common. PSA anxiety is common. Sexual changes are common. But common does not mean meaningless, and it does not mean a man should simply live with symptoms until the bladder fails, sleep collapses, or cancer risk is ignored.

The modern approach is different. Measure first. Understand the anatomy.

Protect the bladder. Interpret PSA intelligently. Preserve sexual function whenever possible.

Choose treatment based on the patient, not the procedure. That is the purpose of this book.

The prostate is a small organ, but it can control a man's life if it is ignored. It can affect sleep, confidence, travel, sex, relationships, energy, and peace of mind. It can create fear when PSA rises. It can create embarrassment when urination changes. It can create frustration when men are told they are "fine" even though they do not feel fine.

Men deserve better than vague reassurance. They deserve clear answers. How large is the prostate?

Is it growing into the bladder opening? How much urine is left behind? How fast does the urine come out?

Is the bladder safe? Is PSA being interpreted correctly? Is medication enough?

Is PAE an option? Is Rezūm appropriate? Is cancer low-risk or dangerous?

Is sexual function being protected? These are not complicated questions, but they are often not asked directly enough.

My goal is for men to become more informed, more proactive, and less afraid. A man does not need to become his own doctor, but he should become an intelligent participant in his care. The future of prostate care is smarter, earlier, and less destructive.

That future starts with information. A modern man should not fear his prostate. He should understand it before it controls his life.

It is not a substitute for medical evaluation, diagnosis, treatment, or individualized advice from a licensed physician or other qualified healthcare professional. Prostate symptoms, urinary problems, PSA changes, erectile dysfunction, testosterone concerns, pelvic pain, infections, blood in the urine, and prostate cancer risk can have many different causes. The right evaluation and treatment depend on the patient's age, medical history, physical examination, laboratory results, imaging, prostate anatomy, bladder function, medications, goals, and overall health.

Nothing in this book creates a doctor-patient relationship. Readers should not start, stop, or change medications, supplements, hormone therapy, prostate treatment, cancer treatment, or any medical plan based only on this book. Seek prompt medical attention for urgent symptoms such as inability to urinate, fever with urinary symptoms, severe pain, blood clots in the urine, worsening kidney function, or other concerning changes.

Medical knowledge changes over time. New research, guidelines, technologies, and treatment options may become available after publication. Use this book as a guide to ask better questions, understand your options, and participate more intelligently in your care. Final decisions should be made with your physician.

ABOUT THE AUTHOR

David Shusterman, MD is a board-certified urologist and the founder of Modern Urologist, a New York-based urology practice focused on advanced prostate, bladder, sexual health, and men's longevity care. Dr. Shusterman has spent more than two decades treating men with prostate enlargement, urinary symptoms, PSA concerns, erectile dysfunction, testosterone issues, prostatitis, kidney stones, bladder problems, and prostate cancer risk. His clinical philosophy is built around one central idea: men deserve clear answers before they are placed on medication indefinitely, rushed into procedures, or told their symptoms are simply part of aging.

His approach emphasizes objective testing, prostate measurement, bladder-safety evaluation, urine-flow analysis, PSA interpretation, MRI-guided cancer-risk evaluation, and anatomy-based treatment planning. He is especially focused on modern BPH care, including prostate artery embolization, or PAE, and Rezūm for properly selected patients. Dr. Shusterman also founded UroLongevity, a men's healthspan platform connecting prostate care with testosterone, erectile function, sleep, metabolism, cardiovascular risk, and long-term male performance.

For patient resources, visit: Dr. Shusterman's message to men is simple: Do not ignore the prostate. Do not fear the prostate. Understand it early, measure it properly, and treat it intelligently.

A FURTHER RESOURCE

For readers who want to go further, I maintain 1Prostate.com, where I explain PAE, BPH, Rezūm, and other prostate treatment options in patient language. It is my site and it describes my practice. Read it the way you should read this book: as one urologist's view, offered to help you ask better questions of whichever doctor you choose.

This book was written for men who know something is changing but have not yet been given clear answers. Many men live for years with urinary symptoms, poor sleep, sexual changes, PSA anxiety, or prostate enlargement without understanding what is happening. They are told to wait, take another pill, repeat the same plan, or accept their symptoms as aging.

I wrote this book because men deserve better. I want to thank the patients who have trusted me with their care over the years. Every office visit, every difficult question, every frustrating symptom, every delayed diagnosis, and every successful recovery has helped shape the way I think about prostate health.

I also want to acknowledge the staff, clinicians, technicians, nurses, physician assistants, nurse practitioners, interventional radiology partners, anesthesia teams, and medical colleagues who make modern prostate care possible. Good outcomes do not come from one person alone. They come from accurate testing, careful planning, proper technique, strong follow-up, and a team that takes the patient seriously.

I am especially grateful to the men who were willing to ask uncomfortable questions. Questions about urination. Questions about erections. Questions about PSA. Questions about cancer. Questions about testosterone. Questions about aging. Those questions matter, and they deserve direct answers.

This book is also a reflection of my belief that urology must keep moving forward. Prostate care should not be trapped in old assumptions, vague reassurance, or one-size-fits-all treatment. Men should know their prostate size, their bladder safety, their PSA risk, their treatment options, and their sexual-function risks before major decisions are made.

To every man reading this: the purpose of this book is not to make you afraid of your prostate. It is to make you informed. A modern man should not fear his prostate. He should understand it before it controls his life.

SELECTED MEDICAL SOURCES

This reader-facing source section is intentionally compact. It identifies high-level sources used for final medical proofing; it is not a complete clinical bibliography.

National Institute of Diabetes and Digestive and Kidney Diseases. Enlarged Prostate (Benign Prostatic Hyperplasia). Last reviewed June 2024.

National Cancer Institute. Prostate Cancer Screening (PDQ) - Patient Version. Updated December 10, 2024.

National Cancer Institute. Prostate Cancer Treatment (PDQ) - Patient Version.

U.S. Preventive Services Task Force. Prostate Cancer: Screening.

A NOTE FROM THE AUTHOR

If this book helped you understand your prostate, your options, or your care, please consider leaving a brief review. Your feedback helps other men find this information.

For bulk purchases, foreign rights, speaking inquiries, or review copies, please contact: info@urolongevity.com

THE UROLOGIST'S GUIDE

The Urologist's Guide This book is part of The Urologist's Guide series — patient-education books written by a practicing urologist for men who want to understand their bodies, their options, and their care. Other titles in the series include: • The Urologist's Guide to Erectile Dysfunction • Below the Belt • Beyond the Pill • UTI Unlocked • Hard Evidence • Restoring Intimacy • Finish When You Want • Shrink the Prostate • Redefining Longevity For more information, visit www.urolongevity.com.

www.ingramcontent.com/pod-product-compliance
Lightning Source LLC
LaVergne TN
LVHW010709061126
851857LV00014B/1115
* 9 7 9 8 9 0 6 4 9 0 0 5 6 *